GASTROENTEROLOGY AND HEPATOLOGY

The Comprehensive Visual Reference

GASTROENTEROLOGY AND HEPATOLOGY

The Comprehensive Visual Reference

series editor
Mark Feldman, MD

Southland Professor and Vice Chairman
Department of Internal Medicine
University of Texas Southwestern
    Medical Center at Dallas

Chief, Medical Service
Veterans Affairs Medical Center
Dallas, Texas

volume 5

Esophagus and Pharynx

volume editor
Roy C. Orlando, MD

Professor of Medicine and Chief
Department of Medicine
Tulane University Medical Center
New Orleans, Louisiana

With 16 contributors

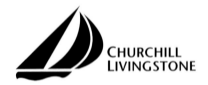

CHURCHILL
LIVINGSTONE

Developed by Current Medicine, Inc.
Philadelphia

Current Medicine, Inc.

400 Market Street
Suite 700
Philadelphia, PA 19106

Managing Editor	*Lori J. Bainbridge*
Development Editors	*Ira D. Smiley and Raymond Lukens*
Editorial Assistant	*Scott Thomas Hurd*
Art Director	*Paul Fennessy*
Design and Layout	*Robert LeBrun*
Illustration Director	*Ann Saydlowski*
Illustrators	*Wieslawa Langenfeld, Beth Starkey, Lisa Weischedel, Debra Wertz, and Gary Welch*
Typesetting Supervisor	*Brian Tshudy*
Production	*David Myers and Lori Holland*
Indexer	*Maria Coughlin*

Esophagus and pharynx / Roy Orlando, volume editor.
 p. cm. — (Gastroenterology and hepatology; v. 5)
 Includes bibliographical references and index.
 ISBN 0-443-07855-6
 1. Esophagus—Atlases. 2. Pharynx—Atlases. 3. Esophagus—Diseases—
Atlases. 4. Pharynx—Diseases—Atlases I. Orlando, Roy C., 1942- .
II. Series.
 [DNLM: 1. Esophageal Diseases—atlases. 2. Esophagus—atlases.
3. Pharynx—atlases. WI 17 G257 1997 v. 5]
QP146.E86 1997
612.3'1—dc20
DNLM/DLC
for Library of Congress   96-18669
                                                             CIP

Library of Congress Cataloging-in-Publication Data
ISBN 0-443-07855-6

Printed in Singapore by Imago Productions (FE) Pte Ltd.

10 9 8 7 6 5 4 3 2 1

DISTRIBUTED WORLDWIDE BY CHURCHILL LIVINGSTONE, INC.

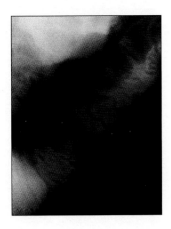

Series Preface

In recent years dramatic developments in the practice of gastro-enterology have unfolded, and the specialty has become, more than ever, a visual discipline. Advances in endoscopy, radiology, or a combination of the two, such as endoscopic retro-grade cholangiopancreatography and endoscopic ultrasonography, have occurred in the past 2 decades. Because of advanced imaging technology, a gastroenterologist, like a dermatologist, is often able to directly view the pathology of a patient's organs. Moreover, practicing gastroenterologists and hepatologists can frequently diagnose disease from biopsy samples examined microscopically, often aided by an increasing number of special staining techniques. As a result of these advances, gastroenterology has grown as rapidly as any subspecialty of internal medicine.

Gastroenterology and Hepatology: The Comprehensive Visual Reference is an ambitious 8-volume collection of images that pictorially displays the gastrointestinal tract, liver, biliary tree, and pancreas in health and disease, both in children and adults. The series is comprised of 89 chapters containing nearly 4000 images accompanied by legends. The images in this collection include not only traditional photographs but also charts, tables, drawings, algorithms, and diagrams, making this collection much more than an atlas in the conventional sense. Chapters are authored by experts selected by one of the eight volume editors, who carefully reviewed each chapter within their volume.

Disorders of the gastrointestinal tract, liver, biliary tree, and pancreas are common in children and adults. *Helicobacter pylori* gastritis is the most frequent bacterial infection of humans and is a risk factor for peptic ulcer disease and gastric malignancies. Colorectal carcinoma is the second leading cause of cancer mortality in the United States, with nearly 60,000 deaths in 1990. Pancreatic cancer resulted in an additional 25,000 deaths. Liver disease is also an important cause of morbidity and mortality, with more that 25,000 deaths from cirrhosis alone in 1990. Gallstone disease is also common in our society, with increasing reliance on laparoscopic cholecystectomy in symptomatic individuals. Inflamma-tory bowel diseases (ulcerative colitis, Crohn's disease) are also widespread in all segments of the population; their causes still elude us.

The past few decades have also witnessed striking advances in the therapy of gastrointestinal disorders. Examples include "cure" of peptic ulcer disease by eradicating *H. pylori* with antimicrobial agents, healing of erosive esophagitis with proton pump inhibitor drugs, remission of chronic viral hepatitis B or C with interferon-α2b, and hepatic transplantation for patients with fulminant hepatic failure or end-stage liver disease. Therapeutic endoscopic techniques have proliferated that ameliorate the need for surgical procedures. Endoscopic advances include placement of peroral endoscopic gastrostomy tubes for nutritional support, insertion of stents in the bile duct or esophagus to relieve malignant obstruction, and the use of injection therapy, thermal coagulation, or laser therapy to treat bleeding ulcers and other lesions, including tumors. *Gastroenterology and Hepatology: The Comprehensive Visual Reference* will cover these advances and many others in the field of gastroenterology.

I wish to thank a number of people for their contributions to this series. The dedication and expertise of the other volume editors—Willis Maddrey, Rick Boland, Paul Hyman, Nick LaRusso, Roy Orlando, Larry Schiller, and Phil Toskes—was critical and most appreciated. The nearly 100 contributing authors were both creative and generous with their time and teaching materials. And special thanks to Abe Krieger, President of Current Medicine, for recruiting me for this unique project, and to his talented associates at Current Medicine.

The images contained in this 8-volume collection are available in print as well as in slide format, and the series is soon being formatted for CD-ROM use. All of us who have participated in this ambitious project hope that each of the 8 volumes, as well as the entire collection, will be useful to physicians and health professionals throughout the world involved in the diagnosis and treatment of patients of all ages who suffer from gastrointestinal disorders.

Mark Feldman, MD

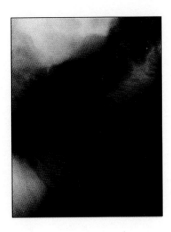

Volume Preface

The esophagus is a long, tubular organ designed to actively transmit ingested material from mouth to stomach. To do this it is constructed of two bundles of muscle—an inner circular bundle and an outer longitudinal bundle—for peristalsis, and an inner lining of moist stratified squamous epithelium for protection. These structures are remarkable for their capacity to effect safe passage of materials to the stomach whether hot or cold, rough or smooth, hypertonic or hypotonic, acidic or alkaline, or direct chemical irritants (*eg*, alcohol). When diseased, organ dysfunction becomes clinically manifest by symptoms of dysphagia, chest pain, heartburn, or regurgitation.

This volume of *Gastroenterology and Hepatology: The Comprehensive Visual Reference* provides an 11-chapter visual panorama of the esophagus in both health and disease.

Beginning with a chapter on esophageal anatomy and physiology, whose content is self-explanatory, this volume takes us through chapters that encompass the role of endoscopy and manometry, pH-monitoring, and Bernstein testing in patient assessment, as well as reviews of gastroesophageal reflux disease, acute esophagitis, esophageal motor disorders, the pharynx, esophageal tumors, noncardiac chest pain, therapeutic endoscopy, and concludes with a chapter detailing surgery of the esophagus. The quality of the chapters in this volume is excellent, and for this I am personally indebted to each of the authors for so generously expending the time and effort necessary to bring this work to fruition.

Roy C. Orlando, MD

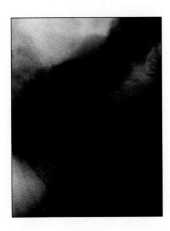

Contributors

Matthew S.Z. Bachinski, MD
Assistant Professor
Department of Medicine
Uniformed Services University of
    Health Sciences
Bethesda, Maryland

Eugene M. Bozymski, MD
Professor of Medicine and Chief
    of Endoscopy
Department of Internal Medicine
Division of Digestive Disease
    and Nutrition
University of North Carolina
Chapel Hill, North Carolina

Donald O. Castell, MD
Clinical Professor of Medicine
Department of Medicine
University of Pennsylvania
Philadelphia, Pennsylvania

Gulchin A. Ergun, MD
Assistant Professor of Medicine
Department of Gastroenterology
    and Hepatology
Northwestern University
Chicago, Illinois

Salima Haque, MD
Assistant Professor
Department of Pathology and
    Laboratory Medicine
Tulane University School of Medicine
New Orleans, Louisiana

Bernard M. Jaffe, MD
Professor and Vice Chairman
Department of Surgery
Tulane University School of Medicine
New Orleans, Louisiana

Bronwyn Jones, MB, BS
Professor of Radiology
Radiology and Radiological Science
Johns Hopkins University School
    of Medicine
Baltimore, Maryland

Peter J. Kahrilas, MD
Professor of Medicine
Department of Gastroenterology
    and Hepatology
Northwestern University
Chicago, Illinois

Louis P. Leite, DO
Division of Gastroenterology
The Graduate Hospital
Philadelphia, Pennsylvania

R. Lee Meyers, BA, MD
Clinical Instructor
Department of Medicine
Division of Digestive Diseases
University of North Carolina
Chapel Hill, North Carolina

Ravinder K. Mittal, MD
Associate Professor
Department of Internal Medicine
University of Virginia
Charlottesville, Virginia

Roy C. Orlando, MD
Professor of Medicine and Chief
Department of Medicine
Tulane University Medical Center
New Orleans, Louisiana

William J. Ravich, MD
Associate Professor
Department of Medicine
Johns Hopkins University School
    of Medicine
Baltimore, Maryland

Richard I. Rothstein, MD
Associate Professor of Medicine
Department of Medicine
Dartmouth Medical School
Hanover, New Hampshire

Roy K.H. Wong, MD
Professor of Medicine
Department of Medicine
Uniformed Services
    University of the Health Sciences
Bethesda, Maryland

Wallace C. Wu, MB, BS
Professor
Department of Medicine
Bowman Gray School of Medicine
Winston-Salem, North Carolina

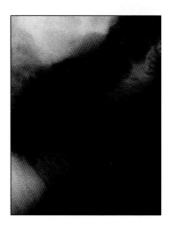

Contents

Chapter 6

Esophageal Motor Disorders

RAVINDER K. MITTAL

Chapter 7

The Pharynx

WILLIAM J. RAVICH AND BRONWYN JONES

Chapter 8

Tumors of the Esophagus

SALIMA HAQUE

Chapter 9

Esophageal Causes of Noncardiac Chest Pain

RICHARD I. ROTHSTEIN

Chapter 1

Esophageal Anatomy and Physiology

GULCHIN A. ERGUN
PETER J. KAHRILAS

The major function of the esophagus is to transport food from the mouth to the stomach while preventing retrograde movement of gastric contents. It is, in essence, a hollow muscular tube that is closed at the proximal portion by the upper esophageal sphincter (UES) and by the lower esophageal sphincter (LES) at the bottom. The pharynx and the proximal esophagus contain striated muscle controlled by the swallowing center in the brain stem through the vagus nerves. The lower two thirds of the esophagus contain smooth muscle with peristalsis controlled primarily by an intrinsic neural network located between the longitudinal and circular muscle layers and is modulated by central mechanisms in the swallowing center. Proximal esophageal function is complex because the oral cavity and pharynx must serve multiple functions, not only as a food conduit, but also as a respiratory conduit, thereby requiring precise control and efficient coordination of swallowing and respiration.

Swallowing has been traditionally divided into four phases: (1) the preparatory phase, which involves mastication, sizing, shaping, and positioning of the bolus on the tongue with saliva; (2) the oral phase, during which the bolus is propelled from the oral cavity into the pharynx; (3) the pharyngeal phase, during which the bolus is transported from the oral cavity into the pharynx with adequate airway protection; and (4) the esophageal phase, during which the bolus is propelled down the length of the esophagus [1]. This seemingly simple task requires coordination of over 100 muscles that are under voluntary and reflexive control during a period of a few seconds. Dysfunction at the proximal portion may result in poor formation of a bolus with misdirection caused by lingual abnormalities, nasal regurgitation if velopharyngeal closure is poor, incomplete UES opening with impaired hyoid or laryngeal excursion, aspiration with poor laryngeal closure, and choking if hypopharyngeal residue with poor pharyngeal clearance is present.

After the pharyngeal contraction traverses the UES, the peristaltic contraction moves from the proximal striated muscle to the distal smooth muscle of the esophagus at 2 to 4 cm per second. Primary peristalsis is controlled by extrinsic innervation whereas secondary peristalsis is an intramural process [2]. Deglutitive inhibition occurs when a second swallow is initiated during a still-continuing peristaltic contraction and causes rapid and complete inhibition of the contraction induced by the first swallow. Similarly, LES tone is inhibited with swallowing concurrently with deglutitive inhibition.

Physiologic control mechanisms that govern the striated and the smooth muscles of the esophagus are different. The striated muscle esophagus receives excitatory vagal innervation exclusively, and the peristaltic contraction results from sequential activation of motor units in a craniocaudad sequence. Vagal control of the smooth muscle esophagus is more complex, with vagal fibers synapsing directly on myenteric plexus neurons. Vagal stimulation can either excite or inhibit esophageal musculature. Finally, two types of effector neurons exist within the esophageal myenteric plexus: (1) excitatory neurons that mediate contraction of both longitudinal and circular muscles through cholinergic receptors [3]; and (2) inhibitory neurons that affect the circular muscle layer through nitric oxide nerves [4,5].

■ OROPHARYNGEAL MUSCULATURE

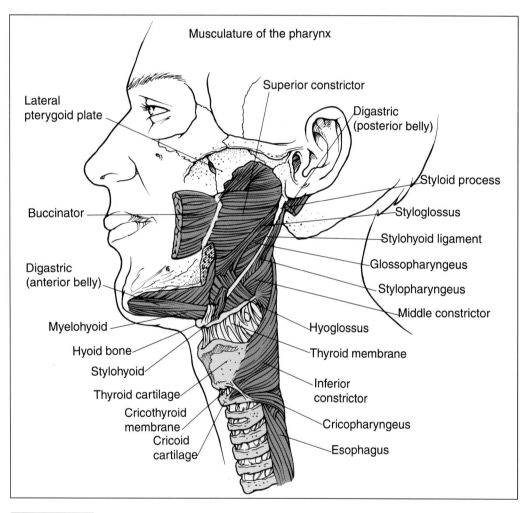

Musculature of the pharynx

Superior constrictor
Lateral pterygoid plate
Digastric (posterior belly)
Styloid process
Buccinator
Styloglossus
Stylohyoid ligament
Glossopharyngeus
Digastric (anterior belly)
Stylopharyngeus
Middle constrictor
Myelohyoid
Hyoglossus
Hyoid bone
Thyroid membrane
Stylohyoid
Thyroid cartilage
Inferior constrictor
Cricothyroid membrane
Cricoid cartilage
Cricopharyngeus
Esophagus

pterygoid hamulus, pterygomandibular raphe, mandible, and tongue, passes posteromedially, and inserts into the posterior median raphe. The middle constrictor arises from the hyoid bone and stylohyoid ligament, passes posteromedially, and also inserts into the posterior median raphe. The inferior constrictor is composed of the thyropharyngeus superiorly and the cricopharyngeus inferiorly. The thyropharyngeus arises from the thyroid cartilage and passes posteromedially to insert into the median raphe. The cricopharyngeus, however, has superior and inferior components that arise from both sides of the cricoid lamina such that the superior fibers course posteromedially to the median raphe and the inferior fibers loop around the esophageal inlet without a median raphe. The cricopharyngeus muscle separates the pharynx from the esophagus.

The pharyngeal walls are supported by attachments to the epiglottic, arytenoid, cuneiform, corniculate, and cricoid cartilages. The larynx and trachea are suspended in the neck between the hyoid bone superiorly and the sternum inferiorly. The laryngeal strap muscles contribute to this suspension and the intrinsic elasticity of the trachea permits the larynx to be elevated and lowered. The hyoid bone serves as the base for the tongue and is positioned as a fulcrum, crucial in directing forces anteriorly and superiorly toward the larynx, and hence, esophageal inlet. Laryngeal movement is critical in permitting the swallow response as the laryngeal inlet is closed and physically removed from the bolus path during the course of the swallow. Failure to achieve laryngeal elevation can result in aspiration of solids and liquids. (*Adapted from* Kahrilas [6].)

FIGURE 1-1.

Musculature of the oral cavity, pharynx, larynx, and proximal esophagus as displayed in a cutaway view. The oral cavity, pharynx, and larynx are all involved in transferring food from the mouth to the esophagus. Within the oral cavity, the lips, teeth, tongue, soft palate, mandible, and floor of the mouth serve various functions in chewing and manipulating food to create a bolus that is suitable for transfer to the pharynx. The walls of the oropharynx are composed of the superior, middle, and inferior constrictors posteriorly and the base of the tongue, which opposes constrictors anteriorly. The superior constrictor arises from the

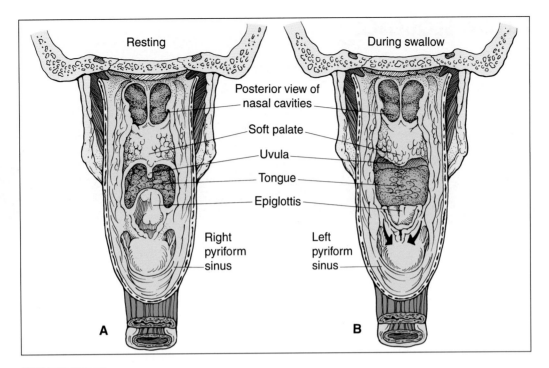

Resting — **During swallow**

Posterior view of nasal cavities

Soft palate

Uvula

Tongue

Epiglottis

Right pyriform sinus — Left pyriform sinus

A B

FIGURE 1-2.

Posterior view of the pharynx showing the oropharyngeal anatomic configuration at rest (**A**) and during swallow (**B**). The pharyngeal constrictors are cut at the midline and laid open to reveal the anterior pharyngeal wall. The spaces formed between the lateral insertion of the inferior constrictor and the lateral walls of the thyroid cartilage are the pyriform sinuses. **Panel B** shows the anatomic configuration during swallow illustrating laryngeal elevation and closure (arrows show the bilateral path taken around the epiglottis by the swallowed material). (*Adapted from* Kahrilas [6].)

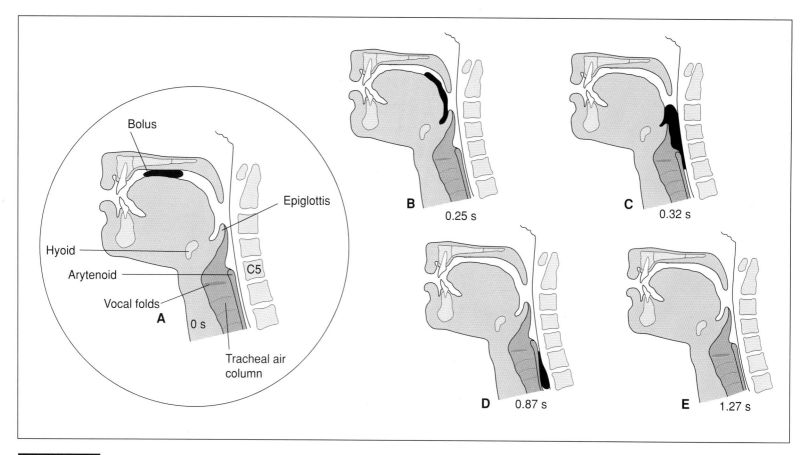

FIGURE 1-3.

Sequence of a normal swallow. Swallowing can be divided into an oral phase and a subsequent pharyngeal phase. The pharyngeal phase is a complex motor event referred to as the *swallow response*. The oral phase of the swallowing is highly voluntary and variable, depending on taste and motivation. It is functionally accomplished by manipulation of the bolus by the tongue to contain the food in the mouth until ready to swallow and the propulsion of the bolus by the posterior tongue squeezing the tongue against the palate with the central groove exhibiting centripetal then centrifugal motion [6]. Close to the time that the bolus reaches the posterior tongue, the pharyngeal swallow is triggered. There is then simultaneous apposition of the muscular soft palate to the posterior pharyngeal wall to prevent nasal regurgitation and elevation of the larynx and hyoid bone to close the airway and pull open the upper esophageal sphincter (UES) [7]. This is followed by clearance of any remaining hypopharyngeal residue by the pharyngeal constrictors [7]. After the pharyngeal swallow has been initiated, the sequence of events is involuntary.

A, At 0 seconds (*A*), the bolus is in the oral cavity, resting on the tongue, with the laryngeal vestibule open and the UES closed. **B**, At 0.25 seconds into the swallow the bolus has been pushed back into the valleculae by the posterior tongue, the nasopharynx has been sealed off, and the larynx has begun to elevate. **C**, By 0.32 seconds the hyoid is maximally elevated, the UES is opened, and the tongue base has been fully retracted against the posterior pharyngeal wall. **D**, Structures are beginning to return back to the rest position 1.27 seconds after the initiation of the swallow. **E**, The rest position. (*Adapted from* Kahrilas *et al.* [9].)

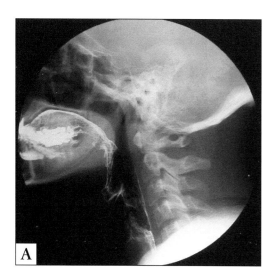

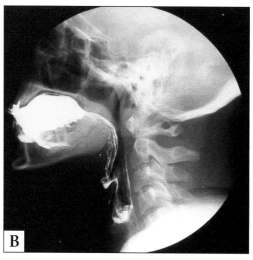

FIGURE 1-4.

Progression of a normal swallow imaged by cineradiography. **A**, Normal preswallow tongue and pharyngeal surface contour are shown before administration of bolus. **B**, With administration of barium, bolus propulsion begins with the loading phase of the tongue and bolus containment through adaptation of the lingual central groove. **C**, Bolus is propelled into the pharynx with the tongue central groove exhibiting centripetal then centrifugal motion. **D**, Nasopharyngeal closure is achieved by soft-palate elevation and apposition to the posterior pharyngeal wall.

(continued on next page)

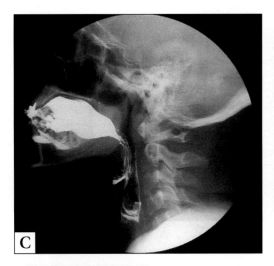 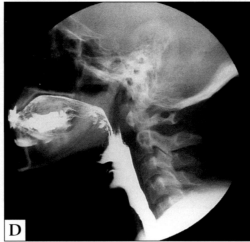 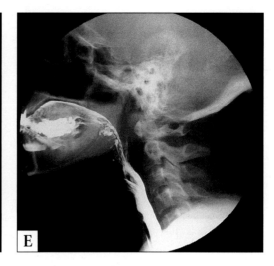

FIGURE 1-4. (CONTINUED)

Airway protection is achieved by laryngeal elevation, vocal cord closure, and arytenoid tilting. Upper esophageal sphincter opening occurs through relaxation of the sphincter and anterior hyoid traction with laryngeal elevation. E, Pharyngeal clearance of ingested contents is achieved by profound shortening of the pharynx, eliminating bolus access to the larynx and the propagating pharyngeal contraction. After the bolus has passed into the proximal esophagus the epiglottis returns upright, the larynx reopens, and the resting positions are resumed (not shown).

NEUROPHYSIOLOGY

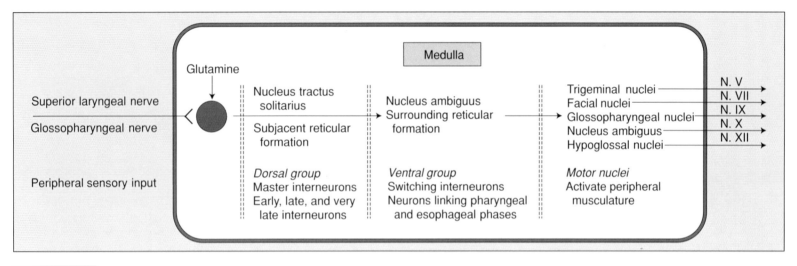

FIGURE 1-5.

Central nervous system organization of the swallow response. Afferent information from the periphery enters into the solitary tract. This sensory information can initiate deglutition and modify ongoing motor activity within reflexes affecting the esophageal body and sphincters independent of swallowing. Sensory information from the oropharyngeal area enters through the extravagal cranial nerves (trigeminal, facial, hypoglossal, and glossopharyngeal) and vagal nerve pathways. Sensory information from the entire esophagus, including the sphincters, is carried in the vagus nerve with the cell bodies in the nodose ganglion. Sensory information also passes by way of the sympathetics to the spinal cord segments C1 to L3.

The portion of the swallowing center that programs the entire swallowing sequence is located in the solitary tract nucleus and the neighboring reticular substance. The dorsal portion within this center is involved in the initiation of the swallow and the organization of the entire swallowing sequence. The ventral portion appears to serve as a connecting pathway to the various motor neuron pools involved in the swallowing sequence, such as integration of the swallowing sequence with the respiratory center in the medulla.

The motor neurons involved in the efferent output of the swallowing sequence lie mainly in the trigeminal, facial, and hypoglossal nuclei, the nucleus ambiguus of the vagus (for esophageal striated muscle), and the dorsal motor nuclei of the vagus (for esophageal smooth muscle) with some input to striated muscle. (*Adapted from* Castell [10].)

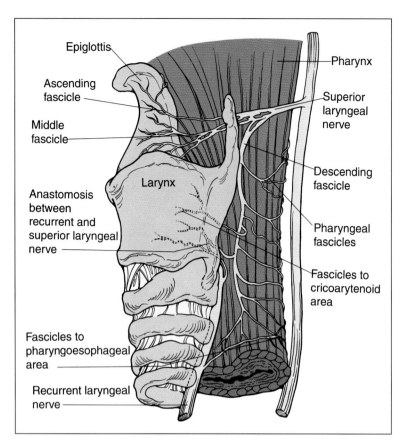

FIGURE 1-6.

Epiglottis

Ascending fascicle

Middle fascicle

Larynx

Anastomosis between recurrent and superior laryngeal nerve

Fascicles to pharyngoesophageal area

Recurrent laryngeal nerve

Pharynx

Superior laryngeal nerve

Descending fascicle

Pharyngeal fascicles

Fascicles to cricoarytenoid area

FIGURE 1-6.

Sensory field of the superior laryngeal nerve in humans. Electrical stimulation of the superior laryngeal nerve (SLN) elicits the pharyngeal swallow response. The structures innervated by the SLN are relatively distal, supporting the notion that in vivo afferents initiating swallowing probably also travel through the glossopharyngeal nerve. More than likely, reflexive swallows aimed at keeping the pharynx clear of secretions are initiated by stimulation of SLN afferents whereas deglutitive swallows are initiated by proximal stimulation or volition (*Adapted from* Kahrilas [6].)

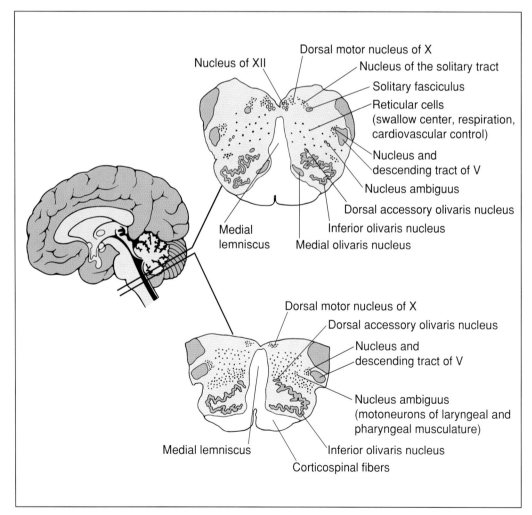

Nucleus of XII

Dorsal motor nucleus of X

Nucleus of the solitary tract

Solitary fasciculus

Reticular cells (swallow center, respiration, cardiovascular control)

Nucleus and descending tract of V

Nucleus ambiguus

Dorsal accessory olivaris nucleus

Inferior olivaris nucleus

Medial olivaris nucleus

Medial lemniscus

Dorsal motor nucleus of X

Dorsal accessory olivaris nucleus

Nucleus and descending tract of V

Nucleus ambiguus (motoneurons of laryngeal and pharyngeal musculature)

Medial lemniscus

Inferior olivaris nucleus

Corticospinal fibers

FIGURE 1-7.

Neuroanatomy of the swallow response. The location of the swallowing center is estimated to be in the reticular substance about 1.5 mm from the midline and 1 to 3 mm dorsal to the inferior olive at a level between the rostral pole of the inferior olive and caudal pole of the facial nucleus. A swallowing center exists bilaterally in each atmosphere, which is capable of independently coordinating swallowing activity, although both sides are extensively interconnected. The swallow center has dominant access to motoneurons and exerts strong inhibitory influence on centers competing for access to these motoneurons. Therefore, an apneic pause of 0.5 to 3.5 seconds occurs to accompany swallowing.

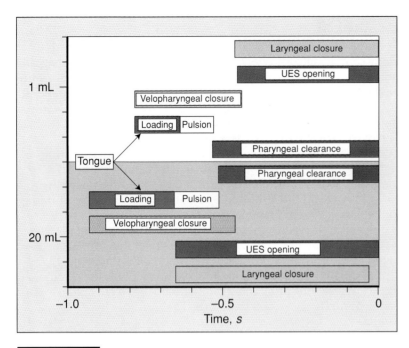

analysis concentrates on the swallowed bolus and how the bolus is manipulated by oropharyngeal structures. Therefore, in biomechanical terms the pharyngeal swallow encompasses several closely coordinated actions: elevation and retraction of the soft palate with the closure of the nasopharynx, upper esophageal sphincter opening, laryngeal closure at the level of the laryngeal vestibule, tongue loading (ramping), tongue pulsion, and pharyngeal clearance. These biomechanical events that comprise the swallow response exhibit systematic variability with the volume of the swallowed bolus.

This figure shows time lines of 1 and 20 mL swallows. The unshaded area depicts time relationships among swallow events during 1 mL swallows whereas the shaded area below depicts time relationships during 20 mL swallows. In both cases, time 0 is the end of the swallow, determined by the timing of the UES closure, and all other events are given negative timing values. When viewed in this way, the apparent prolongation of the 20 mL swallow is associated with an earlier mechanical configuration of the pharynx from a respiratory to a swallowing conduit. This earlier configuration is associated with a prolonged tongue loading phase which starts earlier and takes longer [6]. UES opening along with the associated closure of the laryngeal vestibule also commences sooner and persists longer [8]. Propulsive events occur with a very similar time frame, resulting from more vigorous expulsion of a larger boluses. The mechanics and timing of the pharyngeal contraction, important in pharyngeal clearance and in UES closure, on the other hand, is extraordinarily constant among swallow volumes [7]. (*Adapted from* Kahrilas [12].)

FIGURE 1-8.

Time lines of 1- and 20-mL swallows viewed in biomechanical terms. In addition to neurophysiologic electromyographic patterns, deglutition can also be described in biomechanical terms. Biomechanical

▌UPPER ESOPHAGEAL SPHINCTER

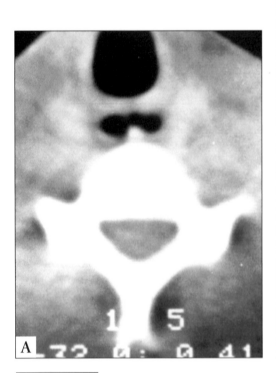

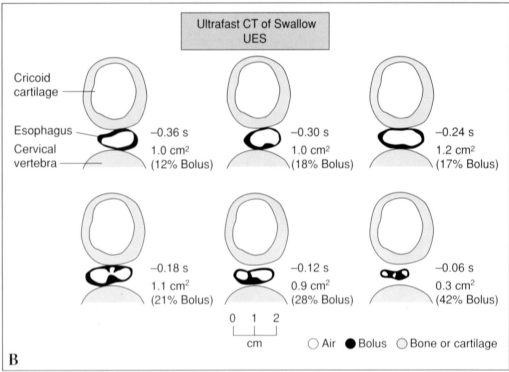

FIGURE 1-9.

Upper esophageal sphincter (UES) imaged by ultrafast computed tomography (CT). The muscular elements of the UES are striated muscle with the cricopharyngeus as well as the adjacent portion of the cervical esophagus and the inferior pharyngeal constrictor contributing to sphincteric function. The cricopharyngeus receives its motor nerve supply through the pharyngeal branch of the vagus. The zone of maximal intraluminal pressure is approximately 1 cm in length axially, and when viewed in cross-section, the closed sphincter has a slitlike configuration with the lamina of the

cricoid cartilage anterior and the cricopharyngeus attached in a C configuration making up the lateral and posterior walls.

A, Representative cross-sectional image at the level of the UES as imaged by ultrafast CT. The tracings (B) illustrate the dynamic changes of the bolus cavity during the course of the swallow, ending with luminal closure at time zero. Note how the sphincter is tightly confined between the cricoid cartilage and cervical vertebrae. Despite this confinement, the opened sphincter maintains an ovoid rather than a dumbbell configuration. (*From* Ergun *et al.* [13]; with permission.)

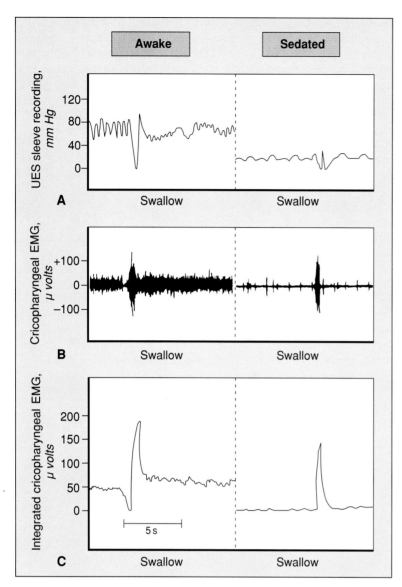

A

Swallow   Swallow

B

Swallow   Swallow

C

Swallow   Swallow

FIGURE 1-10.

Continuous cricopharyngeal electromyography (EMG) recording. These sample data tracings from a dog show the upper esophageal sphincter (UES) intraluminal pressure recorded by sleeve sensor in **panel A**, the raw EMG recording of the cricopharyngeus in **panel B**, and the integrated cricopharyngeal EMG activity in **panel C** while the animal was awake (left) and sedated with pentobarbital (right). The most typical EMG activity pattern of the UES is the brief interval of inhibition followed by a pulse of maximal excitation, regardless of the preexisting tone or activity pattern of the UES. In the awake state, the swallow is associated with inhibition of the cricopharyngeal EMG followed by a burst of activity corresponding to the passage of the pharyngeal contraction. While sedated, there is no detectable resting cricopharyngeal EMG activity and therefore no detectable cricopharyngeal inhibition at the time of UES relaxation. These findings suggest that the residual UES pressure (approximately 15 mm Hg) in the sedated animal is the result of passive elastic forces in the neck rather than active cricopharyngeal contraction. (*Adapted from* Jacob *et al.* [14].)

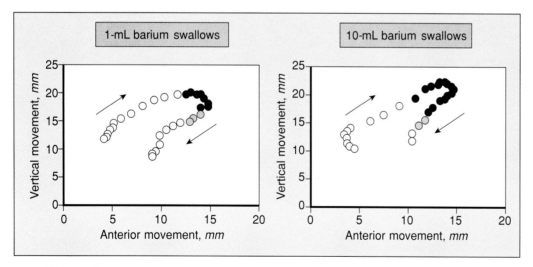

also serves to produce a uniform conduit for directing the bolus into the esophagus.

The contraction of the suprahyoid and infrahyoid musculature that provides the anterior traction for UES opening also results in the characteristic pattern of hyoid displacement shown in this figure. Each circle represents the hyoid position during a single video frame of the recorded fluoroscopic sequence (1/30th second interval) and the arrows indicate the direction of movement. The open circles indicate frames during which the sphincter was closed, closed circles indicate frames when the sphincter was closed, and the gray circles indicate frames during which the sphincter was variably open, depending on the subject. Both the diameter and duration of sphincter opening increase with increased bolus volume. The increased duration of sphincter opening is related to the persistence of the hyoid excursion, whereas changes in the diameter of the opening are related to increased intrabolus pressure with larger volume swallows. (*Adapted from* Jacob *et al.* [11].)

FIGURE 1-11.

Movement pattern of the hyoid bone during 1- and 10-mL barium swallows. The upper esophageal sphincter (UES) is tonically closed at rest because of continuous neural excitation. Within 0.2 seconds after a swallow, excitatory discharge to the UES transiently ceases and laryngeal elevation followed by anterior traction of the hyoid work together to pull open the sphincter. Because the only insertion of the sphincteric musculature is anterior to the cartilages of the larynx, the sphincter and larynx are obliged to move in unison during axial laryngeal movement so that the primary mechanism for opening the relaxed UES

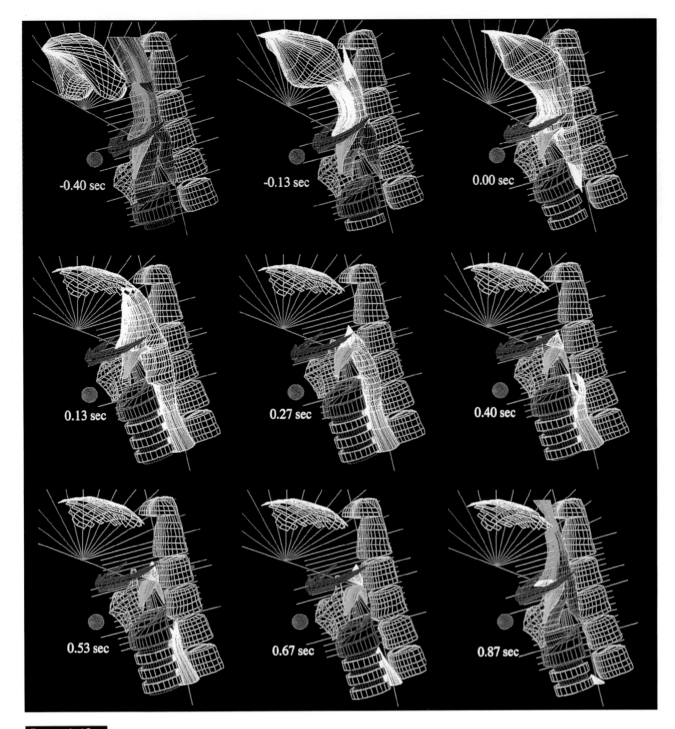

FIGURE 1-12.

Three-dimensional modeling of the oropharynx during swallowing. This figure shows the reconstructions of nine representative pharyngeal configurations during a 10-mL swallow. In each image the bolus chamber is white, the supraglottic airway is blue, the infraglottic airway is purple, the vertebrae are light brown, the hyoid is orange, the epiglottis is yellow, the arytenoid cartilage is dark green, the cricoid cartilage is red, the tracheal rings are cyan, and the hemisected thyroid cartilage is light green. The times next to the images refer to the upper esophageal sphincter (UES) opening (time 0.0 seconds). Many mechanical events are encompassed during the act of deglutition. The preswallow configuration (-0.40 seconds) is characterized by the bolus chamber being segregated from the airway by the sealed glossopalatal junction. At the time of velopharyngeal closure (-0.13 seconds) the nasopharynx is sealed from the bolus chamber by elevation of the soft palate and the bolus chamber expands to the retrolingual space as the glossopalatal junction opens. The central groove of the tongue blade has deepened and the posterior oral portion of the pharyngeal propulsive chamber is forming. The larynx has begun elevating and the arytenoid cartilage is tilting toward the base of the epiglottis. At the instant of UES opening the laryngeal vestibule has been obliterated by contact of the arytenoid cartilage against the epiglottic base. Note that the UES (at the inferior aspect of the cricoid cartilage) has elevated relative to its preswallow position and that the pharyngeal bolus chamber is fully formed. During lingual bolus propulsion (0.13 seconds) the volume of the bolus chamber is reduced by the centrifugal motion of the tongue surface and bolus expulsion results in full distension of the UES and proximal esophagus. The epiglottis is folded over the arytenoid cartilage and there is maximal pharyngeal shortening. The next four reconstructions—pharyngeal clearance (0.27 seconds), midpharyngeal clearance (0.40 seconds), late pharyngeal clearance (0.53 seconds), and UES closure (0.67 seconds)—show the caudal progression of the pharyngeal contraction stripping the residua from the oropharynx into the esophagus. Finally, with airway reopening (0.87 seconds) the pharynx commences its return to the respiratory configuration as the larynx descends, the epiglottis flips up, and the velopharyngeal junction reopens. (*From* Kahrilas *et al.* [15]; with permission.)

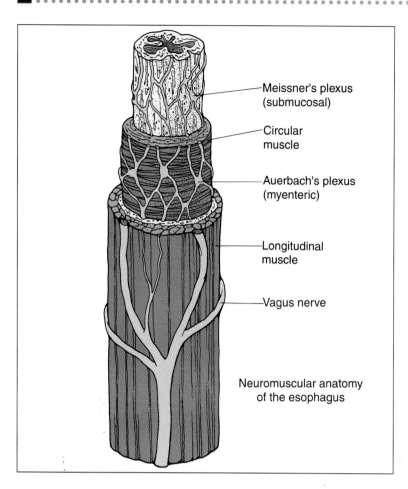

Meissner's plexus (submucosal)

Circular muscle

Auerbach's plexus (myenteric)

Longitudinal muscle

Vagus nerve

Neuromuscular anatomy of the esophagus

FIGURE 1-13.

Cutaway view showing anatomy of the tubular esophagus. The esophagus is a muscular tube that is composed of longitudinal and circular muscle with extensive neural network in between. Auerbach's plexus (myenteric) lies between the longitudinal and circular muscle layers. Another nerve network, Meissner's plexus (submucosal), is situated between the muscularis mucosa and the circular muscle layer. Note that there is no serosa to the esophagus and that the lumen is collapsed and empty. In fact, activity of both esophageal sphincters preserves the vacuum of the esophagus; the upper esophageal sphincter acts to exclude air during respiration and the lower esophageal sphincter excludes gastric contents from refluxing back into the esophagus. (*Adapted from* Kahrilas [6].)

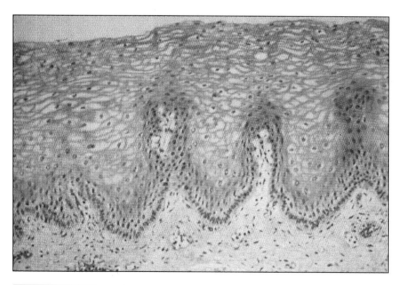

FIGURE 1-14.

Normal histology of the esophagus. The lining of the esophagus is a partially or nonkeratinized stratified squamous epithelium that overlies the connective tissue of the submucosa and the thick circular and longitudinal muscle layers (not shown). (*Courtesy of* Dr. Sambastiva Rao, Northwestern University Medical School.)

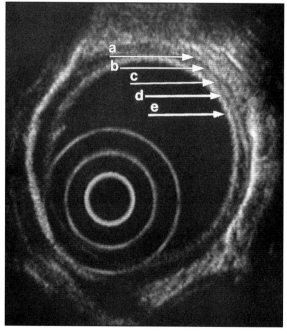

FIGURE 1-15.

Endoscopic ultrasound of the esophagus. This endosonographic image of the esophageal wall demonstrates the five-layer structure that is seen throughout the gastrointestinal tract. These layers correspond to the mucosa adventitia (**a**), muscularis (**b**), submucosa (**c**), and mucosa (**d and e**). Because of balloon filling, the layer structure is not recognizable in all parts of the circumference. (*Courtesy of* Dr. Arvydas Vanagunas, Northwestern University Medical School.)

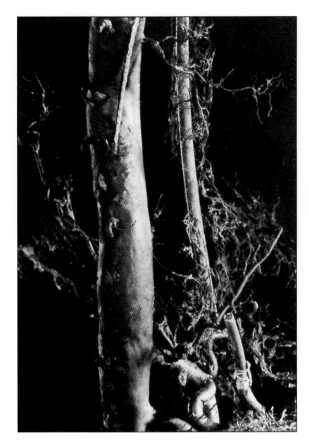

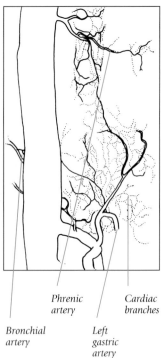

Bronchial artery

Phrenic artery

Left gastric artery

Cardiac branches

FIGURE 1-16.

Arterial supply of the esophagus. Esophageal circulation is in the form of "shared vasculature" [18]. The vasa propria is derived directly from the aorta, but esophageal vessels are small branches of larger-stem vessels intended to supply other organs, such as the thyroid gland, trachea, and stomach, and are thus secondary vessels. They include tracheoesophageal vessels originating from the inferior thyroid artery, tracheobronchial arteries at the level of the carina, esophageal aortic arteries proper, and cardia vessels derived from the celiac axis (the left gastric and splenic artery). These various vascular sources form a dense, continuous submucosal anastomotic network that further subdivides into minute branches before entering the esophageal wall to provide adequate circulation if the nourishing vessel is ligated.

This Beracryl cast of the arterial tree of the middle and lower esophagus shows the tracheobronchial artery originating from the aorta and giving rise to esophageal arteries. These arteries constitute a fine continuous arterial network with vessel diameters of 130 to 150 µm that surround the lumen of the esophagus shown by an intraesophageal probe. the anastomotic network reflects the shape of the esophagus with larger vessels oriented along a longitudinal axis. (*From* Liebermann-Meffert *et al.* [16]; with permission.)

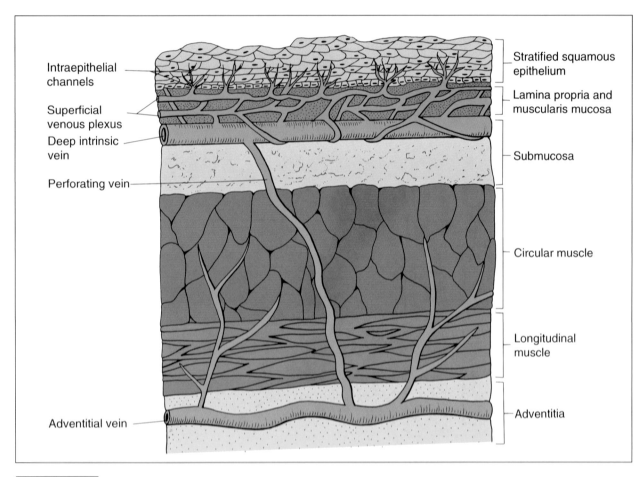

Intraepithelial channels

Superficial venous plexus

Deep intrinsic vein

Perforating vein

Adventitial vein

Stratified squamous epithelium

Lamina propria and muscularis mucosa

Submucosa

Circular muscle

Longitudinal muscle

Adventitia

FIGURE 1-17.

Venous layers of the esophagus. There are three parts of the venous system related to the esophagus: intrinsic veins, associated veins, and extrinsic veins. The two layers of veins in the wall of the esophagus are the superficial venous plexus (located in the lamina propria and muscularis mucosa) and the submucosal plexus (within the circular muscle). In the distal esophagus, venous blood drains first from a superficial mucosal network of small intraepithelial blood vessels into submucosal, longitudinally oriented deep intrinsic veins. Once in the intrinsic veins, blood drains through a system of transverse perforating veins with unidirectional valves into extrinsic serosal and periesophageal veins and ultimately into the left gastric vein inferiorly and the azygos vein superiorly. (*Adapted from* Kitano *et al.* [17].)

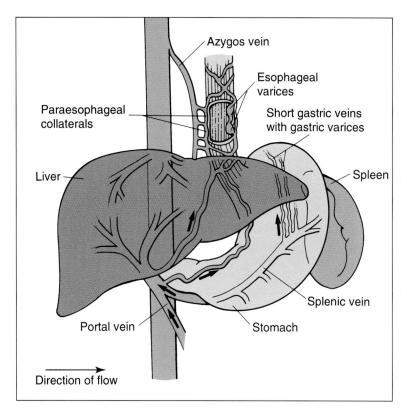

FIGURE 1-18.

Portal venous blood flow observed with esophageal and gastric varices. (*Adapted from* Kitano *et al.* [17].)

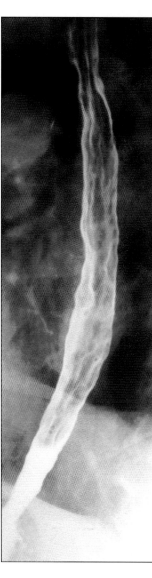

FIGURE 1-19.

Esophageal varices as seen on barium swallow. Portal hypertension results in congestion and dilation with the deep intrinsic veins becoming grossly enlarged, thus displacing the more superficial venous systems. The deep veins eventually occupy a superficial sub-epithelial location and are identified radiographically and endoscopically as esophageal varices. (*Courtesy of* Dr. Frank Miller, Northwestern University Medical School.)

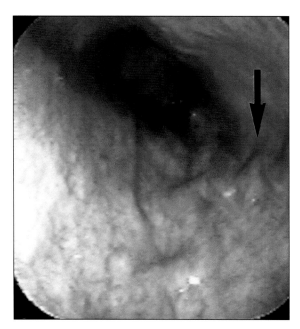

FIGURE 1-20.

Esophageal varices seen endoscopically. The varices appear as slightly bluish dilated vessels (*arrow*).

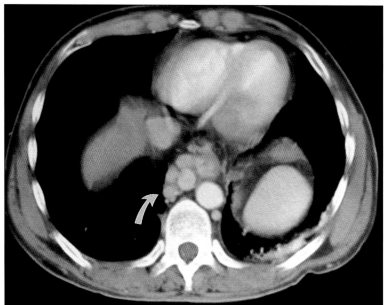

FIGURE 1-21.

Gastroesophageal varices (*arrow*) demonstrated with computed tomography. (*Courtesy of* Dr. Frank Miller, Northwestern University Medical School.)

ESOPHAGEAL PHYSIOLOGY AND PERISTALSIS

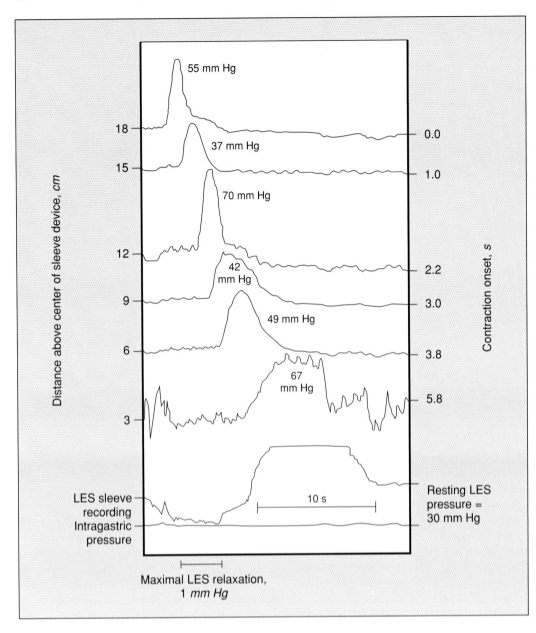

Distance above center of sleeve device, *cm*

55 mm Hg

18 — — 0.0

37 mm Hg

15 — — 1.0

70 mm Hg

12 — — 2.2

42 mm Hg

9 — — 3.0

49 mm Hg

6 — — 3.8

67 mm Hg

3 —

— 5.8

Contraction onset, *s*

LES sleeve recording
Intragastric pressure

10 s

Resting LES pressure = 30 mm Hg

Maximal LES relaxation, *1 mm Hg*

FIGURE 1-22.

Normal manometric recording and primary peristalsis. This figure shows a normal manometric tracing using a sleeve sensor. Distance above the center of the sleeve device positioned in the lower esophageal sphincter (LES) is shown on the left with time of contraction onset on the right. At rest, the esophageal body is quiet and there is no motor activity whereas the upper esophageal sphincter and LES both maintain a contraction that can be measured manometrically and characterized as resting or basal tone. During deglutition the classic coordinated motor pattern of the esophagus, called *primary peristalsis*, is initiated. With transfer of the bolus into the esophagus, a progressive circular contraction begins in the upper esophagus and proceeds down the esophageal body to propel the bolus through a relaxed LES, which subsequently closes with a prolonged contraction.

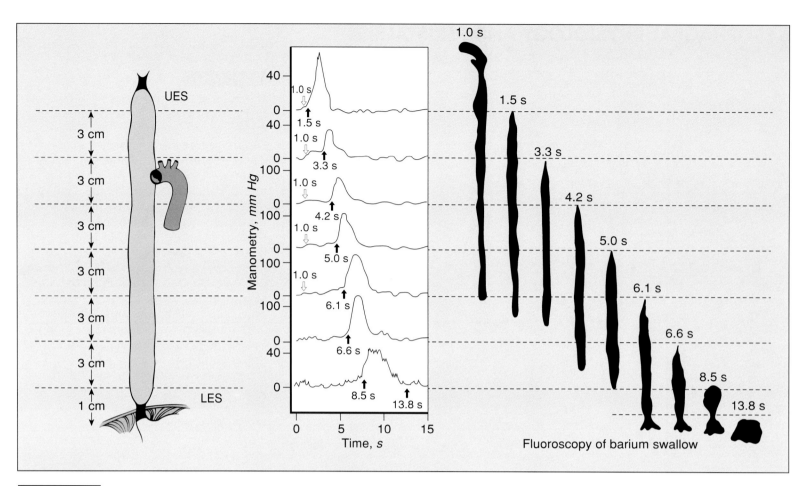

FIGURE 1-23.

Relationship between peristaltic function and esophageal volume clearance. The mechanical equivalent of peristalsis is a stripping wave that clears the esophagus in an aboral fashion. The velocity of the stripping wave corresponds to the manometrically recorded contraction such that the point of the inverted V seen fluoroscopically at each manometric sensor occurs simultaneously to the upstroke of the pressure wave. Data defining the relationship between the amplitude of esophageal peristalsis and the efficacy with which the stripping wave empties the esophagus are demonstrated in this figure.

This figure also shows concurrent manometric and video recordings of a 5-mL barium swallow. The tracings of the sequential fluoroscopic images show the distribution of the barium column at the times indicated above the images and by closed arrows on the manometric tracings. Here, a single peristaltic sequence completely cleared the barium from the esophagus. Administration of the barium occurred at 1.0 second, causing some esophageal distension and slightly increasing intraluminal pressure, shown by the open arrows on the manometric record. With onset of peristalsis, luminal closure is achieved as the tail of the barium bolus passes each recording site concurrent with the onset of the manometric pressure wave. LES—lower esophageal sphincter; UES—upper esophageal sphincter. (*Adapted from* Kahrilas [18].)

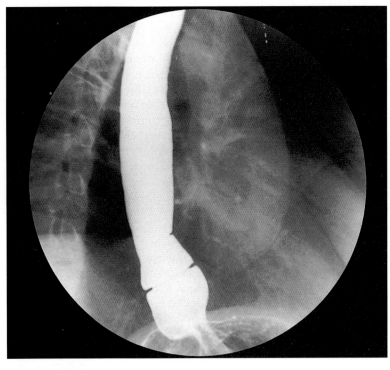

FIGURE 1-24.

Schatzki's ring on barium esophagram. Esophageal webs and rings are thin esophageal stenoses typically composed of only mucosa. Rings formed at the gastroesophageal junction, as described by Schatzki, are usually silent but become symptomatic when the internal diameter is less than 13 mm. (*From* McBride and Ergun [19]; with permission.)

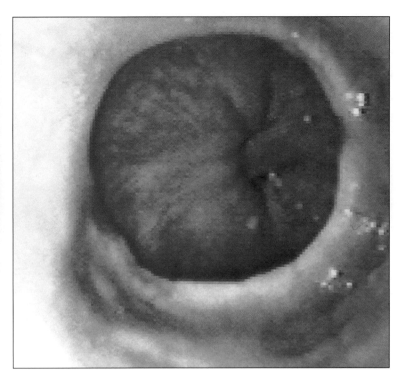

FIGURE 1-25.

Schatzki's ring viewed endoscopically.

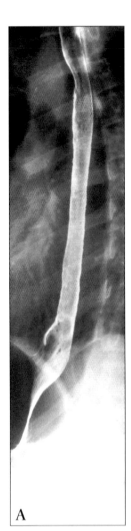

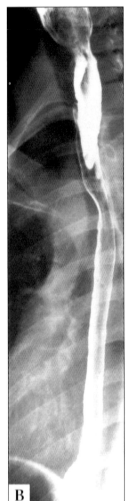

FIGURE 1-26.

A–B, Esophageal stenosis. Congenital esophageal anomalies include atresia, stenosis, webs, and duplications. Three variants of congenital esophageal stenosis exist. The most common type is associated with tracheobronchial remnants in the esophageal wall. The second is associated with multiple esophageal webs. The third type, shown here, is fibromuscular stenosis that is unassociated with webs or tracheobronchial remnants. The esophagogram shows evidence of narrowing in the entire length of the esophagus.

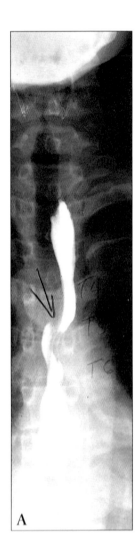

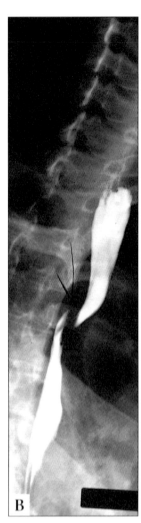

FIGURE 1-27.

Arteria lusoria. Dysphagia lusoria is caused by extrinsic esophageal compression caused by an aberrant right subclavian artery arising from the descending aorta and passing behind the esophagus. A, anterior view; B, oblique view. (*From* McBride and Ergun [19]; with permission.)

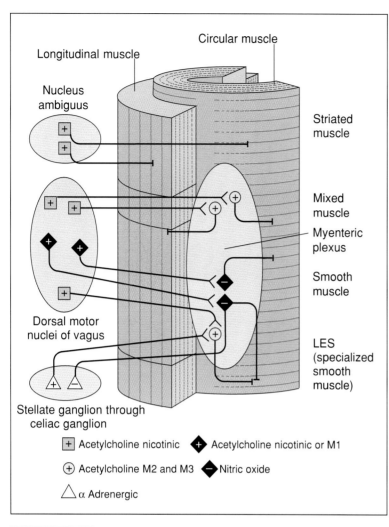

Longitudinal muscle

Circular muscle

Nucleus ambiguus

Striated muscle

Mixed muscle

Myenteric plexus

Smooth muscle

Dorsal motor nuclei of vagus

LES (specialized smooth muscle)

Stellate ganglion through celiac ganglion

- ⊞ Acetylcholine nicotinic
- ◆ Acetylcholine nicotinic or M1
- ⊕ Acetylcholine M2 and M3
- ◆ Nitric oxide
- △ α Adrenergic

FIGURE 1-28.

Extrinsic and intrinsic motor innervation of the esophagus. The control mechanisms that govern the striated and smooth muscu-

lature of the esophagus are distinct. The extrinsic innervation of the esophagus is through the vagus nerve. The striated muscle receives excitatory vagal innervation exclusively from axons of lower motor neurons with cell bodies in the nucleus ambiguus. Peristaltic contraction of this segment results from sequential activation of motor units in a craniocaudad sequence caused by programming by the medullary swallowing center that is potentiated by stimulation of afferent fibers from the esophagus designed to mimic the effect of a bolus being pushed ahead of a peristaltic contraction. Moreover, vagal motor fibers are inhibited during the pharyngeal phase of swallowing, supporting the concept that deglutitive inhibition has a central origin. Similarly, primary peristalsis of the smooth muscle exists following deviation of the bolus path and curarization of the oropharyngeal and cervical esophagus, suggesting that primary peristalsis in the smooth muscle segment is at least partially governed by the medullary swallowing center. Vagal control of the smooth muscle esophagus is more complex, with vagal innervation provided by the dorsal motor nucleus of the vagus and vagal fibers synapsing on myenteric plexus neurons rather than directly on neuromuscular junctions. There is, however, no vagal activity during secondary peristalsis, supporting the notion that the organization of peristalsis in the smooth muscle is an intramural process.

With respect to the intrinsic control of peristalsis, the entire esophagus has an intramural nerve network (*see* Fig. 1-13). Interestingly, the function of the myenteric plexus in the striated esophagus is unknown. The morphology and function in the smooth muscle esophagus have yet to be determined; however, there are two main types of effector neurons within the myenteric plexus. Excitatory neurons mediate contraction of both the longitudinal and circular smooth muscle through cholinergic M2 receptors, and inhibitory neurons affect predominantly the circular muscle layer through a nonadrenergic, noncholinergic neurotransmitter (NANC), now believed to be nitric oxide. Cholinergic excitation of the excitatory neurons is nicotinic whereas cholinergic excitation of the NANC can be muscarinic (M1) as well. LES—lower esophageal sphincter. (*Adapted from* Kahrilas [20].)

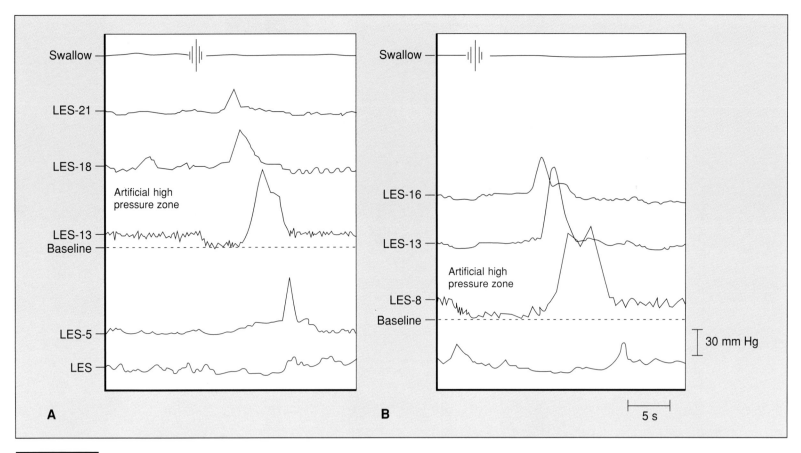

FIGURE 1-29.

Deglutitive inhibition. It has been suggested that swallowing not only induces primary peristalsis but also triggers a wave of inhibition of the smooth muscle that precedes the arrival of the peristaltic contraction (deglutitive inhibition). This idea was based on in vivo experiments in animals but was never studied in humans in detail because inhibition is difficult to visualize. This figure shows resting pressure and deglutitive pressure waves in the human esophagus with an artificial high pressure zone created originally at 13 cm (**A**) and then at 8 cm (**B**) above the lower esophageal sphincter (LES). Note that after swallowing a relaxation of the artificial high pressure zone started simultaneously at 13 cm and 8 cm above the LES. The end of the relaxation coincided with the start of the peristaltic contraction at that level.

This study shows direct evidence that a wave of inhibition precedes a swallow-induced peristaltic contraction in the smooth muscle of the human esophagus. This inhibitory wave was visualized by the appearance, after swallow, of a relaxation of the sustained contraction that was induced by insufflation of a balloon at different levels of the distal esophagus. This relaxation started simultaneously over the entire distal esophageal body but lasted progressively longer in progressively more distal segments. The timing of the relaxation of the artificial high pressure zone strongly suggests that it represents the manometric equivalent of the electrical postdeglutitive smooth muscle membrane hyperpolarization described in animal studies and the esophageal body equivalent of the postdeglutitive LES relaxation (*Adapted from* Sifrim [21].)

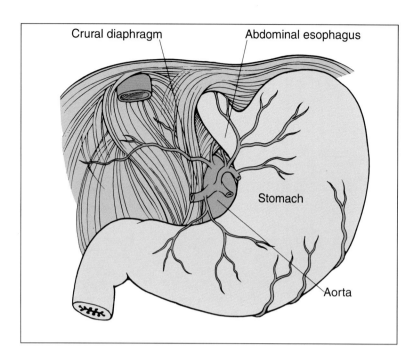

FIGURE 1-30.

Anatomy of the gastroesophageal junction highlighting the relationship between the diaphragm and the lower esophageal sphincter (LES). The esophagus, vagal trunks, and esophageal branches of the left gastric vein traverse the diaphragm through the esophageal hiatus. The crural fibers of the diaphragm encircle the esophagus in such a manner that a contraction of the muscle during inspiration constricts the esophagus.

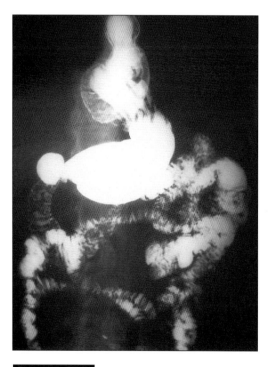

FIGURE 1-31.

Axial hiatus hernia. Most hiatal hernias are classified as axial or sliding. With the axial hiatal hernia there is decreased tethering by the phrenoesophageal ligaments and enlargement of the esophageal hiatus, which allows the gastric cardia to herniate upward into the thorax. The degree of herniation is highly variable. With small hernias only a small amount of the lesser curve and part of the fundus may be apparent, and with large hernias the entire fundus of the stomach may be visible in the thorax.

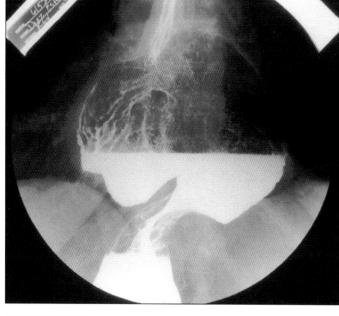

FIGURE 1-32.

Paraesophageal hernia. In patients with paraesophageal hiatal hernias the cardioesophageal junction characteristically maintains normal position because the paraesophageal ligaments are normally arranged around most of the esophagus. A break in the continuity of the phrenoesophageal membrane allows the esophageal hiatus to enlarge, allowing a variable portion of the gastric fundus access into the thorax alongside the esophagus. As the hernia enlarges the body of the stomach is also drawn into the hernial sac whereas the pylorus and duodenum remain in the abdominal cavity, still tethered by their normal attachments.

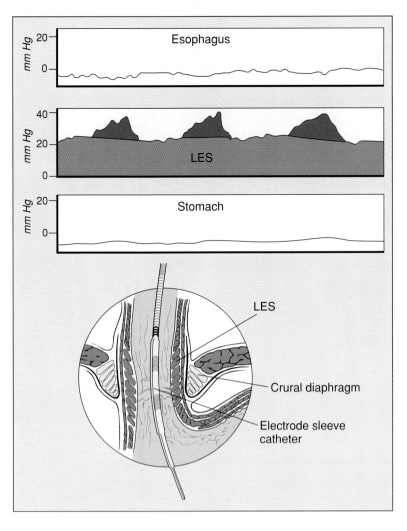

FIGURE 1-33.

Intrinsic lower esophageal sphincter (LES) pressure. The LES is a 3- to 4-cm segment of tonically contracted smooth muscle with a resting tone that varies from 10 to 30 mm Hg relative to gastric pressure. This positive pressure gradient between the stomach and the esophagus can be considered the driving force for gastro-esophageal reflux, with the high pressure zone at the gastroesophageal junction considered a barrier to the prevention of reflux of gastric contents. The high pressure zone has two components: (1) a tonic pressure caused by the LES, which is believed to be caused by a combination of myogenic factors, active tonic neural excitation, and complex interactions of other neural and hormonal factors [22], and (2) superimposed phasic pressure oscillations resulting from contractions of the diaphragmatic crus that encircles the LES [23–26].

This figure shows the contribution of diaphragm contraction (green portion) to basal LES pressure (orange portion). Note that a significant component of LES pressure is contributed by the diaphragm and that augmentation of the LES pressure corresponds temporally and quantitatively with the augmentation of crural electromyographic activity. (*Courtesy of* Dr. R. Mittal, Charlottesville, VA.)

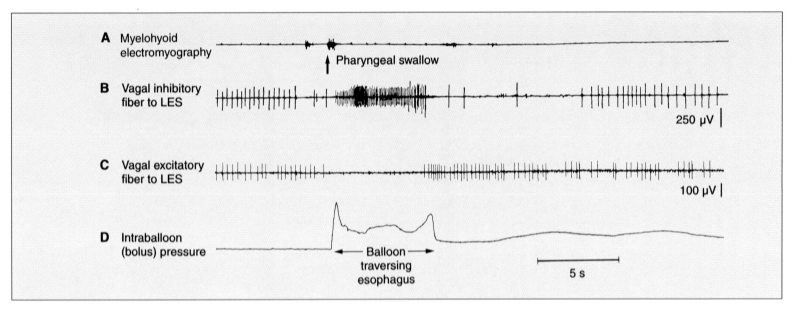

FIGURE 1-34.

Extrinsic control of the lower esophageal sphincter (LES). The LES tone is subject to both vagal and adrenergic influences, with vagal stimulation activating both excitatory (cholinergic) and inhibitory (nitric oxide) myenteric neurons. This figure illustrates the extrinsic control of the LES. A, Myelohyoid electromyography (arrow indicates the time of the pharyngeal swallow). B and C, Activity of the vagal inhibitory and excitatory fibers, respectively, to the LES at the time of swallow. D, Intraballoon (bolus) pressure at time of swallow. Note that the excitatory component is selectively activated under basal conditions and the inhibitory component is activated during swallow and mediates LES relaxation. (*Adapted from* Miolan and Roman [27].)

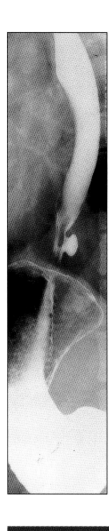

Figure 1-35.

Epiphrenic diverticulum as seen on barium swallow. An esophageal diverticulum is an outpouching of the esophageal wall from the lumen that may contain all portions of the esophageal wall or may lack the muscularis mucosa. Epiphrenic diverticula are usually located within 10 cm of the gastroesophageal junction and are thought to be pulsion-type diverticula. These are hypothesized to result from abnormal pulsion forces associated with abnormal esophageal motility and abnormal lower esophageal sphincter relaxation, producing increased intraluminal pressure, thus allowing outpouching to occur.

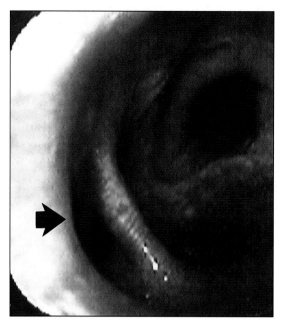

Figure 1-36.

Endoscopic view of an epiphrenic diverticulum. The arrow indicates the opening of the diverticulum. The lumen of the gastroesophageal junction is to the side.

TABLE 1-1. SUBSTANCES INFLUENCING LES PRESSURE

	Increases LES pressure	Decreases LES pressure
Hormones	Gastrin Motilin Substance P	Secretin Cholecytokinin Glucagon Somatostatin Gastric inhibitory polypeptide Vasoactive inhibitory polypeptide Progesterone
Medications	Metoclopramide Domperidone Cisapride Histamine Antacids Prostaglandin F2α	Theophylline Prostaglandins E2 and I2 Serotonin Morphine Meperidine Calcium channel blockers Diazepam
Food	Protein	Fat Chocolate Ethanol Oil of peppermint
Neural agents	α-Adrenergic agonists β-Andrenergic antagonists Cholinergic agonists	α-Adrenergic antagonists β-Adrenergic agonists Cholinergic antagonists

Table 1-1.

Substances influencing lower esophageal sphincter (LES) pressure. Intra-abdominal pressure, gastric distension, food, and many peptides and drugs affect LES pressure.

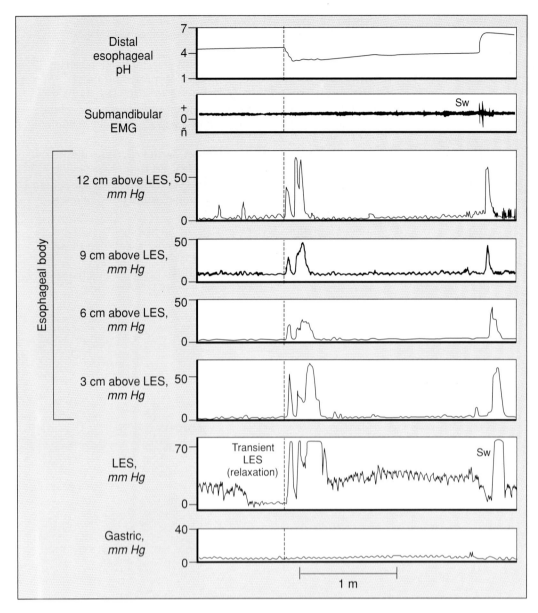

Distal esophageal pH

Submandibular EMG

Esophageal body

12 cm above LES, mm Hg

9 cm above LES, mm Hg

6 cm above LES, mm Hg

3 cm above LES, mm Hg

LES, mm Hg

Transient LES (relaxation)

Gastric, mm Hg

1 m

FIGURE 1-37.

Transient lower esophageal sphincter (LES) relaxation. Individual gastroesophageal reflux events occur by one of three mechanisms: transient LES relaxations, abdominal strain, or free reflux across a patulous LES [28]. Transient LES relaxations occur in both normal individuals and in patients with gastroesophageal reflux; they are the only potential mechanism for reflux during periods in which the LES is normal. These relaxations are part of the reflex that normally allows for gas venting from the stomach and may be triggered by fundic distension with air [29,30].

This example of transient LES relaxation was recorded in an asymptomatic individual. LES pressure is referenced to gastric pressure. Note that the transient LES relaxation persisted for almost 30 seconds whereas the swallow-induced LES relaxation (Sw) lasted for only 5 seconds. Also note the absence of an electromyographic (EMG) signal from a submental electrode during the transient LES relaxation, signifying the absence of a pharyngeal swallow. (*Adapted from* Kahrilas and Gupta [31].)

REFERENCES

1. Dodds WJ, Stewart ET, Logemann JA: Physiology and radiology of the normal oral and pharyngeal phases of swallowing. *AJR Am J Roentgenol* 1990, 154:953–963.

2. Christ J, Gidda JS, Goyal RK: Intramural mechanism of esophageal peristalsis: Roles of cholinergic and noncholinergic nerves. *Proc Natl Acad Sci U S A* 1984, 81:3595.

3. Gilbert RJ, Dodds WJ: Effect of selective muscarinic antagonists on peristaltic contractions in opossum smooth muscle. *Am J Physiol* 1986, 250:G50.

4. Murray J, Du C, Ledlow A, *et al.*: Nitric oxide: Mediator of nonadrenergic noncholinergic responses of opossum esophageal muscle. *Am J Physiol* 1991, 261:G401–G406.

5. Tottrup A, Svane D, Forman A: Nitric oxide mediating NANC inhibition in opossum lower esophageal sphincter. *Am J Physiol* 1991, 260:G385–G389.

6. Kahrilas PJ: The anatomy and physiology of dysphagia. In *Dysphagia, Diagnosis, and Treatment.* Edited by Gelfand DW, Richter JE. New York: Igaku-Shoin; 1989:11–28.

7. Kahrilas PJ, Lin S, Logemann JA, *et al.*: Deglutitive tongue action: Volume accommodation and bolus propulsion. *Gastroenterology* 1993, 104:152–162.

8. Kahrilas PJ, Logemann JA, Lin S, *et al.*: Pharyngeal clearance during swallowing: A combined manometric and videofluoroscopic study. *Gastroenterology* 1992, 103:128–136.

9. Kahrilas PJ, Logemann JA, Gibbons P: Food intake by maneuver: An extreme compensation for impaired swallowing. *Dysphagia* 1992, 7:155–159.

10. Castell DO: *The Esophagus.* Edited by Castell DO. Boston: Little, Brown, and Co; 1995:1–29.

11. Jacob P, Kahrilas PJ, Logemann JA, *et al.*: Upper esophageal sphincter opening and modulation during swallowing. *Gastroenterology* 1989, 97:1469–1478.

12. Kahrilas PJ: Volume accommodation during swallowing. *Dysphagia* 1993, 8:259–265.

13. Ergun GA, Kahrilas PJ, Lin S, *et al.*: Shape, volume, and content of the deglutitive pharyngeal chamber imaged by ultrafast CT. *Gastroenterology* 1993, 105:1396–1403.

14. Jacob P, Kahrilas PJ, Herzon G, *et al.*: Determinants of upper esophageal sphincter pressure in dogs. *Am J Physiol* 1990, 259:G245–G251.

15. Kahrilas PJ, Lin S, Chen J, *et al.*: Three dimensional modeling of the oropharynx during swallowing. *Radiology* 1995, 194:575–579.

16. Liebermann-Meffert D, Luscher V, Neff V, *et al.*: Esophagectomy without thoracotomy: Is there a risk of intramediastinal bleeding? A study on blood supply of the esophagus. *Ann Surg* 1987, 206:184–192.

17. Kitano S, Terblanche J, Kahn D, *et al.*: Venous anatomy of the lower oesophagus in portal hypertension: Practical implications. *Br J Surg* 1986, 73:525–531.

18. Kahrilas PJ: The effect of peristaltic dysfunction on esophageal volume clearance. *Gastroenterology* 1988, 94:73–80.

19. McBride MA, Ergun GA: Role of upper endoscopy in the management of esophageal strictures. *Gastrointest Endosc Clin North Am* 1994, 4:595–621.

20. Kahrilas PJ: Functional anatomy and physiology of the esophagus. In *The Esophagus*. Edited by Castell DO. Boston: Little, Brown, and Co; 1995:1–29.

21. Sifrim D: Inhibition in the human esophageal body: Its role in normal and disordered motility [thesis]. Katholieke Universiteit Leuven, Leuven, Belgium, 1994.

22. Goyal RK, Rattan S: Neurohumoral, hormonal, and drug receptors for the lower esophageal sphincter. *Gastroenterology* 1978, 74:598.

23. Mittal RK, Rochester DF, McCallum RW: Sphincteric action of the diaphragm during a relaxed lower esophageal sphincter. *Am J Physiol* 1989, 256:G139–G144.

24. Boyle JT, Altschuler SM, Nixon TE, *et al.*: Role of the diaphragm in the genesis of lower esophageal sphincter pressure in the cat. *Gastroenterology* 1985, 88:723–730.

25. Mittal RK, Rochester DF, McCallum RW: Electrical and mechanical activity in the human lower esophageal sphincter during diaphragmatic contraction. *J Clin Invest* 1988, 81:1182–1189.

26. Mittal RK, Rochester DF, McCallum RW: Sphincteric action of the diaphragm during a relaxed lower esophageal sphincter in humans. *Am J Physiol* 1989, 256:G139–G144.

27. Miolan JP, Roman C: Activit des fibres vagales efferentes destines la musculature lessé du cardia du chien. *J Physiol Paris* 1978, 74:709–723.

28. Dent J, Dodds WJ, Friedman RH, *et al.*: Mechanism of gastroesophageal reflux in recumbent asymptomatic human subjects. *J Clin Invest* 1980, 65:256–257.

29. Patrikios J, Martin CJ, Dent J: Relationship of transient lower esophageal sphincter relaxation to postprandial gastroesophageal reflux and belching in dogs. *Gastroenterology* 1986, 90:545.

30. Martin CJ, Patrikios J, Dent J: Abolition of gas reflux and transient lower esophageal relaxation by vagal blockade in the dog. *Gastroenterology* 1986, 91:890.

31. Kahrilas PJ, Gupta RR: Mechanisms of acid reflux associated with cigarette smoking. *Gut* 1990, 31:4.

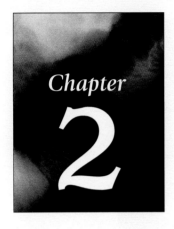

Chapter 2

Diagnostic Esophageal Endoscopy

WALLACE C. WU

Radiology and endoscopy are the two main diagnostic techniques used to evaluate patients with esophageal symptoms. Other methods, such as esophageal manometry, prolonged intraesophageal pH monitoring, Bernstein's test, radionuclide studies, and endoscopic ultrasonography (EUS), play only supplementary roles in these patients. In this chapter the roles of endoscopy, radiology, and EUS in the diagnosis and management of patients with esophageal diseases except gastroesophageal reflux disease are discussed.

Endoscopy of the esophagus with a rigid esophagoscope was first described by Bevan in 1868. Since then the technique has been superceded by fiberoptic endoscopy and later by video endoscopy. Video endoscopy, first introduced in 1983, uses a charge-coupled device to generate electronic images that are then displayed on a monitor. Video endoscopy not only allows for viewing by multiple examiners but also provides better images and superior reporting and storage of data. The images can also be enhanced, modified, and augmented. The full potential of video endoscopy remains to be exploited, however.

EQUIPMENT AND PROCEDURE

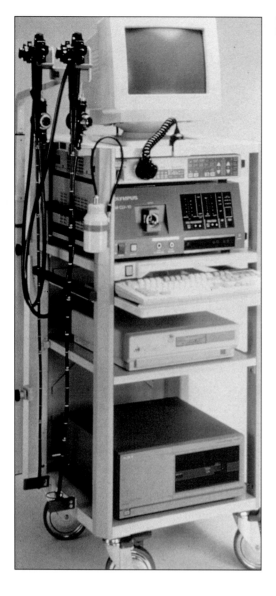

FIGURE 2-1.

Fiberoptic endoscopy is being replaced by video endoscopy. As already stated, video endoscopy not only allows for better images, but more than two examiners can view the images simultaneously. Because images and reports can be stored on disks, video endoscopy provides superior data and image storage. In addition, it is less strenuous for the primary examiner's neck and back! Because the damage-prone fiberoptic image bundle is replaced by a charge-coupled device, it is also cheaper to maintain. One major disadvantage, however, is that it is not as portable as the fiberoptic system.

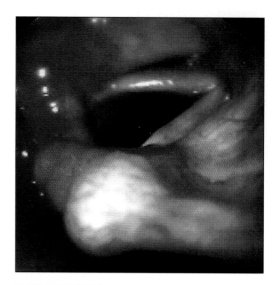

FIGURE 2-2.

Patients undergoing endoscopy in the United States are usually premedicated with intravenous meperidol, diazepam, or midazolam; topical pharyngeal anesthesia is optional. When using video endoscopy the instrument should be passed under direct vision. The epiglottis, larynx, and the vocal cord are identified easily, as illustrated. At this point, when the patient swallows, the cricopharyngeus will relax and the esophagus will be seen between the pyriform sinus and the posterior aspect of the larynx. The instrument can then be inserted at this point.

INDICATIONS AND CONTRAINDICATIONS

TABLE 2-1. INDICATIONS FOR ENDOSCOPY OF THE ESOPHAGUS

Diagnostic

Dysphagia and odynophagia

Certain patients with suspected gastroesophageal reflux disease

Patients with suspected infectious esophagitis

Cancer surveillance (eg, Barrett's esophagus)

Abnormal results of barium esophagogram

Therapeutic

Dilatation of strictures, both benign and malignant

Sclerotherapy and banding of varices

Stent placement in palliative therapy of malignant stricture

Laser therapy of esophageal and gastroesophageal malignancies

Removal of foreign body

TABLE 2-1.

Almost all patients with esophageal symptoms should be evaluated initially with a barium esophagogram and endoscopy. Probably not all patients with suspected gastroesophageal reflux disease require endoscopy. The major advantages of endoscopy over barium esophagogram are that endoscopy not only provides biopsy capabilities but also has other therapeutic potentials. Removal of foreign bodies, esophageal dilatation with a guide wire, sclerotherapy and banding of varices, and palliative treatment of esophageal neoplasms can all now easily be done using the endoscope.

TABLE 2-2. CONTRAINDICATIONS TO ENDOSCOPY

Absolute Contraindications

Patients who are unable to cooperate

Patients who are moribund

Patients with suspected perforated viscus

Patients who are hemodynamically unstable

Relative Contraindications

Patients with large Zenker's diverticulum

Dysphagic patient who has not had an esophagogram recently

TABLE 2-2.

In general, endoscopy can be safely performed in almost all patients. It should, however, not be used in uncooperative and moribund patients. It should also not be performed in patients with a suspected perforated viscus because the nonsterile instrument and air insufflation needed to perform the procedure will more than likely aggravate mediastinal or peritoneal contamination. In a patient with Zenker's diverticulum the endoscope could preferentially enter through the esophagus rather than through the diverticulum. Hence, in this situation the endoscope should be passed carefully under direct vision. Perforation of a Zenker's diverticulum has been reported. As discussed later in this chapter, it may be more appropriate to obtain an esophagogram before endoscopy in a patient with dysphagia.

TABLE 2-3. COMPLICATIONS OF UPPER GASTROINTESTINAL ENDOSCOPY

DIAGNOSTIC	PERCENTAGE
Medication reactions	0.5%
Perforation	0.03–0.1%
Bleeding (with biopsy)	0.03%

TABLE 2-3.

Complications with diagnostic upper gastrointestinal endoscopy are extremely rare. The most common are reactions to conscious sedation that result in cardio-pulmonary complications. Hence, the use of automated blood pressure devices, pulse oximetry, and electro-cardiography in monitoring the patient during and after the procedure is encouraged. Although esophageal perforation may occur with diagnostic endoscopy, it is more likely to result from therapeutic procedures, such as esophageal dilatation and laser therapy.

■ DIAGNOSTIC ENDOSCOPY VERSUS RADIOLOGY

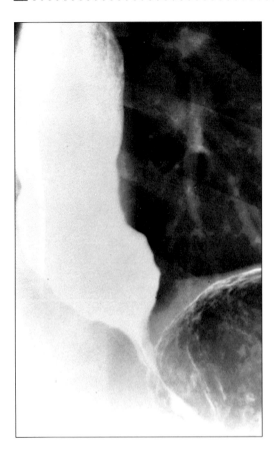

FIGURE 2-3.

Barium esophago-gram and endoscopy are complementary to each other in the diagnosis of esophageal diseases. This figure represents the lower esophagus of a patient with dysphagia. Endo-scopy was thought to be normal. Esophagogram showed a bird's beak appearance of the gastroesophageal junction and total aperistalsis of the esophageal body consistent with the diagnosis of achalasia.

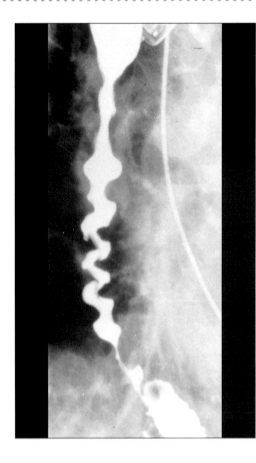

FIGURE 2-4.

Endoscopy is an excellent tool in the diagnosis of mucosal lesions. Unfortunately, it is unable to differen-tiate between normal and abnormal peri-stalsis and hence is insensitive in the diagnosis of motility disorders of the esophagus. This figure depicts the esophagogram of a patient with dysphagia and chest pain. His endoscopy is completely normal. Esophagogram shows classic changes of diffuse esophageal spasm. Esophageal manometry confirms the diagnosis.

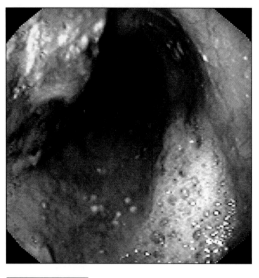

FIGURE 2-5.

Achalasia can occasionally be diagnosed by endoscopy. This image is from a patient who had a markedly dilated esophagus with a large amount of retained ingested food. In a patient with chronic history of dysphagia, this finding is diagnostic for achalasia. In addition, the tightly closed lower esophageal sphincter, which may be difficult to intubate, may show a rosette appearance.

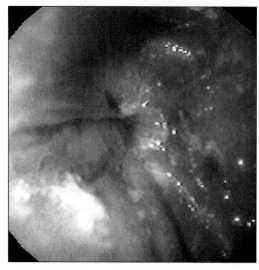

FIGURE 2-6.

Classic rosette appearance of the gastro-esophageal junction in a patient with documented achalasia. This finding is caused by the tightly closed lower esophageal sphincter.

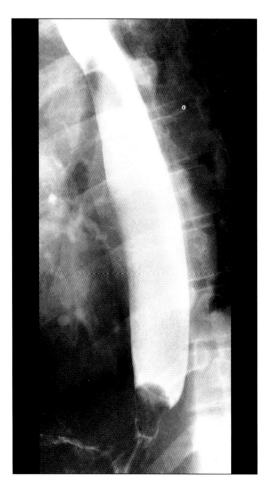

FIGURE 2-7.

Adequate examination of the lower esophagus by both radiology and endoscopy is impossible without adequate distension. For this reason a common lesion, such as lower esophageal mucosal ring, can be missed by both techniques. The radiologist may also challenge the esophagus with a solid bolus such as a marshmallow or a barium tablet. This patient had intermittent solid food dysphagia for many years. Previous evaluation using esophagography, manometry, and endoscopy were normal. The marshmallow distended the lower esophagus and brought out the lower esophageal mucosal ring. In addition, impaction of the marshmallow reproduced the patient's symptom. Esophageal dilatation rendered this patient asymptomatic.

TABLE 2-4. RADIOLOGY VS. ENDOSCOPY IN ESOPHAGEAL DISEASES

	RADIOLOGY	ENDOSCOPY
Oropharyngeal dysphagia	++++	—
Cervical web	++++	++
Extrinsic compression	++++	+
Esophageal diverticula	++++	+++
Carcinoma	++++	++++
Acute caustic injury	—	++++
Pill-induced injury	++	++++
Foreign body	+++	++++
Gastroesophageal reflux disease*	++	+++
Peptic stricture	++++	++++
Barrett's epithelium	++	++++
Lower esophageal mucosal ring	++++	+++
Infectious esophagitis	+++	++++
Varices	+++	++++
Achalasia	++++	++
Diffuse esophageal spasm	++	—
Nonspecific esophageal motor dysfunction	++	—

*As defined by 24-hour pH monitoring.
+—poor sensitivity; ++—fair sensitivity; +++—good sensitivity; ++++—excellent sensitivity;

TABLE 2-4.

Comparison of diagnostic accuracy of radiology with that of endoscopy. Endoscopy is superb for mucosal lesions and has biopsy and therapeutic potentials. On the other hand, the role of endoscopy in the diagnosis of esophageal motor disorders is limited. For this reason, in patients with dysphagia caused by both solids and liquids, it may be more appropriate to obtain an esophagogram as the initial diagnostic procedure. An esophagogram also enables clinicians to rule out oropharyngeal causes of dysphagia that cannot be assessed with endoscopy.

ENDOSCOPIC ULTRASONOGRAPHY

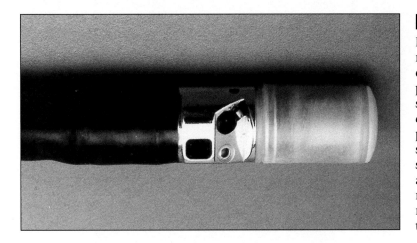

FIGURE 2-8.

Endoscopic ultrasonography (EUS) is performed by a special instrument that consists of mounting an ultrasonic transducer on an endoscope, as illustrated in this figure, or by passing ultrasonic probes through the biopsy channel of an endoscope. The EUS scope is of larger caliber and is slightly more difficult to pass compared with a standard endoscope. Otherwise, the procedure is performed in the same manner as routine endoscopy and ultrasonic examination performed at specific areas of interest. The EUS scope allows for up to 360 degrees of scanning whereas the probe allows for various degrees of sector scanning, depending on the manufacturer of the equipment. In the esophagus a specially mounted balloon is inflated with water so that clinicians can see the esophageal wall in more detail.

TABLE 2-5. ENDOSCOPIC ULTRASONOGRAPHY

Indications

Differential diagnosis of submucosal lesions of the esophagus

Staging of carcinoma of the esophagus

Guided biopsies and cytology of mass lesions

Contraindication

Severe stricture of the esophagus

TABLE 2-5.

In the esophagus, endoscopic ultrasonography (EUS) is most useful in the differential diagnosis of submucosal lesions and tumor staging of malignant neoplasms of the esophagus. Because the instrument is of relatively large caliber, esophageal perforation has been reported during EUS. Therefore, this instrument should always be passed with extreme caution.

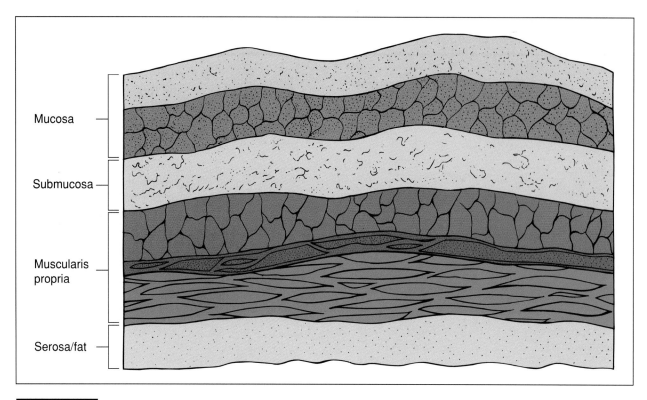

FIGURE 2-9.

Unlike endoscopy, endoscopic ultrasonography allows for the visualization of the wall of the esophagus. This figure depicts the various layers of the esophagus that can be seen with this technique. In addition, immediate surrounding structures, such as lymph nodes, may also be seen.

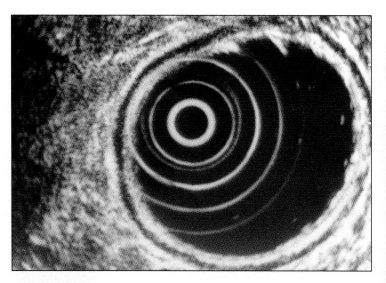

FIGURE 2-10.

This echosonogram of a normal esophagus depicts the five echo layers of the gastrointestinal tract. The first hyperechoic layer represents the balloon mucosal interface; the second layer (hypoechoic) to the mucosal layer; the third (hyperechoic) to the submucosa; the fourth (hypoechoic) to the muscularis propria; and the fifth (hyperechoic) to the serosa.

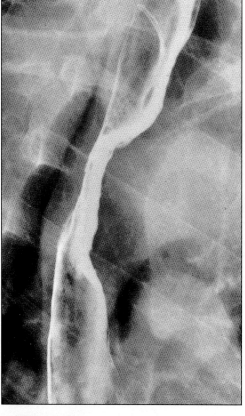

FIGURE 2-11.

This is the esophagogram from a patient who experienced progressive solid-food dysphagia for several months. He also experienced a 20-pound weight loss during that same period. Esophagogram showed a malignant neoplasm involving the esophagus.

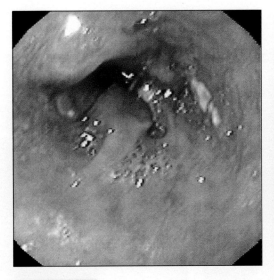

FIGURE 2-12.

Endoscopy of the patient confirmed the presence of an apparently malignant lesion in the esophagus. Biopsies showed a squamous cell carcinoma of the esophagus.

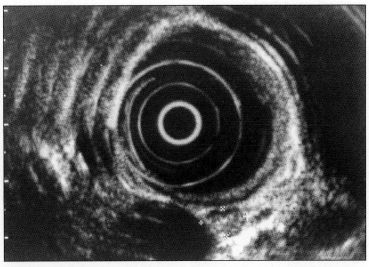

FIGURE 2-13.

Endoscopic ultrasonography was performed for staging. It clearly revealed lymph node metastasis. For this reason, the patient was not considered to be a candidate for primary surgical resection. Instead, he was treated with radiation and chemotherapy.

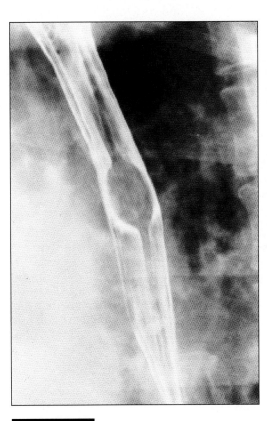

FIGURE 2-14.

A submucosal esophageal lesion was found incidentally during an upper gastrointestinal series performed for the evaluation of dyspepsia. The patient had no esophageal symptoms. Endoscopy confirmed the presence of a submucosal mass lesion covered by apparently normal epithelium.

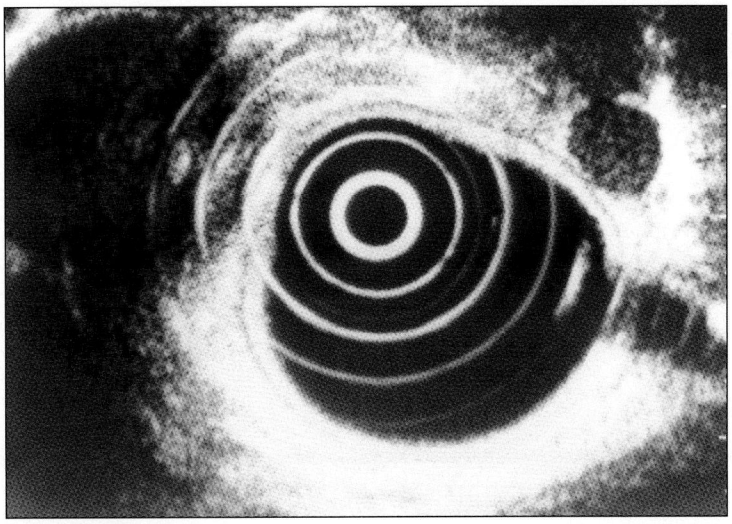

FIGURE 2-15.

Endoscopic ultrasonography of the lesion shown in Figure 2-13 revealed expansion of the fourth layer with complete preservation of the other layers. This finding is consistent with the diagnosis of leiomyoma. Because the patient was asymptomatic and the lesion relatively small, no specific therapy was instituted.

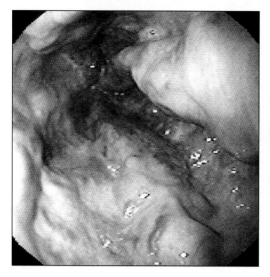

FIGURE 2-16.

This is the endoscopic view of the esophagus of a 79-year-old female. She presented with several episodes of hematemesis on the day before admission. She denied any consumption of alcohol and had no prior history of liver diseases. Her initial hemoglobin was 7.9. Results of all her liver function tests were normal. Endoscopy revealed large esophageal varices. Serologic tests for hepatitis B, hepatitis C, and autoimmune hepatitis were all negative. Liver biopsy showed inactive cirrhosis. Her varices were treated with sclerotherapy and the patient had not bled in a year.

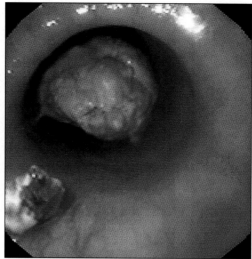

FIGURE 2-17.

Foreign body ingestion with esophageal impaction by items other than food is more common among children. In adults, it tends to occur only in psychiatric patients. Food impaction, particularly of red meat or raw fruits and vegetables, however, may occur in patients with esophageal diseases. This figure is from a patient who is suffering from meat impaction. He had given a history of intermittent solid food dysphagia. The offending bolus was removed endoscopically. The patient was then found to have a lower esophageal ring 9 mm in diameter. After undergoing esophageal dilatation, the patient became completely asymptomatic.

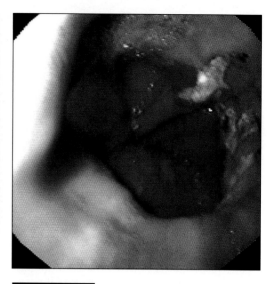

FIGURE 2-18.

Mallory-Weiss tears are usually associated with recent nausea, vomiting, retching, and coughing. The finding is thought to be caused by a sudden increase in intra-abdominal pressure. A strong relationship also exists in patients with heavy alcohol ingestion, which is a common cause of upper gastrointestinal bleeding. This figure showed two tears across the gastroesophageal junction; however, most Mallory-Weiss tears are in the cardia. Treatment is conservative because most bleeding stops spontaneously.

TABLE 2-6. CLASSIFICATION OF ESOPHAGEAL DIVERTICULA

Zenker's diverticulum

Protrusion of hypopharyngeal mucosa between the inferior pharyngeal constrictor and cricopharyngeus

Midesophageal diverticula

Outpouchings of the middle third of the esophagus

Epiphrenic diverticula

Outpouchings in the distal 10 cm of the esophagus

Esophageal intramural pseudodiverticulosis

Multiple pinhead-sized outpouchings of the esophagus

TABLE 2-6.

Esophageal diverticula are outpouchings of the esophagus. They are usually classified according to their anatomic location. Usually caused by pulsion forces, they almost always lack a muscular coat.

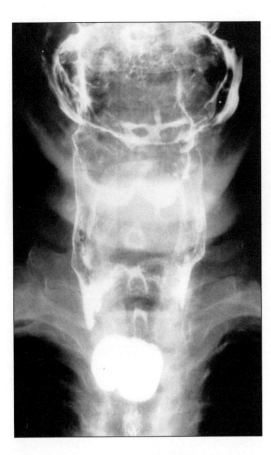

FIGURE 2-19.

Zenker's diverticulum is actually a hypopharyngeal lesion. It is a protrusion of the mucosa between the inferior pharyngeal constrictor and the cricopharyngeus muscle. The pathogenesis of this lesion is controversial, but it appears that pharyngeal and upper esophageal sphincter discoordination may play a role. Many findings are incidental, but dysphagia and regurgitation are the most common symptoms. Treatment, if needed, is by surgical methods.

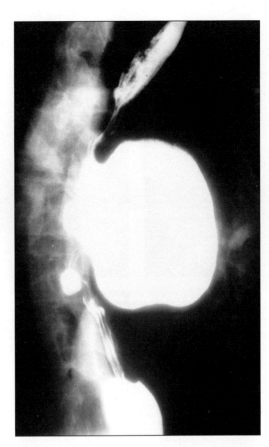

FIGURE 2-20.

The midesophageal diverticulum is usually small and asymptomatic. This figure, however, represents an unusually large midesophageal diverticulum. Most of these lesions are associated with an underlying esophageal motility disorder. In most cases treatment is not needed; however, in the patient whose case is illustrated here, surgery was performed because of severe symptoms of dysphagia and regurgitation.

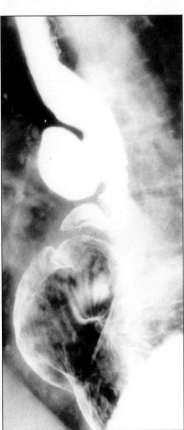

FIGURE 2-21.

A patient with multiple epiphrenic diverticula and achalasia. This is a known association; the diverticulum is presumably caused by the underlying motility disorder. Pneumatic dilatation is thought to be contraindicated in this situation because an increased risk of esophageal perforation may exist. The patient had Heller's myotomy and multiple diverticulectomy.

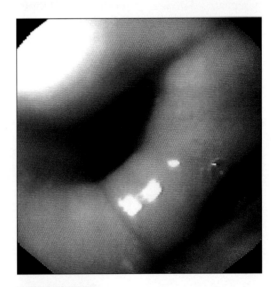

FIGURE 2-22.

Endoscopic view of a patient with a large epiphrenic diverticulum. Two lumen can clearly be seen, one representing the diverticulum and the other the esophageal lumen.

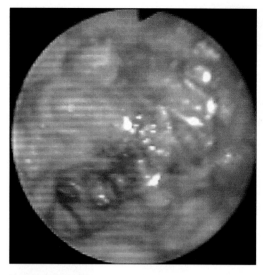

FIGURE 2-23.

This image is from a patient with a long-standing history of symptoms of gastroesophageal reflux disease. Manometry showed a totally aperistaltic esophagus. In addition, he had taken at least eight aspirin a day for many years. Esophagography and endoscopy revealed multiple pseudodiverticula of the lower third of the esophagus. It was postulated that they were formed by repeated damage caused by both acid and aspirin. In addition, the patient's motility disorder probably impaired his esophageal clearance and thus aggravated the situation.

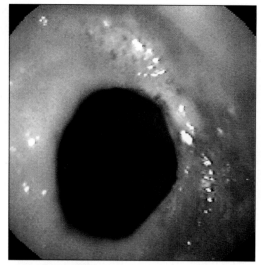

FIGURE 2-24.

The presence of a lower esophageal mucosal ring is one of the most common causes of dysphagia. Its pathogenesis is unknown. Its upper surface is always covered by esophageal (squamous) epithelium, its lower surface by gastric (columnar) epithelium. In general, rings smaller than 13 mm in diameter are always symptomatic and those over 20 mm never produce any symptoms. Intermittent solid food dysphagia is the main presenting symptom. Treatment consists of passing a single large-caliber dilator (*ie*, 15 mm or larger) through the esophagus to disrupt the ring.

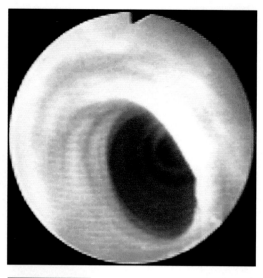

FIGURE 2-25.

Ring-like structures in the esophagus are generally known as *webs*; they can be single or multiple. In most patients no underlying etiology is apparent. It may, however, be associated with graft-versus-host disease in bone marrow transplantation and with some dermatologic diseases, such as epidermolysis bullosa and mucous membrane pemphigoid. This figure is from an otherwise healthy elderly patient with dysphagia. Endoscopic testing revealed multiple esophageal webs. Esophageal dilatation relieved his symptoms.

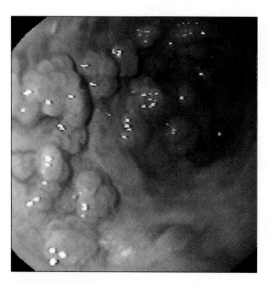

FIGURE 2-26.

Squamous cell papilloma of the esophagus is a rare benign tumor of the esophagus. It usually does not produce any symptoms and appears as a single or multiple wart-like lesion on the esophageal mucosa. This figure comes from a patient who was incidentally found to have multiple squamous cell papilloma. She had no esophageal symptoms, and because of the extent of the lesion endoscopic excision was not contemplated.

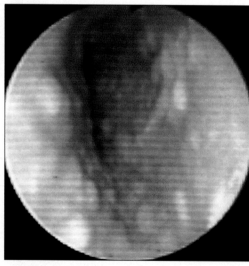

FIGURE 2-27.

Glycogenic acanthosis is represented by single or multiple small white papules, usually found in the distal esophagus. It is relatively common and is not thought to produce any symptoms. Histologically, it represents hyperplastic squamous epithelium with increased glycogen content. Its pathogenesis remains unknown.

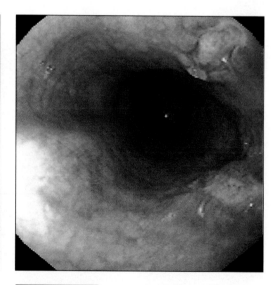

FIGURE 2-28.

A 25-year-old female was prescribed doxycycline for treatment of acne. After she developed dysphagia and odynophagia acutely, she remembered that she had taken a dose of doxycycline just before she went to bed the night before. Endoscopy showed two ulcers in the midesophagus. The history and endoscopic appearance are perfectly compatible with the diagnosis of esophagitis caused by medication in pill form.

TABLE 2-7. COMMON MEDICATIONS CAUSING ESOPHAGEAL INJURY

Antibiotics and antivirals

Doxycycline, tetracyclines, clindamycin, zidovudine

Nonsteroidal anti-inflammatory agents

Doleron, aspirin, indomethacin

Others

Potassium chloride, quinidine, ferrous sulphate and succinate, ascorbic acid

TABLE 2-7.

Esophageal injury caused by medication in pill form is thought to be due to prolonged contact of the offending medication with the normal esophageal mucosa. All medications should therefore be taken with a liberal amount of liquid and never just before retiring to bed. This table lists the most common medications available in the United States that may cause this type of injury.

Chapter 3

Esophageal Investigative Techniques

■ MANOMETRY

Historical perspective

LOUIS P. LEITE
DONALD O. CASTELL

The first manometric studies were performed in 1883 by Kronecker and Meltzer, who used air-filled balloons and an external pressure transducer. Water-filled balloons were first used by Ingelfinger and Abbot in 1940. Because of their inaccuracy and delayed assessment of rapid pressure changes in the esophagus, these methods were later found not to be clinically useful and were abandoned. Studies using water-filled catheters first began in the 1950s and initiated development of the basic knowledge of the physiology and pathophysiology of esophageal motility. The lower esophageal sphincter (LES) was first identified manometrically by Fyke and associates in 1956. Small intraluminal solid-state transducers were introduced in the 1970s.

The devices for measurement of esophageal pressures remain either a water-filled catheter connected to external transducers or a catheter assembly containing small direct intraluminal transducers. Although very slow infusion rates are sufficient (<1.0 mL/min) to record tonic sphincter squeeze, a more vigorous infusion rate within the catheter is required to record accurately the transient high pressures produced during intraesophageal peristaltic activity. Even the best infusion system is incapable of recording the extremely rapid pressure changes (>1000 mm Hg/sec) in the pharynx.

Accurate recording of sphincter pressure and esophageal peristaltic pressure can also be obtained with small direct intraluminal transducers. A comparison of this technique with the best infusion techniques reveals excellent correlation. Increasing numbers of clinical motility laboratories are equipped with this methodology; the resulting lack of dependence on infusion pumps and fluid-filled systems and the ability to record pharyngeal pressures accurately are considered assets. Either system, however, is satisfactory for quantitative clinical studies of esophageal function when properly applied.

Pioneering work with prolonged pH monitoring was first performed by Spencer in 1967 and developed into a clinically applicable technique by Johnson and DeMeester in the mid-1970s. The latter investigators documented that intraesophageal pH could be measured over a 24-hour cycle by using an indwelling pH probe positioned 5 cm above the LES and a standard laboratory physiograph. Reflux was defined as intraesophageal pH below 4; the duration of the reflux episode was the time interval until the pH returned to greater than 4. The value pH 4 was chosen because (1) it is unequivocally distinct from the usual esophageal pH (approximately 7.0) (2) the proteolytic enzyme pepsin is essentially inactive above pH 4 and (3) patients with symptomatic reflux show good association between an intraesophageal pH of 4 and onset and resolution of their symptoms.

Clinical application of esophageal manometric studies

The major value of an esophageal manometry laboratory in clinical practice is in the diagnosis of esophageal (or pharyngeal and upper esophageal sphincter [UES]) motility dysfunction. These conditions can be placed in two types: those in which the motility defect is a primary condition involving only the esophagus and those in which an esophageal abnormality is a secondary aspect of a more generalized disease. The physician using an esophageal manometric laboratory for diagnostic help should recognize these distinctions and note particularly the potential esophageal motility disorders associated with various systemic diseases.

Disease entities in which motility changes are essentially pathognomonic include scleroderma and achalasia. The important manometric feature of sclerodermatous involvement of the esophagus is the marked abnormality in the smooth muscle portion of this organ (ie, lower two thirds) with relative normality of the striated muscle segment (ie, upper third). Achalasia is defined by specific manometric criteria characterized primarily by a poorly relaxing, hypertensive LES and total absence of esophageal peristalsis.

For the clinician the paramount problem is definition of the real value of esophageal manometry for a more precise diagnosis of patients with symptoms potentially of esophageal or pharyngeal origin.

TABLE 3-1. SUGGESTED CLINICAL USES OF ESOPHAGEAL MOTILITY TESTING

Stationary manometry

Evaluation of patients with dysphagia

    Primary esophageal motility disorders (eg, achalasia)

    Secondary esophageal motility disorders (eg, scleroderma)

    Upper esophageal sphincter/pharyngeal manometry for pharyngeal dysphagia

Evaluation of patients with possible gastroesophageal reflux disease

    Identify high-risk patients (lower esophageal sphincter pressure < 10 mm Hg)

    Support diagnosis in a complex case

      Atypical symptoms

      Failed medical therapy

    Evaluate defective peristalsis (particularly before fundoplication)

    Exclude scleroderma

    Assist in placement of pH probe

Evaluation of patients with noncardiac chest pain

    Primary esophageal motility disorders

    Pain response to provocative testing

Exclude generalized gastrointestinal tract disease

    Scleroderma

    Chronic idiopathic intestinal pseudo-obstruction

Exclude esophageal etiology for suspected eating disorder

Ambulatory manometry

Most commonly used in combination with 24-hour pH monitoring

Primarily a research tool

Probably beneficial for unexplained chest pain

Possibly beneficial

    Nonobstructive dysphagia

    Gastroesophageal reflux disease

TABLE 3-1.

Suggested clinical uses of esophageal motility testing. Controversy over the value of esophageal motility testing exists. In some situations esophageal manometry may be particularly helpful, specifically to exclude achalasia or as a preoperative assessment of esophageal motility prior to antireflux surgery. In contrast, the use of esophageal manometry in patients with unexplained chest pain appears to be of limited clinical use and remains a research tool at present.

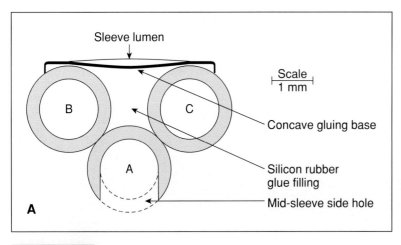

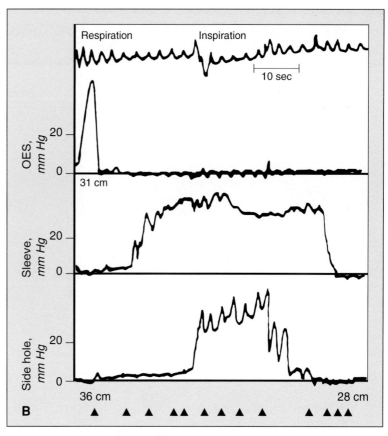

A, Schematic representation of a transverse section of a standard infused catheter modified for construction of the 6-cm long Dent sleeve. The section is cut at the level of the midsleeve position showing the location of the single-site recording orifice at this level. **B,** Lower esophageal sphincter pressure trace from the sleeve illustrated in **panel A** and the midsleeve side hole as the catheter device is pulled through the sphincter. The solid triangles at the base of the figure indicate each 5-mm catheter movement. Note that the sleeve records pressure uniformly over a distance of 4 to 5 cm and that the pressure is similar to the maximal pressure recorded by the single side hole at the midsleeve position. OES—oral esophageal stethoscope. (*Adapted from* Dent *et al.* [1].)

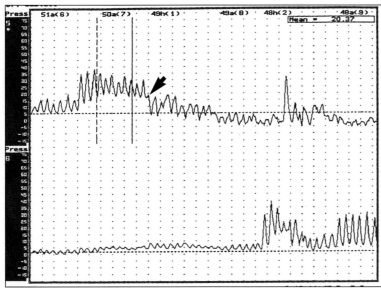

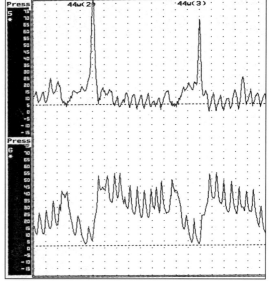

Manometric recording of the "pull through" of a solid-state transducer across the normal lower esophageal sphincter (LES). The upper tracing shows progressive increases in pressure as the catheter is slowly withdrawn across the LES. Maximal average pressure was obtained just distal to the pressure inversion point (*arrow*) before the transducer moved into the esophagus (right side of the graph). Phasic variations in pressure result from respiration. Note that the average intragastric pressure measured before initiation of the pull through is identified on each portion of the graph by a horizontal dotted line. Esophageal pressure is lower than the intragastric pressure, reflecting negative intrathoracic pressure. The lower tracing is recorded from a transducer spaced 3 cm distal to the transducer recording the upper tracing and is shown to begin to enter the high-pressure zone of the LES as the proximal transducer moves into the esophageal body.

Manometric tracing with two recording sites: one in the distal esophageal body (top tracing) and the second in the high-pressure zone of the lower esophageal sphincter (LES) (bottom tracing). Two water swallows are shown, illustrating normal relaxation of the LES. Note that the average resting tone of the LES is approximately 35 mm Hg greater than the gastric baseline pressure (horizontal dotted line) and that during relaxation the pressure falls close to the gastric baseline. Residual pressure, defined as the difference between gastric pressure and the nadir of the relaxation pressure, should not exceed 8 mm Hg in normal patients.

TABLE 3-2. RANGE OF NORMAL VALUES FOR STATIONARY ESOPHAGEAL MANOMETRY

	NORMAL VALUES
Lower Esophageal Sphincter	
Resting pressure, *mm Hg*	10–45
Residual pressure, *mm Hg*	≤8
Sphincter length, *cm*	3–5
Esophageal Body	
Distal (based on ten 5 mL water swallows):	
Peristaltic Waves	
Peristaltic waves, *number*	8–10
Average amplitude, *mm Hg*	30–180
Average duration, *sec*	3–6
Ineffective peristaltic waves	
Simultaneous, *number*	<2
Nontransmitted or low amplitude, *< 30 mm Hg, number*	<3
Triple-peaked peristaltic waves *number*	0
Proximal (based on ten 5 mL water swallows)	
Average amplitude, *mm Hg*	Normal values not established
Continued peristalsis distally	Should be present
Upper esophageal sphincter and pharynx	
UES pressure, *mm Hg*	30–118
UES residual pressure, *mm Hg*	≤8
UES relaxation duration, *msec*	401–689
Pharyngeal contraction pressure, *mm Hg*	60–192
Time from onset UES relaxation until pharyngeal contraction, *msec*	395±37

TABLE 3-2.

Range of normal values for stationary esophageal manometry. UES—upper esophageal sphincter.

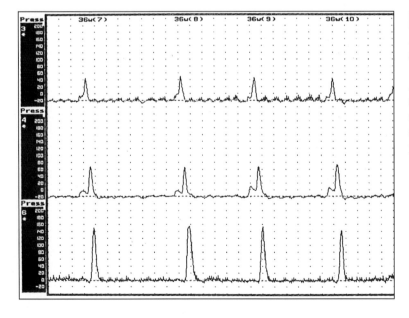

FIGURE 3-4.

Manometric tracing within the esophageal body. Recording sites are located at 3 cm (bottom tracing), 8 cm (middle tracing), and 13 cm (top tracing) above the lower esophageal sphincter (LES). A series of four water swallows is illustrated, demonstrating the sequential contraction pattern of typical peristalsis in the distal esophagus. Amplitudes in the distal two recording sites vary between approximately 60 and 150 mm Hg and represent a typical average pressure of approximately 100 mm Hg.

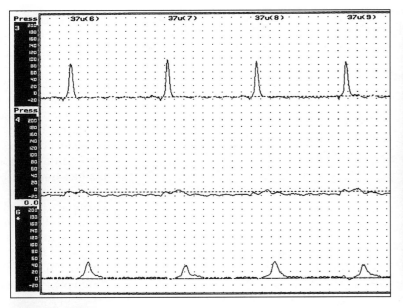

FIGURE 3-5.

Proximal esophageal peristaltic activity of a series of four swallows. Recording sites are located 1 cm (top tracing), 6 cm (middle tracing), and 11 cm (bottom tracing) below the upper esophageal sphincter (UES). Following the four wet swallows a peristaltic wave is initiated in the proximal esophagus transmitted into the midesophagus. Note the more rapid upstroke and shorter duration of the skeletal muscle contraction shown at the proximal recording site and the slower uptake and broader duration shown at the distal recording site. The pressure trough, frequently seen in the transition area between skeletal and smooth muscle, is identified by the nearly flat line at the middle recording site.

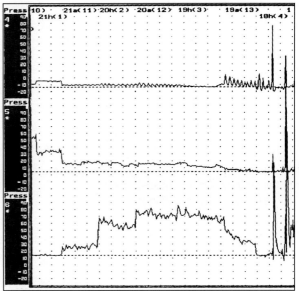

FIGURE 3-6.

Manometric tracing of a slow pull through of the circumferential solid state transducer across the upper esophageal sphincter (UES) (bottom tracing). Note the progressive rise in average resting pressure as the catheter is advanced in 0.5-cm increments. The average maximal UES pressure is 80 mm Hg, approximately the normal average pressure. Note that the middle transducer (spaced 3 cm above the distal transducer) records a tail of the UES pressure as it moves into the pharynx and that the proximal transducer (5 cm above the distal transducer) records pharyngeal pressure.

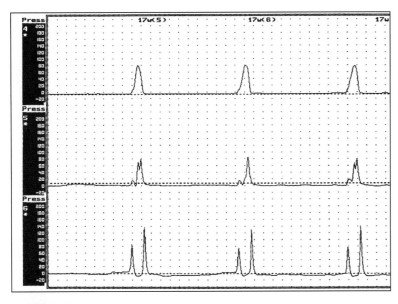

FIGURE 3-7.

Manometric recording of three wet swallows with recording sites at the upper esophageal sphincter (UES) (bottom tracing) and 3 cm

(middle tracing) and 5 cm (top tracing) above the UES. This figure demonstrates the ideal technique to record actual relaxation of the UES. Here, the distal circumferential transducer has been placed just proximal to the UES to allow it to be captured by the sphincter during elevation at the beginning of the swallow (identified by the initial pressure rise in the distal recording site). This is followed by the relaxation and subsequent contraction of the sphincter, which in turn is followed by return of pressure as the UES descends once more to a position below the transducer. This produces the characteristic "M" configuration on the manometric recording. The proximal and middle transducers demonstrate peristaltic pressures in the pharynx and normal coordination of this event with the relaxation phase of the UES. Note that UES residual pressure (nadir of relaxation) is often negative to the esophageal baseline pressure measured before movement of the transducer across the UES and is demonstrated by the horizontal dotted line.

TABLE 3-3A. CLASSIFICATION OF PRIMARY ESOPHAGEAL MOTILITY ABNORMALITIES

TABLE 3-3.

Classification of esophageal motility abnormalities. Traditionally, esophageal motility abnormalities have been divided into primary (occurring without associated diseases), representing abnormalities limited to the esophagus (**A**), or secondary, defined as esophageal involvement in a patient with an associated systemic disease (**B**). LES—low esophageal sphincter; UES—upper esophageal sphincter.

Diagnosis	Motility Findings
Achalasia (the true disorder)	Absent distal peristalsis
	Incomplete LES relaxation (residual pressure > mm Hg)
	Elevated resting LES pressure (> 45 mm Hg)
	Increased baseline esophageal pressure
Abnormal Motility Patterns (nonspecific esophageal dysmotility)*	
Diffuse esophageal spasm	Simultaneous contractions (≥20% wet swallows)
	Intermittent peristalsis
	Repetitive contractions (≥3 peaks)
	Prolonged duration contractions (> 6 sec)
Hypercontracting esophagus	
Hypertensive peristalsis (nutcracker esophagus)	Increased distal peristaltic amplitude (> 180 mm Hg)
	Increased distal peristaltic duration (> 6 sec)
Hypertensive LES	Resting LES pressure > 45 mm Hg
	May be incomplete LES relaxation (residual pressure > 8 mm Hg)
Hypocontracting esophagus	
Ineffective motility[†]	Increased nontransmitted peristalsis (≥ 30%)
	Low distal peristaltic amplitude (< 30 mm Hg)
Hypotensive LES [†]	Resting LES pressure (< 10 mm Hg)
Others	Retrograde contractions
	Triple-peaked contractions
	Isolated incomplete LES relaxation (> 8 mm Hg)

*Defined as exceeding two standard deviations from mean of normal values.
†May be "secondary" to gastroesophageal reflux disease.

TABLE 3-3B. CLASSIFICATION OF SECONDARY ESOPHAGEAL MOTILITY ABNORMALITIES

Diagnosis	Motility Findings
Systemic sclerosis	Loss of distal (smooth muscle) peristalsis
	Weak LES pressure (< 10 mm Hg)
	Normal proximal esophagus and UES (striated muscle)
Chagas' disease	Identical to idiopathic achalasia (see above)
Diabetes mellitus	A variety of motility abnormalities of the esophageal body
Chronic idiopathic intestinal pseudo-obstruction	Loss of distal esophageal motility
Chronic gastroesophageal reflux disease	Ineffective motility
	Hypotensive LES

Achalasia

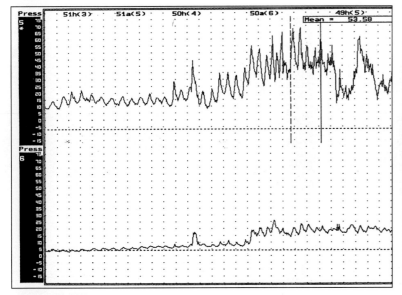

FIGURE 3-8.

Manometric tracing of a pull through into the lower esophageal sphincter (LES) in a patient with achalasia. Note the high resting LES pressure of approximately 54 mm Hg. During water swallows (right side of tracing) relaxation is incomplete, with a residual pressure of approximately 20 mm Hg. The bottom tracing shows the trailing transducer moving into the LES.

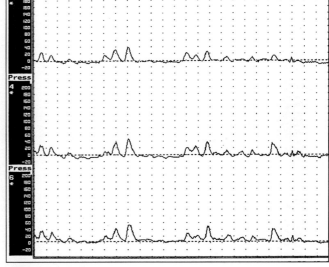

FIGURE 3-9.

Manometric tracing of a patient with achalasia. The transducers are placed at 3 cm (bottom tracing), 8 cm (middle tracing), and 13 cm (top tracing) above the lower esophageal sphincter. Note that a pressure change is identified with each of the water swallows but a peristaltic wave front is completely absent. In fact, the pressure changes noted at each recording site are identical, or *mirror images*. These waves represent pressure transmitted throughout the dilated, nonpropulsive esophagus, and have also been termed *hyperbaric waves*. This is a typical pattern of esophageal body motility in a patient with achalasia.

Diffuse esophageal spasm

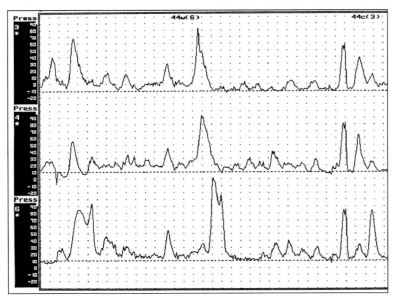

FIGURE 3-10.

Manometric tracing of a patient with diffuse esophageal spasm (DES). Recording sites are located at 3 cm (bottom tracing), 8 cm (middle tracing), and 13 cm (top tracing) above the lower esophageal sphincter. Variations in manometric responses (as shown in this patient) are quite typical of DES. On the left a spontaneously occurring simultaneous contraction is shown. This is followed by a swallow-induced peristaltic wave that appears normal. The final water swallow (on the right) shows simultaneous and repetitive contractions, which are typical of DES. This entity is characterized by increased numbers of simultaneous contractions after wet swallows (20% or more), but with intermittent normal peristaltic responses, as illustrated in this figure.

Hypercontracting esophagus

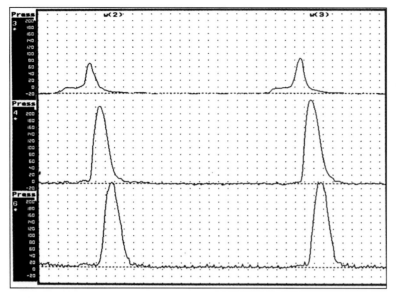

FIGURE 3-11.

Manometric recording from a patient with hypertensive peristalsis (nutcracker esophagus). Recording sites are located at 3 cm (bottom tracing), 8 cm (middle tracing), and 13 cm (top tracing) above the lower esophageal sphincter. The two responses to water swallows show a normally progressive peristaltic wave of excessive amplitude (approximately 240 mm Hg) at the distal two recording sites. Nutcracker esophagus is defined by average peristaltic responses at these two recording sites, exceeding 180 mm Hg.

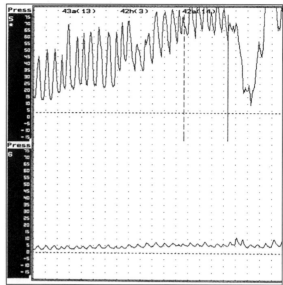

FIGURE 3-12.

Manometric recording of a portion of the lower esophageal sphincter (LES) pull through in a patient with a hypertensive LES. Recordings obtained by two circumferential solid-state transducers spaced at 3-cm intervals are shown. The proximal transducer has moved into the high-pressure zone, showing an average maximal pressure of approximately 71 mm Hg (measured between the solid and dotted vertical lines) above the average intragastric pressure, which is identified by the dotted horizontal line. Relaxation with the swallows at the right shows a residual pressure of 5 mm Hg. Note that the distal transducer is moving from gastric pressure (left) into the distal portion of the LES on the right.

Ineffective esophageal motility

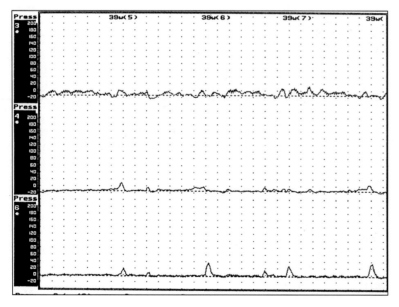

FIGURE 3-13.

Manometric tracing from a patient showing findings previously classified as nonspecific esophageal dysmotility, characterized by essentially nontransmitted contractions following a series of three swallows with only very low amplitude (approximately 20 mm Hg) contractions seen at the distal site. Recording sites are 3 cm (bottom tracing), 8 cm (middle tracing), and 13 cm (top tracing) above the lower esophageal sphincter. This tracing illustrates one of the typical features of what has previously been classified as nonspecific dysmotility, and is probably better classified as *ineffective esophageal motility.*

Systemic sclerosis

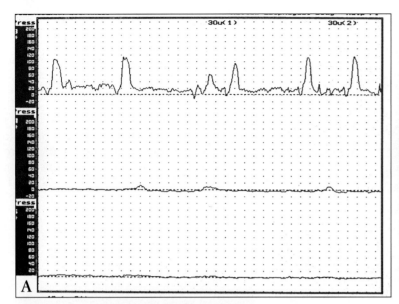

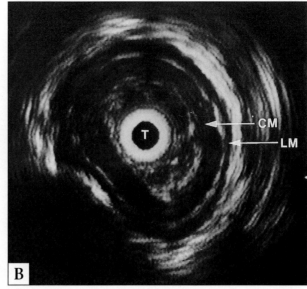

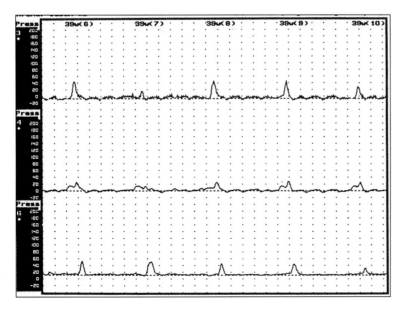

FIGURE 3-14.

A, Manometric tracing from a patient with systemic sclerosis. Recording sites are 1 cm (top tracing), 6 cm (middle tracing), and 11 cm (bottom tracing) below the upper esophageal sphincter. Contraction is regular in the proximal, striated muscle segment of the esophagus with each swallow, but transmission fails in the peristaltic contraction into the distal (smooth muscle) esophagus. Loss of smooth muscle peristalsis is typical of systemic sclerosis being a manifestation of the collagen replacement of the smooth muscle in this portion of the esophagus. Often the resting lower esophageal sphincter (LES) pressure is below normal. This combination of manometric events results in extreme acid reflux, often with markedly prolonged acid clearance because of the loss of peristaltic function in these patients. B–C, High-frequency intraesophageal ultrasound image comparing the normal esophagus (panel B) with the esophagus from a patient with scleroderma and absent distal esophageal peristalsis (panel C). In the normal subject the image clearly demonstrates the dark band of circular muscle (CM) and longitudinal muscle (LM) in this view taken from the distal esophagus. In contrast, the ultrasound image from the patient with scleroderma esophagus demonstrates complete replacement of the entire muscularis with hyperechoic abnormalities in the circular and longitudinal muscles, shown by the broken light areas between the arrows. T—transducer. (*From* Miller *et al.* [2]; with permission.)

Diabetes mellitus

FIGURE 3-15.

Manometric tracing from a patient with diabetes mellitus. Recording sites are located at 3 cm (bottom tracing), 8 cm (middle tracing), and 13 cm (top tracing) above the lower esophageal sphincter. On this tracing a series of water swallows shows peristaltic sequences of low amplitude. Abnormal motility (as shown in this tracing) is common in patients with diabetes mellitus and includes a spectrum from ineffective peristalsis of low amplitude (as shown here) to exaggerated nonperistaltic contractions resembling diffuse esophageal spasm. Interestingly, these patients are often asymptomatic for esophageal symptoms despite often quite marked motility abnormalities.

Chronic idiopathic intestinal pseudo-obstruction

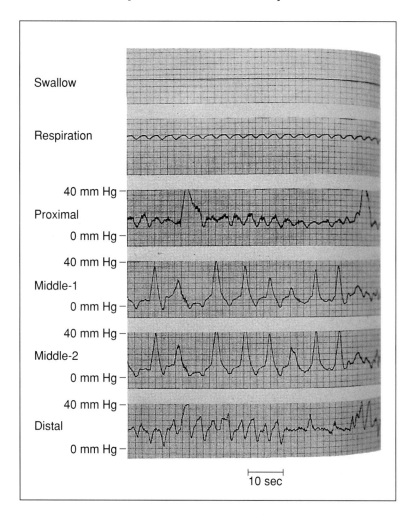

FIGURE 3-16.

Manometric recording from a patient with chronic idiopathic intestinal pseudo-obstruction (CIIP). This tracing demonstrates the degree of unusual motility that may be seen in the esophagus in patients with CIIP showing spontaneous activity of the esophageal body. The proximal tip is 32 cm from the teeth, the two middle tips are both 37 cm from the teeth, and the distal tip is 42 cm from the teeth. The distal tip is located in the upper portion of the lower esophageal sphincter (LES). Most of the pressure variations are related to respiration. Rates of spontaneous contractions vary at 5 cm and 10 cm above the LES. The patient has not swallowed during this interval, as shown by the flat record from the swallow marker. (*From* Schuffler *et al.* [3]; with permission.)

Hypertensive resting upper esophageal sphincter pressure

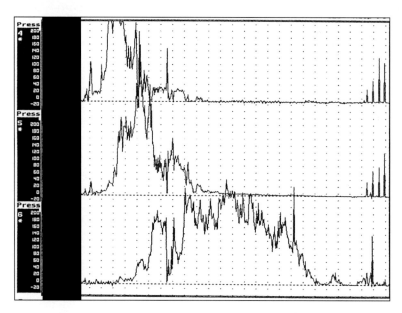

FIGURE 3-17.

Manometric tracing of a patient with a hypertensive resting upper esophageal sphincter (UES) pressure. The distal circumferential transducer is slowly pulled across the UES to identify maximal resting pressure, here reaching approximately 260 mm Hg (normal upper value approximately 115 mm Hg). The middle transducer, located 3 cm proximally, moves out of the UES high-pressure zone and into the pharynx as the distal transducer is drawn into the sphincter. The proximal transducer (5 cm above the distal transducer) records pharyngeal pressures.

Zenker's diverticulum

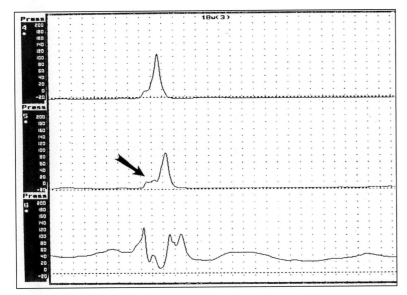

FIGURE 3-18.

Manometric tracing of pharyngeal and upper esophageal sphincter (UES) function during swallowing in a patient with Zenker's diverticulum. Recording sites are at the UES (bottom tracing) and 3 cm (middle tracing) and 5 cm (top tracing) above the UES. Although the pharyngeal contraction sequence is peristaltic and properly coordinated with UES relaxation, relaxation is defective, as indicated by a residual pressure of approximately 15 mm Hg. This abnormal relaxation is associated with defective opening of the UES segment seen radiographically in these patients and results in the large intra-bolus pressure seen preceding the pharyngeal clearing pressure in the middle recording site (*arrow*).

Oculopharyngeal muscular dystrophy

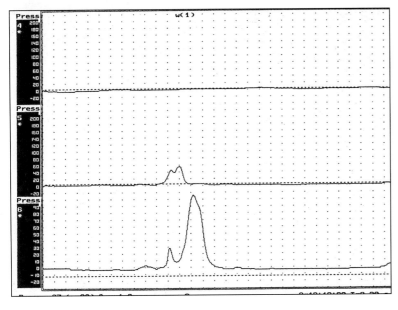

FIGURE 3-19.

Manometric tracing from a patient with oculopharyneal muscular dystrophy. The recording sites are located in the upper esophageal sphincter (UES) (bottom tracing), hypopharynx, 3 cm proximally (middle tracing), and oropharynx, 5 cm proximally (top tracing). During the single wet swallow illustrated, the UES demonstrates defective relaxation, characterized by a residual pressure of approximately 20 mm Hg above the proximal esophageal baseline (dotted horizontal line) and with a very short duration of relaxation of approximately 0.3 seconds. In addition, the pharyngeal contraction is weak (maximal pressure approximately 55 mm Hg) and is not coordinated with the inadequate UES relaxation. This combination of pharyngeal weakness and poor relaxation of the UES is typical of the manometric abnormality in these patients as their dysphagia becomes more progressive. This represents a true example of *cricopharyngeal achalasia*. Such patients have been shown to respond well to a cricopharyngeal myotomy.

Pharyngeal paresis

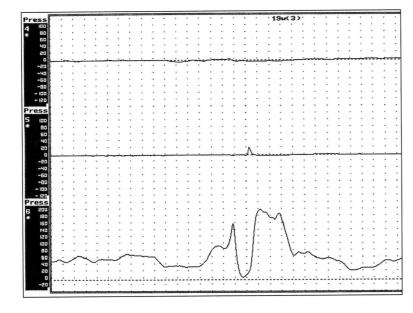

FIGURE 3-20.

Manometric tracing from a patient with pharyngeal paresis secondary to severe neuromuscular disease. Recording sites are located in the upper esophageal sphincter (UES) (bottom tracing) and 3 cm (middle tracing) and 5 cm (top tracing) above the sphincter. During the swallow shown in the tracing, elevation is normal and relaxation of the UES is normal, but there is almost complete absence of pharyngeal contraction with the exception of a weak (20 mm Hg) contraction in the hypopharynx.

Oropharyngeal Dysphagia

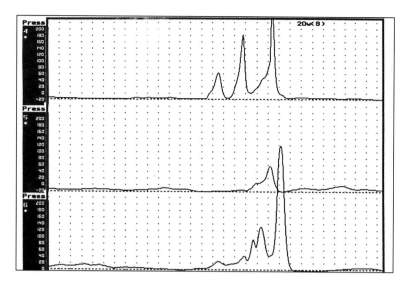

FIGURE 3-21.

Manometric tracing from a patient with severe oropharyngeal dysphagia and marked manometric abnormalities showing both pharyngeal spasm and incomplete upper esophageal sphincter (UES) relaxation. Recording sites are located in the UES (bottom tracing) and at 3 cm (middle tracing) and 5 cm (upper tracing) above the sphincter. Note the early and discoordinated repetitive (spastic) contractions in the oropharynx (top tracing) and the early contraction in the hypopharynx (middle tracing). Relaxation is very short and incomplete in the UES, showing a residual pressure of approximately 40 mm Hg.

Stroke

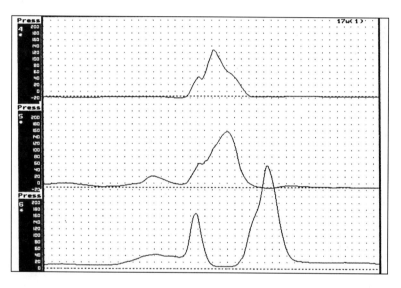

FIGURE 3-22.

Manometric tracing from a patient following a stroke with brain-stem involvement. Recording sites are located at the UES (bottom tracing), at 3 cm (middle tracing), and at 5 cm (upper tracing) above the sphincter. The most striking abnormality involves the simultaneous and broad contraction pattern in the pharyngeal recordings with marked incoordination between the pharynx and the relaxation of the UES.

■ AMBULATORY pH MONITORING

TABLE 3-4. PARAMETERS EVALUATED DURING pH MONITORING

Percentage of recording time when intraesophageal pH was below 4.0 in the upright position or recumbent position
Percentage of recording time with pH below 4.0 for the total 24-hour period
Total number of reflux episodes
Number of episodes longer than 5 minutes
Duration of longest episode

TABLE 3-4.

Johnson and DeMeester [6] developed a scoring system based on six variables to characterize the patterns of reflux. They introduced the concept of *physiologic reflux*, which is defined as a pattern seen in asymptomatic volunteers and characterized by rapidly cleared reflux episodes occurring primarily postprandially in the upright position, with rarer reflux episodes while recumbent (*see* Fig. 3-25). They also called attention to the importance of nocturnal (recumbent) reflux episodes as a risk factor for esophagitis and the associated prolonged clearance of acid during recumbent reflux.

TABLE 3-5. 24-HOUR AMBULATORY pH VALUES FOR NORMAL SUBJECTS*

	MEDIAN	RANGE	95TH PERCENTILE
Total, %	1.10	0–8.6	5.78
Upright, %	1.45	0–12.4	8.15
Supine, %	0.10	0–8.5	3.45
Total episodes (n)	18.0	0–101	46.00
Episodes > 5 min (n)	0	0–7	4.0
Longest episode, min	3.0	0–46	18.45

*n=110 Subjects (47 M, 63 W, mean age = 38 years)
"%" refers to % of 24-hour pH study that distal esophagael pH dropped below 4.0 (measured 5 cm above proximal border of the manometrically located LES)

TABLE 3-5.

Twenty-four hour pH values for normal patients.

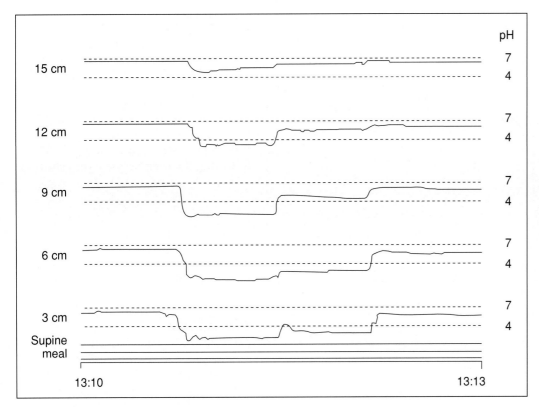

FIGURE 3-23.

This series of pH tracings shows a 3-minute interval, during which a single reflux episode was recorded during a 24-hour, 5-channel pH monitoring. In this example reflux spreads rapidly throughout the esophagus. Clearing of refluxate is stepwise. Note that at 15 cm above the lower esophageal sphincter the fall in pH does not pass the threshold of pH below 4 whereas the curve shows the same overall pattern as in the distal esophagus. This observation by Weusten and co-workers illustrates the importance of accurate placement of the pH probe when testing duration of acid exposure in the esophagus and also suggests that a pH cut off above 4.0 might be preferable to identify proximal reflux. (*Adapted from* Weusten *et al.* [4])

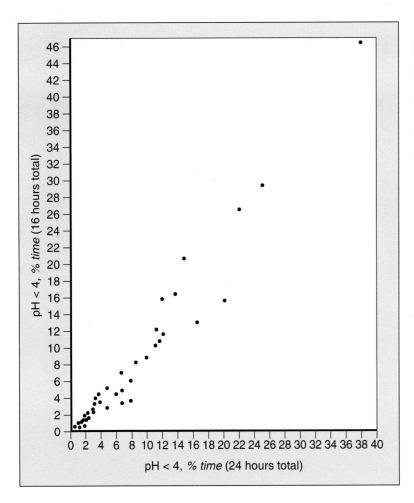

FIGURE 3-24.

Relationship between total percentage of time with pH below 4 comparing the 24-hour study with the 16-hour interval of the same study in the same patients. The excellent correlation ($r=0.98$) indicates that a total recording time of 16 hours can provide information similar to that of a full 24-hour study, particularly if the period studied includes the overnight recumbent phase and an equal portion of upright recording, as was performed in the study shown in the figure. (*Adapted from* Dobhan *et al.* [5].)

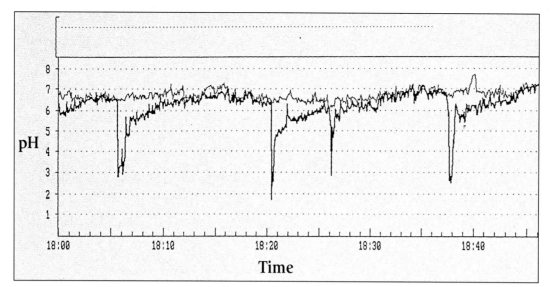

FIGURE 3-25.

Dual electrode pH recording showing distal acid exposure 5 cm above the lower esophageal sphincter (LES) (heavy line) and proximal pH 20 cm above the LES (narrow line) in a normal individual studied postprandially. Note the occasional brief episodes of distal reflux shown in this patient over a 40-minute period following the evening meal (not shown).

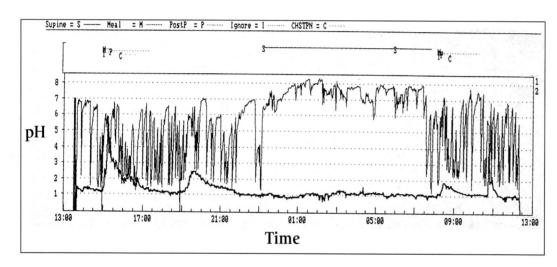

FIGURE 3-26.

Dual electrode pH recording showing esophageal (top tracing) and gastric (bottom tracing) pH in a patient with abnormal upright reflux. During the 24-hour period illustrated in the figure, this patient shows repeated episodes of reflux while awake and in the upright position, many associated with symptoms. In contrast, while in a recumbent position during sleep the patient shows a total absence of reflux. This is a frequent pattern seen in the patient who has reflux only when upright.

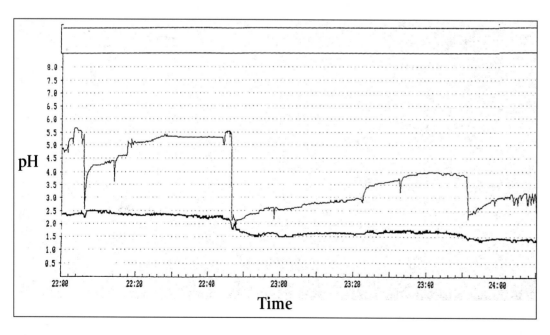

FIGURE 3-27.

Dual electrode pH recording on the computer screen showing esophageal (top tracing) and gastric (bottom tracing) pH in a patient with severe recumbent gastroesophageal reflux. Note the abrupt drop in pH followed by prolonged recovery, itself followed by additional episodes of reflux. This tracing demonstrates the markedly prolonged esophageal acid exposure time that occurs in patients with both recumbent reflux and prolonged acid clearance.

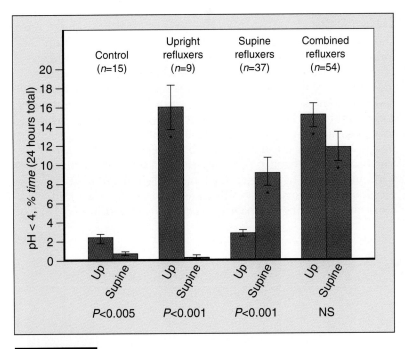

FIGURE 3-28.

Reflux patterns occurring in healthy controls, upright refluxers, supine refluxers, and combined refluxers shown as mean percentage of time pH below 4 during the 24-hour study in these patient groups. Asterisks indicate difference from control by $P<0.005$ to $P<0.001$. (*Adapted from* Johnson and DeMeester [6].)

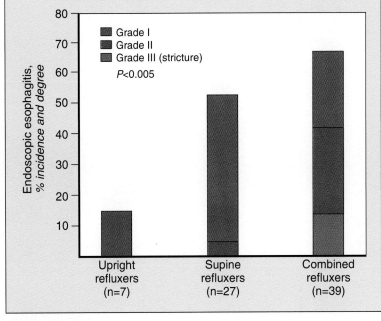

FIGURE 3-29.

This graph shows the relative prevalence and severity of endoscopic esophagitis compared to the reflux patterns identified during pH monitoring as shown in Figure 3-28. The prevalence of reflux and its severity increase with the total duration of acid exposure and, particularly, with the percentage of time of abnormal pH with the patient supine or recumbent. (*Adapted from* Johnson and DeMeester [6]).

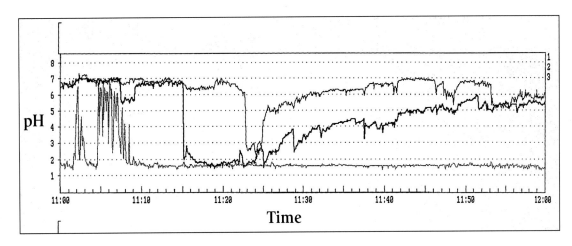

FIGURE 3-30.

Triple electrode pH recording with the proximally placed electrode (top line) placed 20 cm above the lower esophageal sphincter (LES), middle electrode (heavy line) positioned 5 cm above the lower esophageal sphincter, and the distal electrode (bottom line) 15 cm below the LES in the gastric fundus. This tracing demonstrates a typical pattern of distal reflux with the intraesophageal pH falling to the level of the intragastric pH. During the distal acid reflux, proximal acid exposure is also present. Note that proximal reflux occurs later and clears sooner than distal reflux. This tracing demonstrates severe reflux in a patient in the upright position.

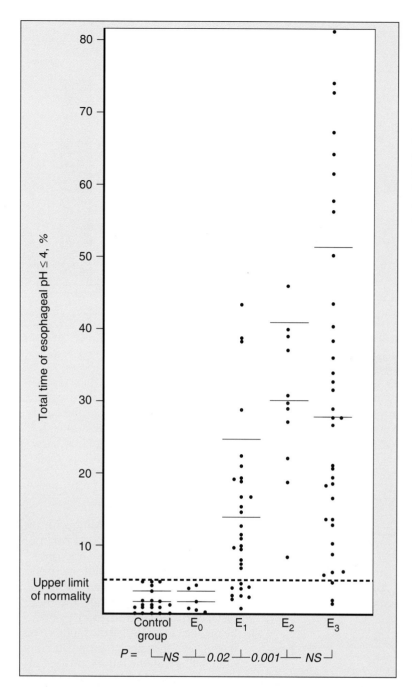

FIGURE 3-31.

Data illustrated on this figure document the rough correlation found between the severity of esophagitis and the total percentage of time pH is less than 4 in the distal esophagus during ambulatory monitoring. Normal acid exposure was found for normal controls and symptomatic patients without evidence of esophagitis. Although considerable overlap of values is noted, there is a definite trend toward greater amounts of acid exposure as the grade of esophagitis progresses from 1 through 3. E_0—abscence of macroscopic or microscopic esophagitis; E_1—microscopic esophagitis with or without mucosal hyperemia or edema; E_2—nonconfluent esophageal erosions; E_3—confluent erosions with or without erosions or Barrett's esophagus. (*Adapted from* Mattioli *et al.* [7].)

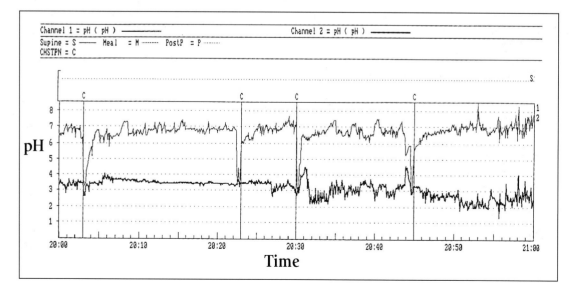

FIGURE 3-32.

Double electrode pH recording with electrodes in the distal esophagus (top tracing) and gastric fundus (bottom tracing). During this 1-hour interval the patient had four episodes of typical chest pain, each precisely related to a reflux event. A strong symptom association of this kind is extremely helpful to confirm the diagnosis of reflux-related symptoms.

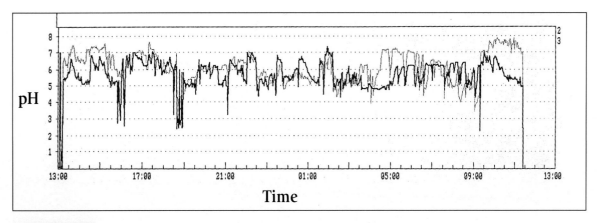

FIGURE 3-33.

Double electrode pH recording with the fainter line indicating distal esophageal pH and the heavier line gastric pH. The patient is taking omeprazole, 20 mg b.i.d. Intragastric pH remains above 4 throughout the 22 hours and 30 minutes of recording with the exception of brief drops in pH during meal periods (indicated by letter M) produced by acidic contents of ingested material. This pH tracing demonstrates the type of total control of intragastric pH that can be achieved with omeprazole, 20 mg b.i.d. S—supine period; O—omeprozole taken.

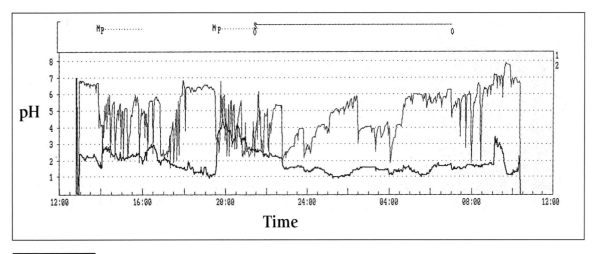

FIGURE 3-34.

In contrast with the prolonged ambulatory pH study demonstrated in Figure 3-33, this dual electrode study of distal esophageal pH (top tracing) and intragastric pH (bottom tracing) while the patient is taking omeprazole, 20 mg b.i.d., demonstrates total lack of control of gastric acid and of reflux. Note that the intragastric pH remains below 4 throughout the study with the exception of the brief period of neutralization following the evening meal (indicated by letter M). Similarly, repeated and frequent esophageal acidification is noted, in particular, showing long periods of slowly cleared acid during the sleeping recumbent period, identified by the letter "S," followed by the broken line above the tracing itself. O—time omeprazole taken.

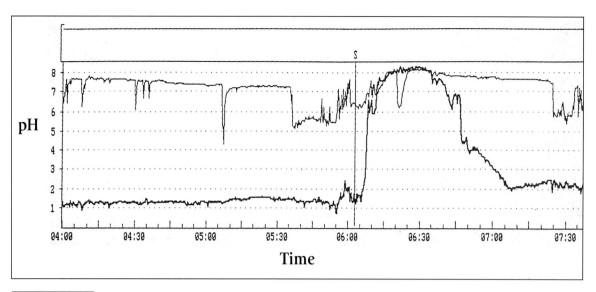

FIGURE 3-35.

Double electrode pH monitoring with distal esophageal (upper tracing) and intragastric (lower tracing) recording. In this figure a classic example of alkaline reflux is seen. There is an abrupt rise in the intragastric pH from the usual baseline level of approximately pH 1.5 to a peak of approximately 8.0. The patient has noted the onset of symptoms with the event marker identified by the letter S above the tracing. Simultaneously, with the abrupt rise in intragastric pH, the esophageal pH rises from its normal level of 6.0 to 7.0 to approximately 8.0 is seen and then gradually recovers as the wave of alkalinity clears. This is an example of duodenogastric esophageal reflux.

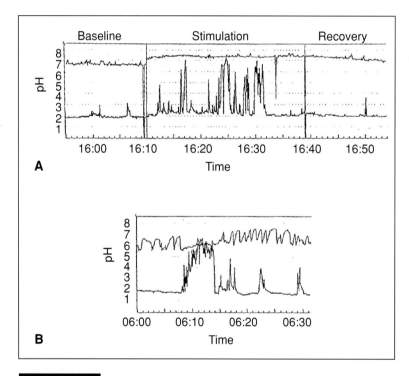

FIGURE 3-36.

The studies illustrated in this figure show double esophageal pH recording in the distal esophagus (**A**) and in the gastric fundus (**B**). The experiment shown includes recording of baseline values, showing the usual level of pH as seen in the esophagus and stomach. This was followed by having this normal volunteer dissolve a neutral lozenge in the mouth to stimulate saliva. Note the rise in distal esophageal pH to a value of approximately 7.5 pH units, with the repeated increases in intragastric pH to a peak value in the same range. In the absence of the lozenge the recovery shows return of the esophageal and gastric pH levels to their usual value. This experiment demonstrates the potential for a false-negative study simulating alkaline reflux, produced by increased salivary flow. (*Adapted from* DeVault *et al.* [8].)

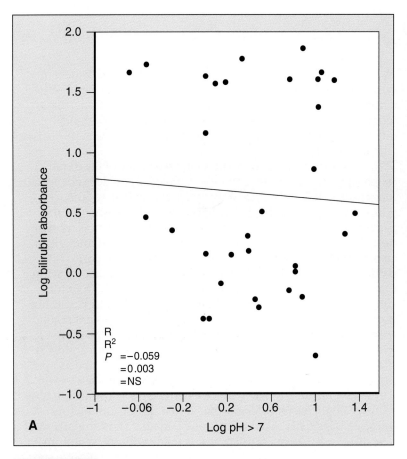

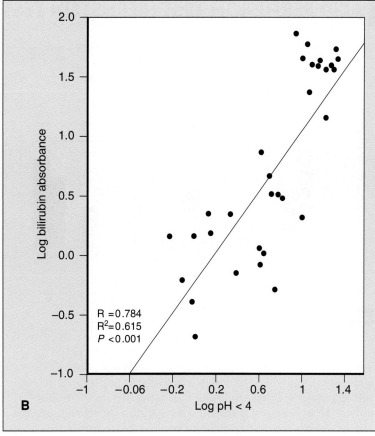

FIGURE 3-37.

A–B, The studies illustrated in these graphs were performed with the direct recording bilirubin probe (Bilitec, Synectics, Inc., Irving, TX) compared with a pH electrode, both placed in the distal esophagus. A group of healthy controls and patients with gastroesophageal reflux disease or Barrett's esophagus is included. The data, presented as a logarithmic transformation of all values, indicate a poor relationship between percentage of time with pH above 7 and bilirubin absorbance, but a strong correlation was seen between percentage of time with pH below 4 and bilirubin absorbance. These data show that duodenogastric esophageal reflux containing bile is much more likely to be nonalkaline than to have a pH above 7 (actual alkaline level). (*Adapted from* Champion *et al.* [9].)

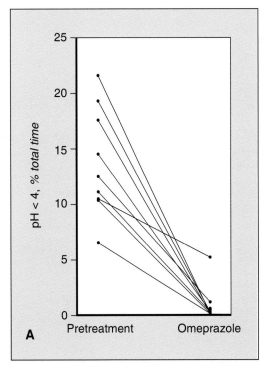

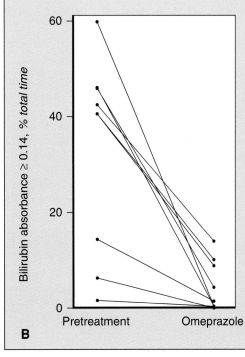

FIGURE 3-38.

A–B, These graphs represent the effect of omeprazole treatment (20 mg b.i.d.) on distal esophageal acid exposure (percentage of time pH < 4) and distal esophageal bilirubin absorption, measured by the Bilitec (Synectics, Inc., Irving, TX) probe in a group of patients demonstrating duodenogastric esophageal reflux in a primarily acid environment. The suppression of bile reflux coincidental with the suppression of gastric acid suggests that most bile reflux occurs as total gastric reflux is mixed with acid. The improvement in bile reflux while on omeprazole therapy is most likely explained by a dramatic decrease in total gastric fluid volume. (*Adapted from* Champion *et al.* [9].)

ACID PERFUSION TEST (BERNSTEIN TEST)

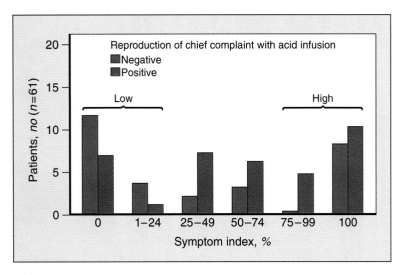

Figure 3-39.

Following its introduction in 1958 by Bernstein and Baker, esophageal acid perfusion was widely accepted and used as a clinical test to identify symptoms resulting from gastroesophageal reflux. The patient sits upright in a chair with a nasogastric tube placed 30 cm from the nares. Normal saline solution is infused for 15 minutes followed by 0.1 sodium hydrochloride solution for 30 minutes or until symptoms are produced. Solutions are infused at a rate of 100 to 120 drops (6 mL to 7.5 mL) per minute in such a manner that changes in solutions can be made unknown to the subject. The test is considered positive when the patient's symptom is twice reproduced during acid perfusion and relieved by saline solution.

The initial report found that 19 of 22 patients with gastroesophageal reflux had a positive test whereas 20 of 21 controls had a negative test resulting in study sensitivity of 85% and specificity of 95%. Over the last 20 years subsequent studies have continued to find a high degree of clinical correlation, with an overall sensitivity of

79% and specificity of 82%. Patients with reflux usually become symptomatic early in the course of the acid infusion, frequently within 7 to 15 minutes, whereas false-positive studies are characterized by symptoms appearing later. This modification may increase the specificity of the acid perfusion test to near 100%, but will also decrease its sensitivity.

The acid perfusion test only shows the sensitivity of the distal esophagus to acid. It is not a test for esophagitis and does not actually measure acid reflux. This test is designed to deliberately produce a symptom (*ie*, pain) through esophageal acid stimulation that the patient can compare with symptoms he or she experiences spontaneously. Therefore, the test is most useful in patients with multiple or atypical symptoms. If results of the acid perfusion test are positive, particularly early in the perfusion, one can be certain that the symptoms are esophageal in origin. A negative test, however, does not eliminate an esophageal source. In the busy clinical setting, this test is particularly attractive because it is simple, rapid, does not require special equipment, and can be easily administered in the office without special personnel and with minimal patient discomfort. It may, however, have been made relatively obsolete by ambulatory pH monitoring, now advocated as an *endogenous* Bernstein test.

The data illustrated here compare Bernstein's acid-infusion test with spontaneous reflux symptoms noted during ambulatory intraesophageal pH monitoring in 61 patients. The comparison of a positive or negative Bernstein test is made with the symptom index recorded as a percentage of reflux symptoms that were specifically associated with a fall in intraesophageal pH below 4.0. These data indicate that the Bernstein test shows rather poor association with the spontaneous relationship between acid reflux and symptoms, even in those patients at the extremes, (*ie*, having a low or high symptom index). Studies of this kind reinforce the suggestion that ambulatory pH monitoring may have made the Bernstein test obsolete, replacing it with an endogenous test of reflux and associated symptoms. (*Adapted from* Wiener et al. [10].)

REFERENCES

1. Dent J, Chir B: A new technique for continuous sphincter pressure measurement. *Gastroenterology* 1976, 71:263–267.

2. Miller LS, Liu JB, Klenn PJ, *et al.*: Endoluminal ultrasonography of the distal esophagus in systemic sclerosis. *Gastroenterology* 1993, 105:31–39.

3. Schuffler MD, Pope CE: Esophageal motor dysfunction in idiopathic intestinal pseudoobstruction. *Gastroenterology* 1976, 70:677–682.

4. Weusten BL, Akkermans LM, vanBerge-Henegouwen GP, *et al.*: Spatiotemporal characteristics of physiological gastroesophageal reflux. *Am J Physiol* 1994, 266(Gastrointest. Liver Physiol. Suppl. 29):G357–G362.

5. Dobhan R, Castell DO: Prolonged intraesophageal pH monitoring with 16-hr overnight recording: Comparison with "24 hour" analysis. *Dig Dis Sci* 1992, 37:857–864.

6. Johnson LF, DeMeester TR: New concepts and methods in the study and treatment of gastroesophageal reflux disease. *Med Clin North Am* 1981, 65:1195–1219.

7. Mattioli S, *et al.*: Reliability of 24-hour home esophageal pH monitoring in diagnosis of gastroesophageal reflux. *Dig Dis Sci* 1989, 34:71–78.

8. DeVault KR, Gorgeson S, Castell DO: Salivary stimulation mimics esophageal exposure to refluxed duodenal contents. *Am J Gastroenterol* 1993, 88:1040–1043.

9. Champion G, Richter JE, Vaezi MF, *et al.*: Duodenogastric reflux: Relationship to pH and importance in Barrett's esophagus. *Gastroenterology* 1994, 107:747–754.

10. Wiener R, Richter JE: The symptom index: Correlation of acid reflux with symptoms. In *Ambulatory Esophageal pH Monitoring: Practical Approach and Clinical Applications*. New York: Igaku-Shoin; 1991:93–100.

11. Richter JE, Bradley LA, DeMeester TR, *et al.*: Normal 24-hr ambulatory esophageal pH values: Influence of study center, pH electrode, age and gender. *Dig Dis Sci* 1992, 37:849–856.

Chapter 4

Gastroesophageal Reflux Disease

ROY C. ORLANDO

Gastroesophageal reflux (GER) is by definition a process in which gastric contents move spontaneously and passively into the esophagus. This process in itself is for the most part benign in that it occurs in everyone, many times every day and without producing symptoms or injuring tissue [1]. *Gastroesophageal reflux disease* (GERD) is the term used to encompass the circumstance with which GER is associated with symptoms or signs of tissue injury. Predictably, the organ most commonly damaged by regular exposure to gastric contents is the esophagus. For instance, GER reportedly produces heartburn on a regular basis in up to 40% of the adult U.S. population, and in approximately 10% of this population, heartburn is experienced daily. Further, in an estimated 2% of this population, the esophageal epithelium is damaged to the extent that it is visually apparent on upper endoscopy. When GER is associated with symptoms but without evidence of tissue injury on endoscopy and esophageal biopsy, the individual is described as having "symptomatic" reflux, whereas an individual with evidence of tissue injury is described as having "reflux esophagitis." GER may also be associated with damage to the oropharynx, larynx, or bronchopulmonary structures; such damage may occur with or without concomitant damage to the esophagus.

The fundamental cause for the development of reflux esophagitis is at present unclear and likely to be multifactorial. Conceptually, however, the factors that contribute to its development or perpetuation include one or more of the following: defective antireflux barriers; defective luminal clearance; defective epithelial tissue resistance; increased noxious quality of the refluxate. The effect of these defects in esophageal defense or increases in noxious quality of the refluxate is to produce disease by enabling contact of the esophageal epithelium with gastric (hydrochloric) acid and pepsin for a period of time sufficient to overcome the tissue's intrinsic defenses, thereby leading to disease [1]. Notably, what constitutes sufficient time to cause disease varies greatly among individuals, making reliance on pH monitoring an inaccurate means for diagnosis. And despite state-of-the-art technology, the most accurate means of diagnosis is a history of recurrent heartburn with or without the presence of typical histopathologic changes within the lower esophagus on endoscopy.

The natural history of reflux esophagitis is poorly defined because it remains unclear with what frequency individuals with symptomatic reflux progress to develop erosive esophagitis or complications such as stricture formation or a columnar-lined lower (Barrett's) esophagus. Nonetheless, it is clear that approximately 5% to 20% of patients with erosive esophagitis have an esophageal stricture and 5% to 15% have

Barrett's esophagus, the latter a premalignant lesion [2]. More rarely, reflux esophagitis may be complicated by esophageal ulceration with subsequent hemorrhage or perforation. Although a chronic disease with associated morbidity, reflux esophagitis rarely causes death.

The treatment of reflux esophagitis is initially medical. Medical therapy has two components: lifestyle modification and pharmacotherapy—both of which are aimed at either reducing the noxious quality of the refluxate or increasing the strength of the esophageal defenses. In some instances reflux esophagitis may be severe enough to warrant surgery for either control of symptoms or maintenance against lesion relapse [1].

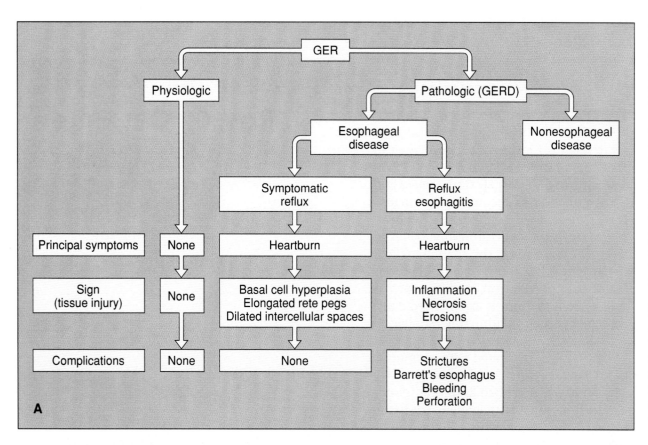

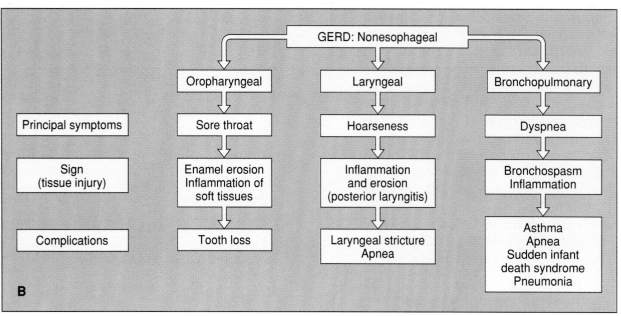

FIGURE 4-1.

A, The presumed relationship between the phenomenon of gastroesophageal reflux (GER) and gastroesophageal reflux disease (GERD) is depicted. GERD encompasses both nonesophageal and esophageal pathology, with esophageal pathology being subdivided into patients with "symptomatic reflux" and patients with "reflux esophagitis," based on the endoscopic or histologic demonstration of inflammation and necrosis. **B**, The range of nonesophageal signs, symptoms, and complications attributed to GERD is depicted.

EPIDEMIOLOGY

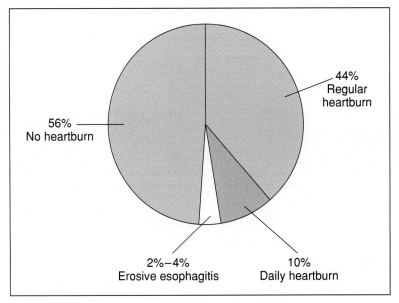

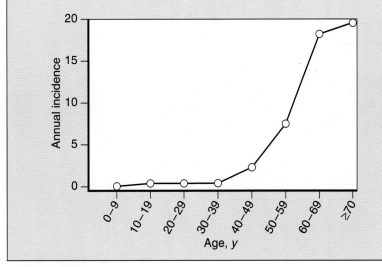

Epidemiology: prevalence. The prevalence figures for symptomatic reflux (heartburn) and reflux (erosive) esophagitis for the adult U.S. population were extrapolated from data provided in the Gallup Organization National Survey, in reports by Nebel and associates, and by Rasmussen [3–5]. GERD has a 2–3:1 male:female predominance, and although common in whites, is uncommon in African Americans [2].

Epidemiology: incidence. Data from a population in northeast Scotland [6] indicate a rapid rise in incidence of symptomatic reflux beginning in the fourth decade of life. (*Adapted from* Brunnen *et al.* [6].)

PATHOPHYSIOLOGY AND ETIOLOGY

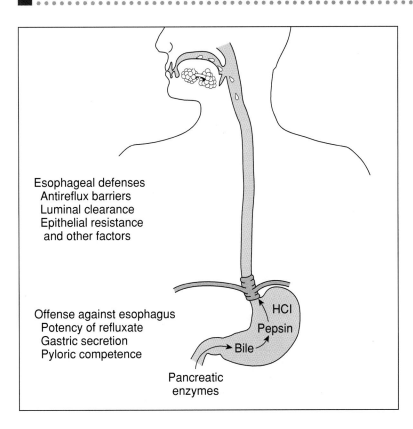

Although the cause of reflux-induced esophageal disease is unknown, it involves abnormalities in one or more of the elements depicted this figure. These elements include antireflux barriers to minimize reflux frequency, luminal clearance mechanisms to minimize duration of contact between epithelium and contents of the refluxate, and factors compromising tissue resistance to minimize damage during contact of epithelium with refluxate. HCl—hydrochloric acid. (*Adapted from* Orlando [1].)

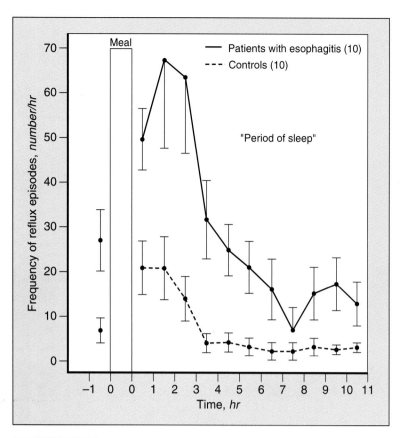

FIGURE 4-5.

Pathogenesis: antireflux mechanisms. The frequency of reflux is shown to be increased in patients with gastroesophageal reflux disease compared with healthy controls. This observation indicates that the esophageal epithelium is exposed more frequently to acidic gastric contents and therefore has a greater statistical likelihood of having this contact lead to injury. Injury, however, is not predictable from any given reflux event because of the existence of luminal acid clearance mechanisms that limit the duration of acid contact and tissue resistance, which limits the potential for damage during the contact of acid and pepsin with esophageal tissues. (*Data from* Dodds *et al.* [7].)

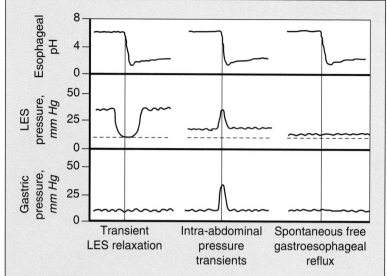

FIGURE 4-6.

Pathophysiology: antireflux mechanisms. Three different mechanisms are shown to account for all reflux events in healthy controls and patients with gastroesophageal reflux disease (GERD). All episodes in healthy controls and the majority (approximately 75%) of episodes in patients with GERD are associated with the phenomenon of transient lower esophageal sphincter (LES) relaxation. Transient LES relaxations are non–swallow-related reflex relaxations of the LES; they produce a common cavity phenomenon and therefore predispose to acidic reflux events. A minority of reflux episodes in patients with GERD are associated with other phenomena, such as increases in intra-abdominal pressure that overcome the barrier effect of the LES and spontaneous free reflux that occurs when the LES is so weakened as to produce no high-pressure zone. (*Adapted from* Dodds *et al.* [7].)

TABLE 4-1. MECHANISMS OF ESOPHAGEAL LUMINAL ACID CLEARANCE

Bolus Clearance
    Gravity
    Peristalsis
Acid Clearance
    Swallowed salivary bicarbonate-rich secretions
    Secreted bicarbonate-rich fluid from esophageal
        submucosal glands

TABLE 4-1.

Physiology: mechanisms of esophageal luminal acid clearance. This depicts the four major mechanisms available to the esophagus to clear refluxed gastric contents from its lumen. Bolus clearance is achieved by gravity and primary (swallow-initiated) or secondary (distension-initiated) peristalsis. Acid clearance is achieved by dilution and titration of acidity by swallowing the aqueous bicarbonate-rich salivary secretion and by the direct secretion of aqueous bicarbonate-rich secretion from esophageal submucosal glands into the lumen.

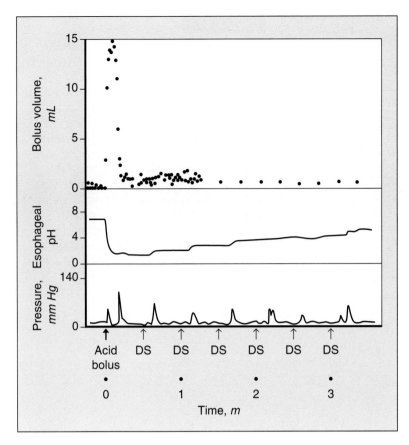

FIGURE 4-7.

Physiology: luminal acid clearance. Two active mechanisms for the clearance of luminal acid from the esophagus are depicted after the injection of 15 mL of hydrochloric acid, with a pH of 2, into the esophagus. One mechanism, peristalsis, is elicited by dry swallows (DS), which is shown to clear the bolus of acid after one to two swallows. Bolus clearance, however, is not synonymous with acid clearance in that luminal acidity remains until the continued swallowing of bicarbonate-rich saliva titrates the residual acidity to a neutral level over the subsequent 3 to 5 minutes. (*Adapted from* Helm *et al.* [8].)

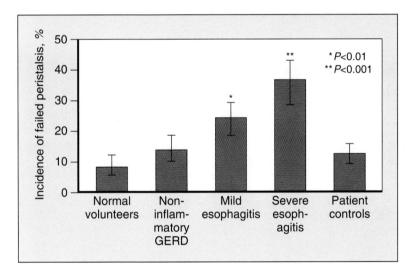

FIGURE 4-8.

Pathophysiology: luminal acid clearance. An increased frequency of failed peristaltic sequences following swallows is present in patients with increasing grades of gastroesophageal reflux disease (GERD). This phenomenon is one means by which luminal acid clearance may be delayed, and this in turn increases the risk that the reflux episode may result in damage to the esophageal epithelium. (*Adapted from* Kahrilas [9].)

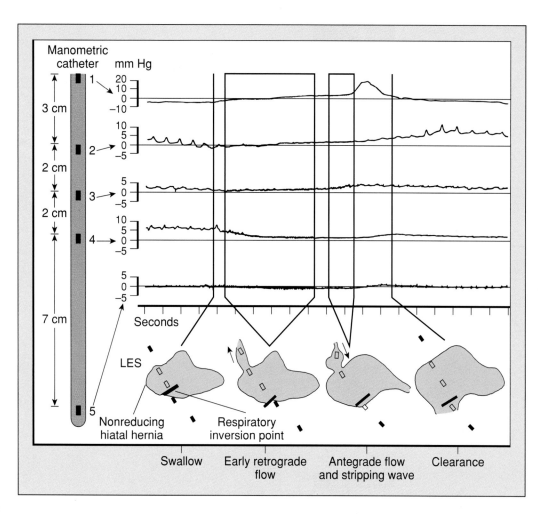

FIGURE 4-9.

Pathophysiology: luminal acid clearance. Although the presence of a hiatal hernia is not enough for the development of reflux disease, there is an association between the presence of a hiatal hernia and erosive esophagitis. This association appears to occur in part because hernias distort the supportive relationship between the diaphragm and the lower esophageal sphincter (LES), and in part because some nonreducing hernias predispose to delayed esophageal luminal acid clearance by producing "early retrograde reflux" (*ie*, reflux early during the swallow-initiated relaxation phase of the LES) [10]. (*Adapted from* Sloan and Kahrilas [10].)

TABLE 4-2. POTENTIAL COMPONENTS OF TISSUE RESISTANCE AGAINST ACID INJURY IN THE ESOPHAGUS.

Preepithelial defenses
  Mucous layer
  Unstirred water layer
  Surface bicarbonate ion concentration
Epithelial defenses
  Physical barriers
    Cell membranes
    Intercellular junctional complex
      Tight junctions
      Intercellular lipid or mucin
  Functional components
    Cellular defense against acidification
      Epithelial transport (*eg*, NA^+/H^+ exchange)
      Intracellular buffering
      •Basic proteins
      •Bicarbonate ions
  Epithelial repair
    Epithelial restitution
    Cell replication

Postepithelial defense
  Blood flow
    Delivery of protective agents
      Oxygen
      Metabolic substrates (nutrients)
      Bicarbonate ions (extracellular buffering)
    Removal of noxious agents
      CO_2
      H^+
      Metabolic byproducts
      Cellular debris

TABLE 4-2.

Physiology: tissue resistance. This is not a single factor but a series of epithelial structures and functions that together produce a dynamic state with the capacity to resist injury upon contact with a variety of noxious luminal materials. (*Adapted from* Orlando [11].)

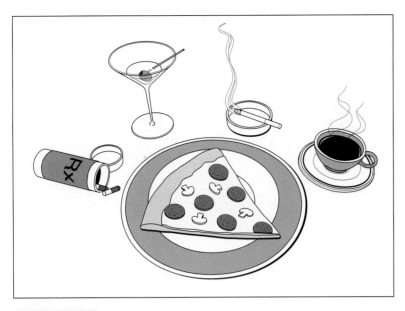

Figure 4-10.

Pathophysiology: tissue resistance. A number of possible factors may alter the ability of the esophageal mucosa to defend itself against refluxed gastric acid, including smoking, excessive alcohol use, exposure to hot beverages, exposure to foods producing hypertonic luminal contents, and exposure to medications with topical irritant effects (*eg*, tetracycline, potassium chloride, and nonsteroidal anti-inflammatory drugs, among others).

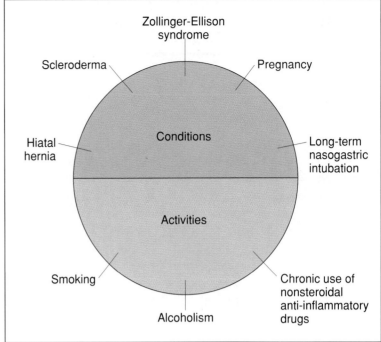

Figure 4-11.

Conditions and activities reported in association with reflux-induced gastroesophageal disease. This figure depicts those conditions and activities for which epidemiologic data suggest a relationship with the development of reflux esophagitis.

Figure 4-12.

Diagnosis: heartburn. Heartburn is a symptom complex characterized by substernal (burning) pain radiating toward the mouth, which is worsened by meals and recumbency and ameliorated by antacid ingestion. When typical, recurrent heartburn is adequate for the diagnosis of gastroesophageal reflux disease (GERD). Regurgitation of bitter material into the mouth and "water brash," the latter the spontaneous appearance of a salty fluid within the mouth, are symptoms of GERD that frequently accompany the symptoms of heartburn. Noteworthy is that odynophagia, or pain on swallowing, is uncommon in GERD and usually reflects esophagitis secondary to pills or infectious causes.

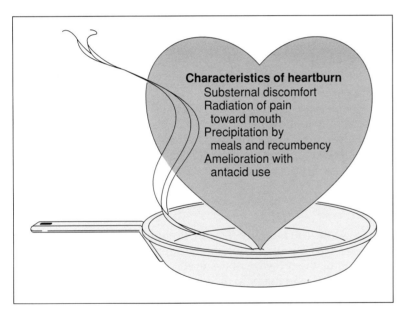

Characteristics of heartburn
Substernal discomfort
Radiation of pain toward mouth
Precipitation by meals and recumbency
Amelioration with antacid use

TABLE 4-3. ESOPHAGEAL PATHOLOGY IN GASTROESOPHAGEAL REFLUX

Noninflammatory changes
    Basal cell hyperplasia
    Increased papillary height

Inflammatory changes
    Acute
        Vascular congestion with or without stasis
        Mucosal edema
        Polymorphonuclear leukocytic infiltration (neutrophils
           and eosinophils)
    Chronic
        Mononuclear leukocyte infiltration (macrophages)
        Increased macrophage activity
        Proliferation of fibroblasts
        In-growth of vascular endothelium

Epithelial necrosis
    Erosion
    Ulceration

Epithelial repair
    Granulation tissue
    Fibrosis (stricture formation)
    Epithelial regeneration
        Squamous replication
        Columnar metaplasia (Barrett's esophagus)

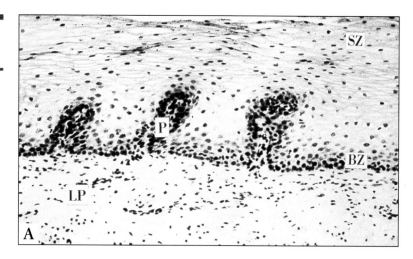

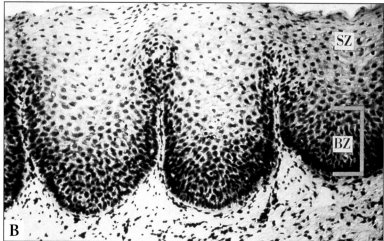

FIGURE 4-13.

A–B, Histopathology: noninflammatory changes. The microscopic changes most commonly reported in association with reflux damage to esophageal epithelium are basal cell hyperplasia and rete peg proximity to the lumen [13]. Although sensitive, these features have a low specificity for the disease, being identified in the lower 2.5 cm of the esophagus in up to 20% of healthy subjects [14]. (*From* Ismail-Beigi *et al.* [13]; with permission.)

TABLE 4-3.

Esophageal pathology in gastroesophageal reflux. The variety of abnormalities associated with injury to the esophageal epithelium is shown. They range from noninflammatory to inflammatory changes and from normal epithelial (squamous) repair to aberrant repair in the form of Barrett's esophagus. (*Adapted from* Orlando [12].)

FIGURE 4-14.

Histopathology: acute inflammation. The presence of acute inflammation within the esophageal epithelium, which is depicted on this section of an esophageal biopsy, is specific for esophagitis. It is characterized by the presence of tissue edema, polymorphonuclear (or eosinophilic) leukocyte infiltration, and injury to the vasculature. Although specific for esophagitis, these microscopic changes are not pathognomonic for reflux-induced injury occurring in esophagitis from other causes (*eg*, infectious esophagitis) [10]. (*From* Mitros [12a]; with permission.)

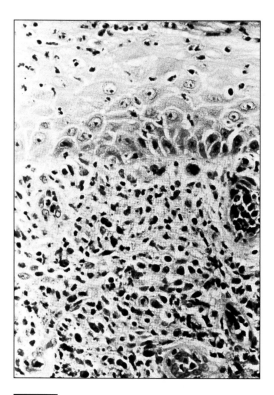

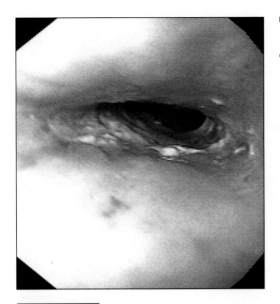

TABLE 4-4. SAVARY-MILLER NEW ENDOSCOPIC GRADING

Grade I	Single, erosive or exudative lesion, oval or linear, taking only one longitudinal fold
Grade II	Noncircular multiple erosion or exudative lesion taking more than one longitudinal fold, with or without confluence
Grade III	Circular erosive or exudative lesion
Grade IV	Chronic lesions: ulcer(s), stricture(s), or short esophagus, isolated or associated with lesions of grades I, II, or III
Grade V	Islands, fingerlike forms or circumferential distribution of Barrett's epithelium isolated or associated with a lesion of grades I through IV

FIGURE 4-15.

Erosive esophagitis: endoscopic view. The hallmark of reflux esophagitis on endoscopy is the presence of one or more erosions within the distal esophagus [15]. Although the finding of such lesions is neither sensitive, (being found in less than 50% of those whose heartburn is explored endoscopically) nor specific (because they can occur with other esophageal injuries), the diagnosis is established by the chronicity of symptoms coupled with the typical nature of the lesions in the absence of other definable causes (*eg*, infectious or pill-induced esophagitis.)

TABLE 4-4.

Endoscopic grading of reflux esophagitis. The most common system for grading reflux esophagitis determined by endoscopy is known as the Savary-Miller classification [16]. It is often used in controlled clinical trials for assessing the efficacy of various treatment regimens. Despite its utility, differences between middle grades (II–IV) may at times be difficult to distinguish. (*Adapted from* Ollyo *et al.* [16].)

TABLE 4-5. ESOPHAGEAL COMPLICATIONS OF REFLUX ESOPHAGITIS

COMPLICATION	PREVALENCE, %
Esophageal stricture	4–20
Barrett's esophagus	8–20
Hemorrhage	<5
Perforation	<1

TABLE 4-5.

Prevalence of the major complications of reflux esophagitis [2]. Each is likely preceded by gross (erosive) disease on endoscopy. Nonetheless, many patients seeking medical care present with complications, which therefore affords less opportunity to prevent them by effective antireflux treatment.

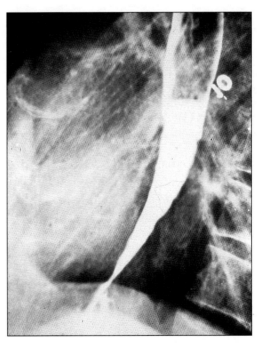

FIGURE 4-16.

Esophageal stricture: Radiologic pathology. A barium esophagogram demonstrates the presence of a partially obstructing smooth-walled distal esophageal stricture secondary to reflux esophagitis [1]. Patients with this complication may note amelioration of heartburn when a new symptom (*ie*, dysphagia for solid foods) becomes more pronounced. (*From* Orlando [1]; with permission.)

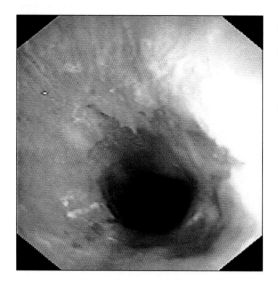

FIGURE 4-17.

Barrett's esophagus: endoscopic pathology. The endoscopic appearance of a columnar-lined lower esophagus (*ie,* Barrett's) is shown for a patient with reflux esophagitis. The typical red coloration of the columnar epithelium is readily distinguished from the lighter pink or orange stratified squamous epithelium [15]. For a specific diagnosis, however, endoscopic biopsy is required for histologic confirmation of the nature of the epithelium lining the lower esophagus.

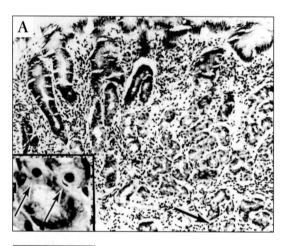
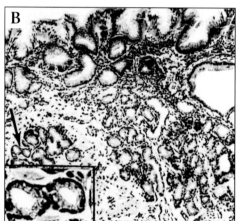
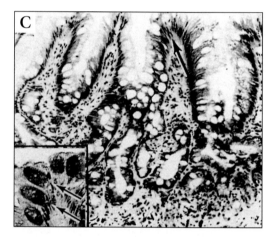

FIGURE 4-18.

Barrett's esophagus: histopathology. Three types of columnar epithelium have been identified within the lower esophagus: junctional (**A**)—looks like the columnar epithelium of the gastric cardia; atrophic gastric fundic (**B**)—looks like the columnar epithelium of the gastric fundus; specialized columnar (**C**)—looks like a small intestine with its characteristic villiform surface, microvilli, goblet cells, and Paneth cells [17]. The detection of specialized columnar epithelium on esophageal biopsy is diagnostic for Barrett's esophagus.

Further, specialized columnar epithelium is, unlike the others, a metaplastic epithelium and therefore carries the risk of malignant degeneration. Arrow in **panel A** shows location of inset scope (original magnification × 100); inset depicts parietal cells in glandular layers (original magnification × 5000). Arrow in **panel B** depicts inset (original magnification × 100; inset × 425). **C,** Original magnification × 100. Inset shows goblet cells using Alcian blue staining (original magnification × 350). (*From* Paull [17]; with permission.)

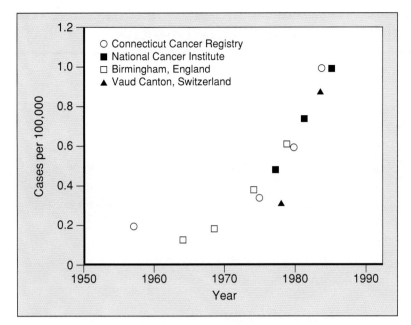

FIGURE 4-19.

Rising incidence of adenocarcinoma of the esophagus. Concern about malignant potential of Barrett's esophagus has been growing due to evidence that the incidence of adenocarcinoma of the esophagus is increasing at rates that exceed all other cancers in both the United States and Europe. (*Adapted from* Pera [18].)

TABLE 4-6. TESTS FOR DIAGNOSTIC ASSESSMENT OF GASTROESOPHAGEAL REFLUX DISEASE, ITS MECHANISMS, AND ITS CONSEQUENCES

Tests for reflux
    Upper gastrointestinal series
    Tuttle's (standard acid reflux) test
    Continuous intraesophageal pH monitoring
    Radionuclide (^{99}Tc) scintigraphy
Tests to assess symptoms
    Bernstein's (acid-perfusion) test
    Continuous intraesophageal pH monitoring
Tests to assess esophageal damage
    Barium esophagogram or upper gastrointestinal series
    Upper endoscopy
    Esophageal biopsy
    Esophageal potential difference measurement*
Tests to assess pathogenesis of esophagitis
    Acid clearance test*
    Radionuclide (^{99}Tc) scintigraphy*
    Esophageal manometry
    Gastric analysis

Principally investigational.

TABLE 4-7. MODIFICATIONS OF LIFESTYLE TO LESSEN REFLUX ESOPHAGITIS

Elevate the head of the bed 6"
Stop smoking
Stop consuming excessive alcohol
Reduce fat in diet
Reduce size of meals
Avoid eating at bedtime
Lose weight (if overweight)
Foods to avoid:
Chocolate
Carminatives (spearmint, peppermint)
Coffee (caffeinated and decaffeinated)
Tea
Cola beverages
Tomato juice
Citrus juices
Drugs to avoid, when possible:
Anticholinergics
Theophylline
Diazepam
Narcotics
Calcium channel blockers
β-Adrenergic agonists (isoproterenol)
Progesterone (some contraceptives)
α-Adrenergic antagonists (phentolamine)

TABLE 4-6.

Diagnostic testing in gastroesophageal reflux disease (GERD). Testing falls into four categories, depending on whether designed to document: (1) the presence and degree of reflux, (2) the relationship between reflux and atypical chest pain, (3) the type and extent of reflux-induced esophageal damage, or (4) the pathophysiology of reflux-induced disease [1]. (*Adapted from* Orlando [1].)

TABLE 4-7.

Medical management: lifestyle modifications. The commonly recommended lifestyle modifications are listed [14]. All patients will likely gain some benefit by elevating the head of the bed and by changing diet. The benefit-to-risk ratio of reducing or stopping medications prescribed for other active diseases should be carefully considered because reductions in lower esophageal sphincter pressure in most cases are modest; these agents have not been shown to produce reflux symptoms independently. (*Adapted from* Orlando [19].)

TABLE 4-8. MANAGEMENT OF GASTROESOPHAGEAL REFLUX DISEASE BY PHARMACOTHERAPY.

CONVENTIONAL DRUGS	DOSE	MECHANISM(S) OF ACTION*
Antacid: liquid (*eg,* Mylanta II/Maalox TC) (HCl neutralization, capacity 25 mEq/5 mL)[†]	15 mL/q.i.d. 1 h after meals and at bedtime	Buffer HCl ↑ LESP
Gaviscon (Al hydroxide, Mg trisilicate, NaHCO$_3$, Alginic acid)	2–4 tablets, q.i.d. after meals and at bedtime	↓ Reflux by viscous mechanical barrier Buffer HCl in esophagus
H$_2$-receptor antagonists		
Cimetidine (Tagamet)	800 mg b.i.d.	↓ HCl secretion ⎫ by inhibiting ↓ Gastric volume ⎭ H$_2$-receptor
Ranitidine (Zantac)	150 mg q.i.d./300 mg b.i.d.	
Famotidine (Pepcid)	20 mg b.i.d.	Same as cimetidine
Nizatidine (Axid)	150 mg b.i.d.	
Prokinetics		
Bethanechol (Urecholine)	25 mg q.i.d. 1/2 h before meals and at bedtime	↑ LESP ↑ Esophageal acid clearance
Metoclopramide (Reglan)	10 mg q.i.d.	↑ LESP
Cisapride	10 mg t.i.d. or q.i.d. 1/2 h before meals and at bedtime	↑ LESP, ↑ gastric emptying
Mucosa Protectant		↑ Gastric emptying
Sucralfate (Carafate)	1 g q.i.d. 1 h after meals and at bedtime	↑ Tissue resistance Buffer HCl in esophagus Bind pepsin and bile salts
Inhibitors of H$^+$-K$^+$-ATPase		
Omeprazole (Prilosec)	20 mg/day	↓ HCl secretion, ↓ gastric volume
Lansoprazole (Prevacid)	30 mg/day	↓ HCl secretion, ↓ gastric volume

*LESP—lower esophageal sphincter pressure; ↑—increase; ↓—decrease.
[†]Note: Patients with reflux are generally not known to be hypersecretors of gastric acid. Therefore, therapeutic doses of antacids are based on capacity to buffer basal HCl secretion of approx. 1–7 mEq/hr (mean 2 mEq/hr) and peak meal-stimulated HCl secretion of approx. 10–60 mEq/hr (mean 30 mEq/hr).

TABLE 4-8.

Medical management: pharmacotherapy. Commonly prescribed classes of medications used in the treatment of reflux esophagitis include antacids that act by buffering gastric acid, either within the esophageal lumen or stomach; H$_2$-receptor antagonists or proton pump inhibitors that act by inhibiting gastric acid secretion, thereby making the refluxate less noxious to the esophageal epithelium; prokinetics that act to increase smooth muscle contractility, thereby increasing lower esophageal sphincter pressure, amplitudes of esophageal peristaltic contractions, and the rate of gastric emptying; and mucosal protective agents that act on the epithelium to reduce the damaging action of acid and pepsin [1]. (*Adapted from* Orlando [1].)

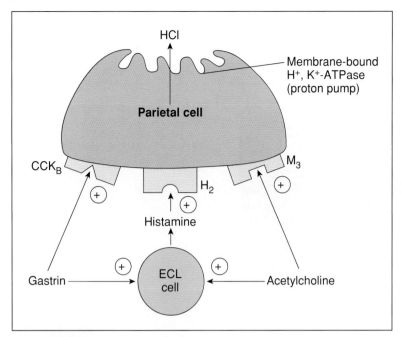

FIGURE 4-20.

Physiology of gastric parietal cell acid secretion. One of the most effective means of treating patients with gastroesophageal reflux disease is to inhibit gastric acid secretion. This can be achieved pharmacologically by the administration of H_2-receptor antagonists, anticholinergics, or proton pump inhibitors because each type of medication inhibits an important pathway that mediates acid secretion by the gastric parietal cell. Notably, anticholinergic agents, which are limited in use by problematic side effects, and H_2-receptor antagonists inhibit only one of three basolateral membrane pathways by which the parietal cell is stimulated to secrete acid. For this reason, they possess only moderate power in lowering gastric acid secretion. In contrast, proton pump inhibitors, by blocking the apical membrane H^+, K^+–ATPase and the final common pathway for acid secretion, are more potent as inhibitors of gastric acid secretion. ECL—enterochromaffin-like; CCK_B—cholecystokinin type B receptor; M_3—cholinergic receptor M_3 type; H_2—histamine-2 receptor.

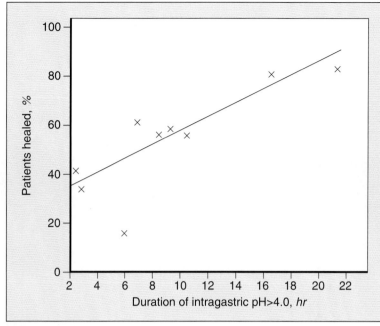

FIGURE 4-21.

Relationship of gastric acid secretion to healing of erosive esophagitis. There is an almost linear relationship between the length of time that gastric acid secretion is inhibited to a pH above 4 and the degree of success in healing patients with erosive esophagitis. This is because reduction in acid secretion is paralleled by elevation of intraluminal esophageal pH, and elevation of esophageal pH provides time for epithelial healing to take place. Because it is the proton pump inhibitors that provide the greatest control over gastric acidity, they achieve higher rates of success than do the H_2-receptor antagonists for the treatment of erosive esophagitis. (*Adapted from* Wilkinson and Hunt [20].)

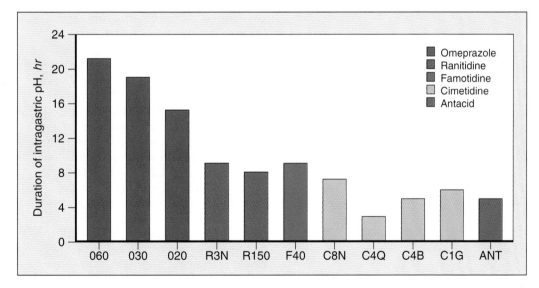

FIGURE 4-22.

Pharmacotherapy and acid inhibition. The relationship between the use of various pharmacologic agents and the ability to control gastric acidity (to pH >4) is depicted. Note that antacid regimens are the least effective, H_2-receptor antagonists moderately effective, and proton pump inhibitors the most effective in controlling gastric acidity. This pattern also parallels their success in healing patients with erosive esophagitis. 060 = omeprazole, 60 mg/day; 030 = omeprazole, 30 mg/day; 020 = omeprazole, 20 mg day; R3N = ranitidine, 300 mg at bedtime; R150 = ranitidine, 150 mg twice daily; F40 = famotidine, 40 mg at bedtime; C8N = cimetidine, 800 mg at bedtime; C4Q = cimetidine, 400 mg four times; daily C4B = cimetidine, 400 mg at bedtime; ANT = antacid 450 mmol seven times daily. (*Adapted from* Wilkinson and Hunt [20].)

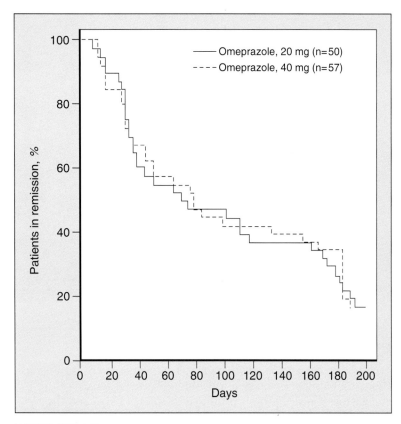

FIGURE 4-23.

Relapse rates after healing erosive esophagitis. Patients with erosive esophagitis healed by treatment with proton pump inhibitors are shown to have a very high rate of relapse. Because it is this group that is at greatest risk for complications (stricture formation, Barrett's esophagus), medical and surgical strategies for maintenance have been advocated. (*Adapted from* Hetzel [21].)

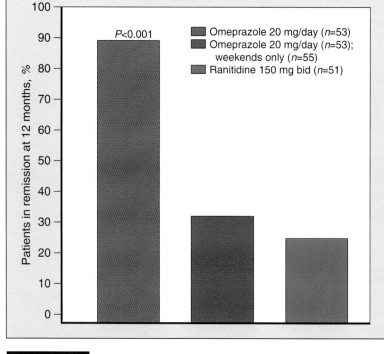

FIGURE 4-24.

Medical maintenance of healing in erosive esophagitis. The continued daily, but not weekend only, use of proton pump inhibitors has been shown to be superior to placebo and standard dose H^2-receptor antagonists for maintenance of the healed state in patients with erosive esophagitis. Currently, three oral medications are approved by the Food and Drug Administration for medical maintenance: ranitidine 150 mg b.i.d., lansoprazole 15 mg q.d., and omeprazole 20 mg q.d. (*Adapted from* Dent *et al.* [22].)

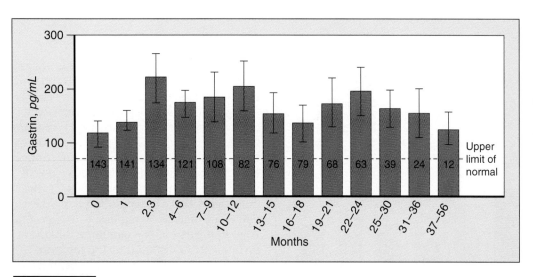

FIGURE 4-25.

Long-term therapy with proton pump inhibitors (PPIs) increases basal serum gastrin levels. The potent acid-inhibiting properties of the proton pump inhibitors (and to a lesser

extent, high-dose H^2-receptor antagonists) are associated with hypergastrinemia, the latter due to persistently high antral pH (pH > 3). It is important to note that when antral pH is acidic, somatostatin is released. This, in turn, inhibits the release of gastrin by antral G cells. Early on the hypergastrinemia was of concern because this correction was accompanied in experimental animals (rats) by the development of enterochromaffin-like cell hyperplasia and subsequent gastric carcinoids. At present, however, and after 5 years of surveillance of patients requiring continuous therapy with PPIs, no evidence has appeared to suggest that the PPI-induced hypergastrinemia produces gastric carcinoids in humans. Numbers in parentheses indicate total patients. (*Adapted from* Brunner *et al.* [23].)

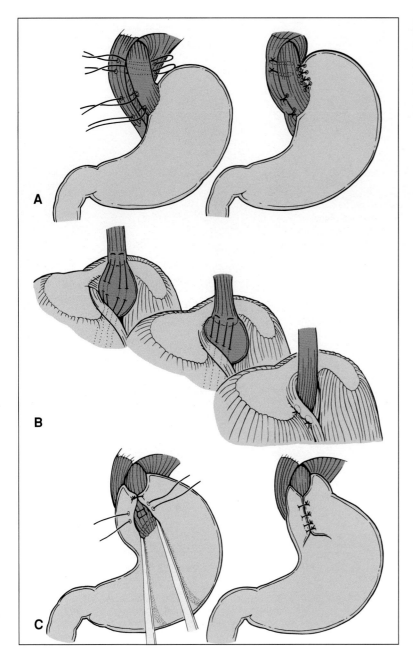

FIGURE 4-26.

Surgical management. The most commonly performed surgical procedures for gastroesophageal reflux disease include Hill's gastropexy (**A**), Belsey's fundoplication (**B**), and Nissen fundoplication (**C**) [15]. The Nissen procedure can be performed either as an open procedure or using a laparoscopic approach. (*Adapted from* Pope [24].)

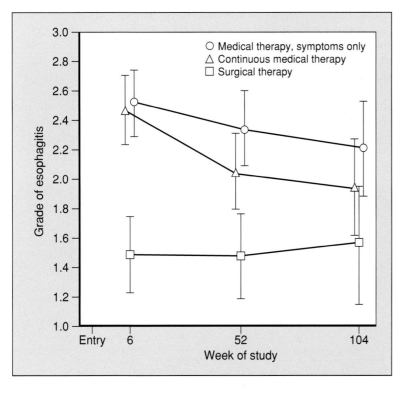

FIGURE 4-27.

Surgical maintenance of healing in erosive esophagitis. Surgery (fundoplication) has previously been shown to be superior to medical therapy (*eg*, antacids, H^2-receptor antagonists, prokinetic drugs, mucosal protectants) for maintenance of healing in patients with erosive esophagitis. Notably, this study was performed before the availability of the more potent proton pump inhibitors, therefore no comparison with this form of therapy is available. (*Adapted from* Spechler *et al.* [25].)

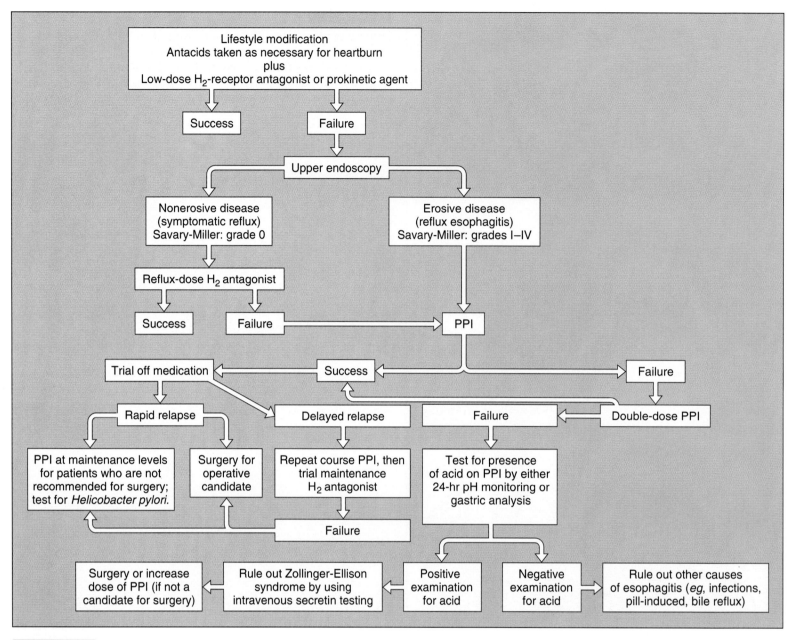

FIGURE 4-28.

Strategy for the management of esophagitis. This strategy uses a stepped approach to the treatment of heartburn. When patients require more than standard-dose H_2-receptor antagonists regularly for control of symptoms, endoscopy is recommended to evaluate for the presence of erosive disease, complications of reflux, such as Barrett's esophagus, and the presence of *Helicobacter pylori* gastric infection. Those with erosive esophagitis are treated with a proton pump inhibitor (PPI), and those without erosive disease are managed by increasing doses of the H_2-receptor antagonist. If antireflux doses of H_2-receptor antagonist are unsuccessful, a PPI is used. Failure of PPIs at twice their standard dose to control symptoms

or heal lesions should prompt an assessment of whether they have effectively controlled gastric acid secretion (gastric analysis on therapy) or esophageal acidity (24-hr pH monitoring on therapy). Those that remain acid producers should have Zollinger-Ellison syndrome ruled out, and those that are achlorhydric should have other causes for esophageal disease ruled out (*eg*, infectious or pill-induced esophagitis). All patients on protracted therapy with high-potency acid suppressive medication should be evaluated for *H. pylori* infection, and if positive, therapy for its eradication should be employed to prevent the development of gastric atrophy.

TABLE 4-9. EFFECTS OF THERAPY ON NEED FOR SUBSEQUENT DILATATIONS IN PATIENTS WHO HAVE ESOPHAGITIS WITH STRICTURE AT THE END OF 6 MONTHS OF THERAPY

	OMEPRAZOLE ($N = 17$)	H$_2$RA ($N = 15$)	P VALUE
Patients needing follow-up dilatations, %	41%	73%	0.07
Dilatation sessions, no	0.6 + 0.9 (standard deviation)	2.1 + 1.6	<0.01
Dilatation sessions, total	11	31	

TABLE 4-9.

Esophageal stricture. Proton pump inhibitors (PPIs) are shown to be more effective than histamine$_2$ receptor antagonists (H$_2$RA) in reducing the number of dilatations for control of dysphagia in patients with esophageal strictures. Because lumen-narrowing strictures result from both fibrotic and nonfibrotic (inflammatory) reactions, the PPIs, and to a lesser extent the H$_2$RAs, likely produce their beneficial effect by exerting control over the latter. (*Adapted from* Marks [26].)

TABLE 4-10. MEAN LENGTH AT BASELINE EACH VISIT, AND CHANGE FROM BASELINE (SD) OF BARRETT'S EPITHELIUM (CM)

TREATMENT MONTH	PATIENT NO.	LENGTH OF BARRETT'S EPITHELIUM		
		BASELINE (MEAN [SD])	VISIT (MEAN [SD])	CHANGE* FROM BASELINE (SD)
Month 6	27	5.7 (2.3)	5.6 (2.3)	−0.1 (1.4)
Month 12	27	5.7 (2.3)	5.2 (2.2)	−0.5 (1.4)
Month 18	24	5.8 (2.5)	5.7 (2.3)	0.0 (1.3)
Month 24	22	5.8 (2.4)	5.4 (2.4)	−0.5 (1.4)
Month 30	18	5.9 (2.4)	5.4 (1.9)	−0.5 (1.8)
Month 36	8	4.8 (1.7)	4.8 (2.0)	0.0 (1.8)
Final	27	5.7 (2.3)	5.3 (2.3)	−0.4 (1.7)

*No statistically significant changes from baseline at $P < 0.05$.
SD—Standard Deviation; CM—centimeters.

TABLE 4-10.

Barrett's esophagus. Proton pump inhibitors (PPIs), despite long-term continuous treatment, appear to have little or no ability to reduce the length of Barrett's esophagus. Studies as long as 3 years showed no significant clinical benefit to such therapy, although small islands of squamous epithelium have appeared among the metaplastic Barrett's epithelium. (*Adapted from* Sampliner [27].)

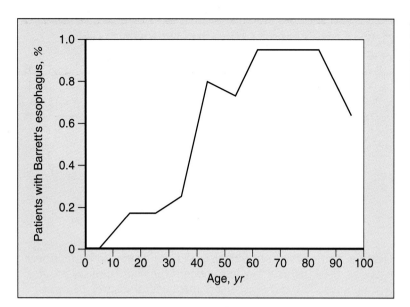

FIGURE 4-29.

Barrett's esophagus. The prevalance with which Barrett's esophagus is present on endoscopy is shown to increase with the patient's age. (*Adapted from* Cameron *et al.* [28].)

TABLE 4-11. ESOPHAGEAL CANCER: SMOKING AND ALCOHOL AS RISK FACTORS BY HISTOLOGIC TYPE

TABLE 4-11.

Barrett's esophagus. Adenocarcinoma developing in Barrett's esophagus, as with esophageal squamous cell carcinoma, is shown to be increased by smoking and excessive alcohol consumption. (*Adapted from* Kabat *et al.* [29].)

| | HISTOLOGIC TYPE OF ESOPHAGEAL CARCINOMA | |
	ADENOCARCINOMA ODDS RATIO	SQUAMOUS CELL CARCINOMA ODDS RATIO
Smoking		
Never smoked	1.0	1.0
Current smoker	2.3	4.5
Alcohol use		
Less than 1 drink/week	1.0	1.0
More than 4 oz of whiskey equivalent/day	2.3	10.9

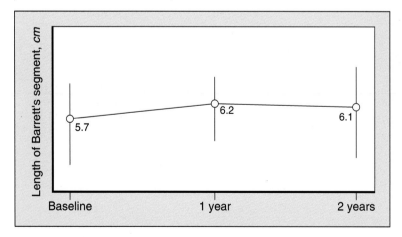

FIGURE 4-30.

Barrett's esophagus. Antireflux surgery (fundoplication) is shown to have no effect on the length of Barrett's esophagus over a 2-year period. This indicates that no therapy, either medical or surgical, has been able to reliably reverse its presence, and thus the risk of adenocarcinoma associated with Barrett's esophagus. (*Adapted from* Kim *et al.* [30].)

REFERENCES

1. Orlando RC: Reflux esophagitis. In *Textbook of Gastroenterology*. Edited by Yamada T, Alpers DH, Owyang C, *et al*. Philadelphia: JB Lippincott; 1991:1123–1147.

2. Spechler SJ: Epidemiology and natural history of gastro-oesphageal reflux disease. *Digestion* 1992, 51(suppl 1):24–29.

3. A Gallup Organization National Survey: *Heartburn Across America*. Princeton: The Gallup Organization; 1988.

4. Nebel OT, Fornes MF, Castell DO: Symptomatic gastroesophageal reflux: Incidence and precipitating factors. *Am J Dig Dis* 1976, 21:953.

5. Rasmussen CW: A new endoscopic classification of chronic esophagitis. *Am J Gastroenterol* 1976, 65:409.

6. Brunnen PL, Karmody AM, Needham CD: Severe peptic oesophagitis. *Gut* 1969, 10:831.

7. Dodds WJ, Dent J, Hogan WJ, *et al*.: Mechanisms of gastroesophageal reflux in patients with reflux esophagitis. *N Engl J Med* 1982, 307:1547.

8. Helm JF, Dodds WF, Pela LR, *et al*.: Effect of esophageal emptying and saliva on clearance of acid from the esophagus. *N Engl J Med* 1984, 310:284.

9. Kahrilas PJ: Esophageal peristaltic dysfunction in peptic esophagitis. *Gastroenterology* 1986, 91:897.

10. Sloan S, Kahrilas PJ: Impairment of esophageal emptying with hiatal hernia. *Gastroenterology* 1991, 100:596.

11. Orlando RC: Esophageal epithelial resistance. In *Gastroesophageal Reflux Disease: Pathogenesis, Diagnosis, Therapy*. Edited by Castell DO, Wu WC, Ott DJ. Mt. Kisco, NY: Futura; 1985.

12. Orlando RC: Pathology of reflux esophagitis and its complications. In *Surgery of the Oesophagus*. Edited by Jamieson GG. Edinburgh: Churchill Livingstone; 1988:189–200.

12a. Mitros FA: Inflammatory and Neoplastic Diseases of the Esophagus. In *Pathology of the Esophagus, Stomach, and Duodenum*. Edited by Appleman HD. New York: Churchill Livingstone; 1984:1–9.

13. Ismail-Beigi F, Horton PF, Pope CE: Histological consequences of gastroesophageal refluxes in man. *Gastroenterology* 1970, 58:163.

14. Weinstein WM, Goboch ER, Bowes KL: The normal human esophageal mucosa: A histologic reappraisal. *Gastroenterology* 1975, 68:40.

15. Tytgat GNJ: Upper gastrointestinal endoscopy. In *Textbook of Gastroenterology*. Edited by Yamada T, Alpers DH, Owyang C, *et al*. Philadelphia: JB Lippincott; 1991:435–436.

16. Ollyo JB, Lang F, Fontollet CH, *et al*.: Savary's new endoscopic grading of reflux-oesophagitis: a simple, reproducible, logical, complete and useful classification. *Gastroenterology* 1990, 89:A100.

17. Paull A, Trier JS, Dalton MD, *et al*.: The histologic spectrum of Barrett's esophagus. *N Engl J Med* 1976, 295:476.

18. Pera M, Trastek VF, Pairolero PC, *et al*.: Barrett's disease: Pathophysiology of metaplasia and adenocarcinoma. *Ann Thorac Surg* 1993, 56:1191.

19. Orlando RC: Gastroesophageal reflux. In *Current Therapy in Gastroenterology and Liver Disease*, edn 3. Edited by Bayless TM. Philadelphia: BC Decker; 1990:7.

20. Wilkinson J, Hunt RH: Appropriate acid suppression for the management of gastroesophageal reflux disease. *Digestion* 1992, 52(suppl 1):59.

21. Hetzel DJ, Dent J, Reed WD, *et al*.: Healing and relapse of severe peptic esophagitis after treatment with omeprazole. *Gastroenterology* 1988, 95:903.

22. Dent J, Yeomans ND, Mackinnon M, *et al*.: Omeprazole versus ranitidine for prevention of relapse in reflux oesophagitis: A controlled double blind trial of the efficacy and safety. *Gut* 1990, 35:590.

23. Brunner GHG, Lamberts R, Creutzfeldt W: Efficacy and safety of omeprazole with long-term treatment of peptic ulcer and reflux oesophagitis resistant to ranitidine. *Digestion* 1990, 47(Suppl 1):64.

24. Pope CE II: Gastroesophageal reflux disease (reflux esophagitis). In *Gastrointestinal Disease: Pathophysiology, Diagnosis, Management*. Edited by Sleisenger MH, Fordtran JS. Philadelphia: WB Saunders; 1983:449.

25. Spechler SJ and the Department of Veteran's Affairs Gastroesophageal Reflux Disease Study Group: Comparison of medical and surgical therapy for complicated gastroesophageal reflux disease in veterans. *N Engl J Med* 1992, 326:786.

26. Marks RD, Richter JE, Rizzo J, *et al*.: Omeprazole versus H2-receptor antagonists in treating patients with peptic stricture and esophagitis. *Gastroenterology* 1994, 106:907.

27. Sampliner RE: Effect of up to 3 years of high-dose lansoprazole on Barrett's esophagus. *Am J Gastroenterol* 1994, 89:1844.

28. Cameron AJ, Lomboy CT: Barrett's esophagus: Age prevalence and extent of columnar epithelium. *Gastroenterology* 1992, 103:1241.

29. Kabat GC, Ng SK, Wynder EL: Tobacco, alcohol intake, and diet in relation to adenocarcinoma of esophagus and gastric cardia. *Cancer Causes and Controls* 1993, 4:123.

30. Kim SL, Waring JP, Spechler SJ, *et al*.: Diagnostic inconsistencies in Barrett's esophagus. *Gastroenterology* 1994, 107:945.

Chapter 5

Acute Esophagitis

With the spread of the AIDS epidemic and the more general use of immunosuppressive agents for cancer chemotherapy and autoimmune disease, acute infectious esophagitis is a more frequent finding. Less commonly, other forms of acute esophageal injury result from toxins, radiation, or from foreign body penetration of the esophagus. This chapter systematically reviews the endoscopic, radiographic, and histologic findings in addition to discussing the epidemiology, pathogenesis, and treatment of these entities.

MATTHEW S.Z. BACHINSKI
ROY K.H. WONG

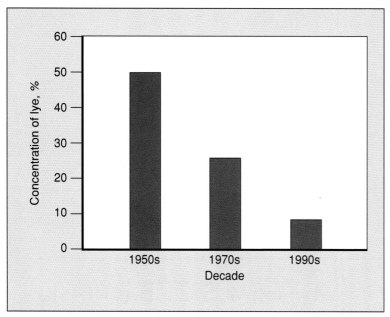

FIGURE 5-1.

Epidemiology. Chemical ingestion remains an important problem in the United States despite improved packaging, child-proof containers, and labeling. Approximately 5000 ingestions of caustic material occur per year. In the 1950s the concentration of lye in drain cleaners was greater than 50%; by the 1970s, it was reduced to 25% to 26%, and at present most lye products contain less than 10% NaOH. Hence, acute injuries have become less devastating although long-term esophageal stricture formation is still common. Crystalline solid preparations generally cause oral, pharyngeal, and laryngeal injury because of difficulty swallowing solid particles and local pain. Liquid products can be more readily swallowed and therefore cause more extensive esophageal injury.

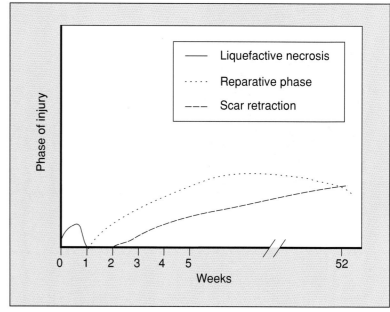

FIGURE 5-2.

Pathology. The acute and chronic sequelae of ingestion of caustic matter relate to the severity of esophageal injury and are histologically proportional to the depth of tissue necrosis. Experimentally, three phases of caustic injury occur: (1) liquefactive necrosis (0 to 5 days), (2) reparative phase (5 days to months), (3) scar retraction (2 weeks to months).

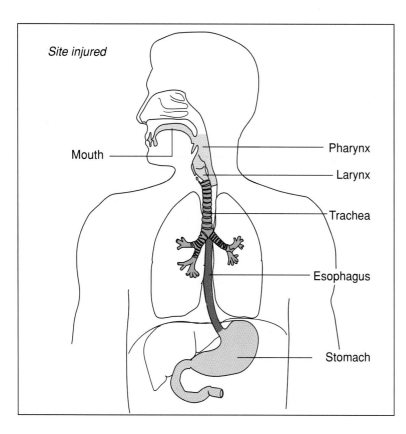

FIGURE 5-3.

Clinical presentation. Patients may present with uncomplicated ingestion manifested by acute oral burns, pain, and dysphagia. This is followed by latent phase without esophageal symptoms. A final retractive phase occurs when 10% to 30% of patients have scar and stricture formation, usually within 2 to 8 weeks. Complications include acute dysphagia, acute respiratory compromise, laryngeal edema, tracheitis and pneumonitis, esophageal perforation, septicemia, mediastinitis, peritonitis, empyema, hemorrhage, and death.

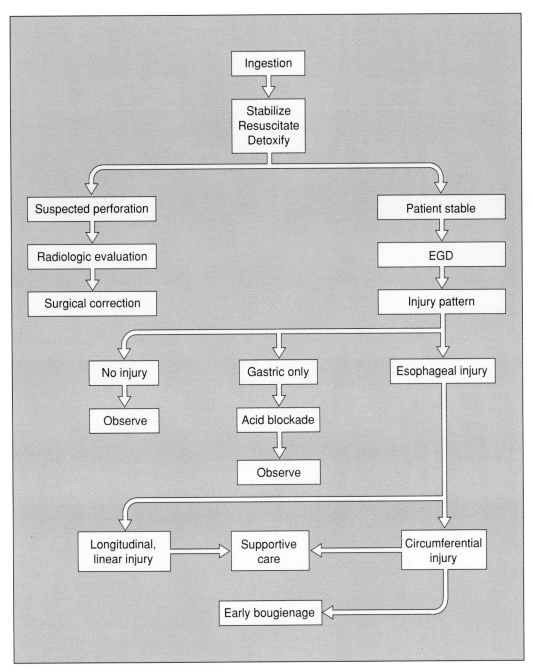

FIGURE 5-4.

Algorithm for the treatment of ingestion of caustic material. Endoscopy is not generally part of the acute evaluation. Initially, neutralization of ingested chemicals should be attempted. Patients should be stabilized by protecting the airway and resuscitated hemodynamically as appropriate. After the patient is stable and surgery has been ruled out, patients should undergo a gentle and careful upper endoscopy to determine the severity of the injury. There are four common esophagogastroduodenoscopy (EGD) findings: (1) no injury, (2) gastric only, (3) longitudinal, linear esophageal injury, and (4) circumferential esophageal injury with risk of stricture.

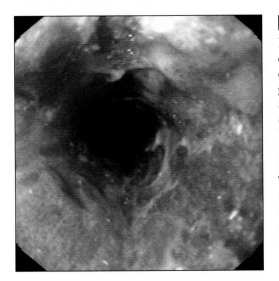

FIGURE 5-5.

Endoscopic view of caustic injury. This endoscopic photograph demonstrates a desquamated esophageal epithelium from the middle to the distal esophagus. The likelihood of stricture formation in this patient with circumferential injury is high.

TABLE 5-1. GRADING OF CORROSIVE ESOPHAGEAL AND GASTRIC BURNS

GRADE	PATHOLOGIC FINDINGS
1st degree	Superficial mucosal involvement
2nd degree	Transmucosal involvement with or without mucosal involvement
	No extension into periesophageal or perigastric tissue
3rd degree	Full thickness injuries with extension into periesophageal or perigastric tissue
	Possible mediastinal or intraperitoneal organ involvement

TABLE 5-1.

In general there is little indication for biopsy of lye-induced esophagitis, but if performed, there is a grading system based on the level of invasion. (*Adapted from* Fenoglio-Preiser *et al.* [1].)

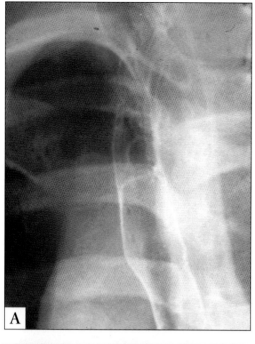

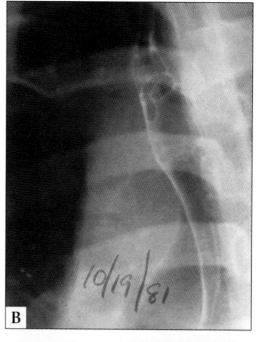

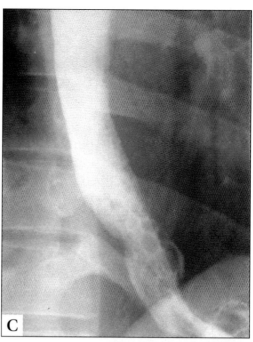

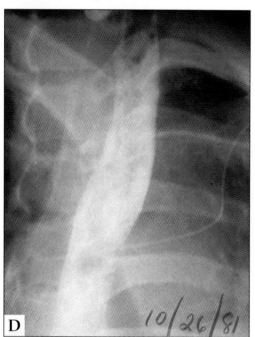

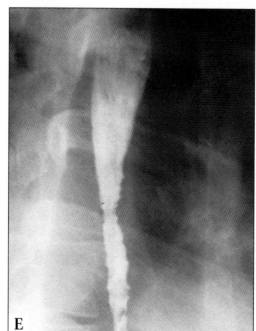

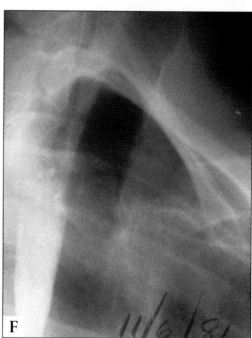

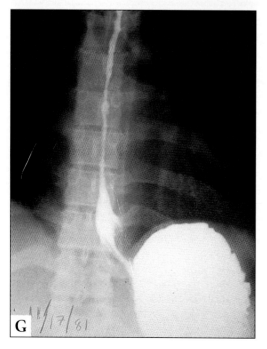

Figure 5-6.

Radiology. Radiologic studies are used during the initial evaluation and resuscitation. Chest radiographs to evaluate for pneumonitis and abdominal films to look for free air signifying hollow viscus perforation should be done. Esophagogram with water-soluble contrast is reserved for patients with suspected perforation.

This series of radiographs are from a patient who had four separate barium swallows over a 5-week period following lye ingestion. They demonstrate the progression from acute lye injury to esophageal mucosal repair followed by scarring and stricture formation. In **panel A** and **panel B**, taken October 19, proximal esophageal ulceration is seen without evidence of narrowing. In **panel C** and **panel D**, taken October 26, there is increased ulcerative changes seen best in the midesophagus. There is some evidence of early narrowing. In **panel E** and **panel F**, taken November 6, midesophageal stricture with proximal dilation is also seen. Note in **panel G**, taken November 17, the long middle to distal esophageal stricture diagnostic for lye stricture. To date no good evidence shows that steroids or antibiotics alter the long-term outcome from lye ingestion except antibiotics in cases of infection. Supportive care and watchful anticipation of possible complication remain the most important aspects of care. Early careful bougienage may be necessary to maintain patency of the esophageal lumen and to prevent future esophagectomy.

HIV

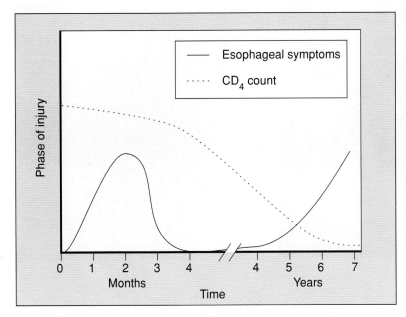

FIGURE 5-7.

Epidemiology and pathophysiology. HIV-1 is a 100-nm, single-stranded, diploid RNA retrovirus that preferentially infects CD-4 surface antigen presenting lymphocytes. Patients with HIV infection can be subject to acute esophageal symptoms at two points during their infection: first following acute seroconversion and later when the immune status becomes compromised. This second illness may be associated with an unrecognized cause, such as cytomegalovirus (CMV) and herpes simplex virus (HSV), but is currently termed *HIV-associated idiopathic esophageal ulceration*. HIV-positive patients with esophageal ulcers should have biopsies done for tissue culture, histopathology, and special stains to exclude other causes of esophagitis. Electron microscopy of esophageal biopsies has shown viral particles of similar morphology to those of retroviruses. In one study, polymerase chain reaction to the HIV genome was positive in 80% of tissue from HIV-associated idiopathic ulcers. Esophageal biopsies in HIV patients *without* esophageal ulcer, however, have revealed HIV virus, raising the question of whether it was an active invasion or simply a "carrier" status. About a third of patients with AIDS and esophageal symptoms have been found to harbor HSV, CMV, and *Candida*.

AIDS AND CLINICAL PRESENTATION

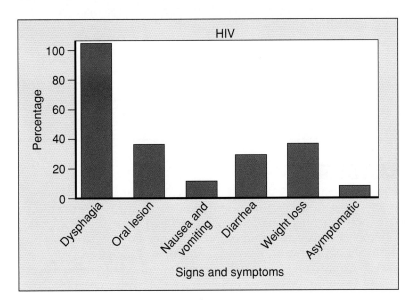

FIGURE 5-8.

Seroconverters have acute onset of flu-like illness lasting 2 to 14 days, characterized by fever, diarrhea, rash, and dysphagia or odynophagia. Chronic HIV patients present with acute/subacute dysphagia and odynophagia indistinguishable from other infections.

Endoscopic findings

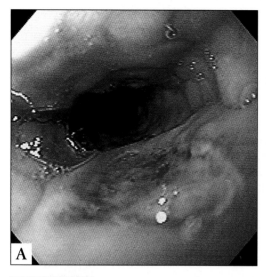 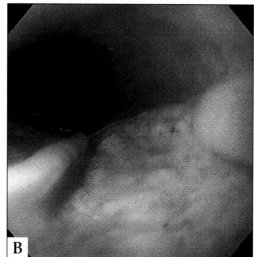 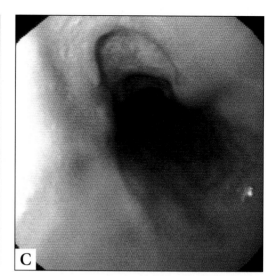

FIGURE 5-9.

The endoscopic characteristics of an esophageal ulcer caused by HIV are variable, ranging from small, superficial shallow aphthous ulcers (0.5 to 1.0 cm) to large, deep ulcers with undermining borders (1 to 5 cm). To be considered as an ulcer caused by HIV other causes of esophageal ulceration must be excluded. **Panel A** demonstrates a large, 2-cm ulceration with some hemorrhage in the midesophagus. **Panel B** and **panel C** demonstrate large 6-cm chronic ulcers with deep undermining edges and nodularity within the ulcer base. Idiopathic HIV-associated ulcers have been treated with intravenous corticosteroid therapy. In one study, 23 of 24 patients (95.8%) improved. Relapses were common after discontinuation of therapy. To maintain remission, long-term therapy was required. Trials of sucralfate four times daily mixed with dexamethasone (0.5) mg given as a slurry have been promising. These results must be tempered by the risk of additional long-term immunosuppressive therapy.

CYTOMEGALOVIRUS

Epidemiology

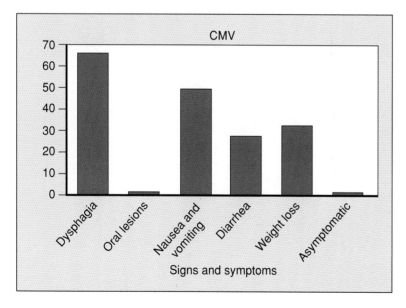

FIGURE 5-10.

Cytomegalovirus (CMV) is a ubiquitous herpesvirus, with approximately 80% of the world's population seropositive. It is the most common viral infection of the esophagus after herpes simplex 1, and is almost exclusively found in the immunocompromised host. Normally, seroconversion occurs during preschool or teenaged years, with latent infections reactivating in the immunocompromised host. About 1% of AIDS patients developed esophagitis caused by CMV.

This figure shows clinical presentation of CMV. Asymptomatic patients shedding viral particles must be differentiated from symptomatic patients with active organ involvement. Both the humoral and the cellular components of immunity are required to prevent reactivation. As with herpes simplex virus (HSV), cytomegalovirus (CMV) may coexist with other viral (*eg*, HSV) or fungal organisms. Patients present with gradual onset of nausea, vomiting, fever, epigastric pain (*ie*, retrosternal pain is less common than with HSV), diarrhea, and weight loss. If untreated, patients may progress to unrelenting dysphagia, secondary to severe esophagitis.

Pathophysiology

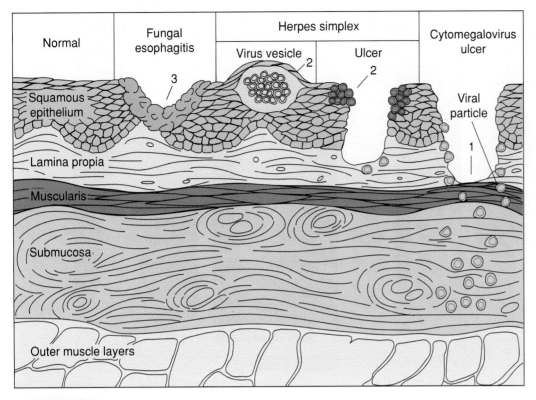

FIGURE 5-11.

The hallmark of active esophagitis caused by cytomegalovirus (CMV) is submucosal injury with ulceration. Cytopathic effects are seen in the glandular epithelium as opposed to the squamous epithelium in HSV, and are present in both endothelial cells and fibroblasts of the granulation tissue. A role for vasculitis caused by CMV has also been implicated.

This figure shows sites of tissue invasion of the esophagus by pathogens. Biopsies with the greatest yield for CMV should be obtained from the ulcer crater (*site 1*). Biopsies for HSV should be obtained adjacent to the ulcer or on a vesicle (*site 2*). Candida is best diagnosed from biopsies obtained from an active ulcer (*site 3*). Appropriate biopsy from the ulcer crater reveals large cells in the subepithelial layer with amphophilic intranuclear inclusions, a halo surrounding the nucleus, and multiple small cytoplasmic inclusions (not seen with HSV). Analysis of tissue samples can rapidly detect CMV by using special techniques such as rapid Giemsa staining or fluorescent antibody staining. Giemsa staining can be done from a touch prep whereas fluorescent antibody staining can be performed on either touch prep or frozen sample. Tissue histology is better than cytologic brushings or tissue culture for the diagnosis, and special techniques, such as rapid Giemsa and fluorescent antibody staining, increase both the sensitivity and specificity of diagnosis.

Pathology

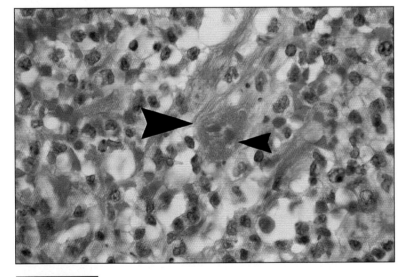

FIGURE 5-12

Viral culture for cytomegalovirus (CMV) can be sensitive if the biopsy is obtained from the correct location. Unfortunately, culturing technique requires long incubation periods (up to 3 weeks) and may not be clinically useful.

This figure shows a photomicrograph with hematoxylin and eosin staining showing typical changes associated with infection caused by CMV. Cells have intranuclear inclusions, halos surrounding the nucleus, and intracytoplasmic inclusions. The large arrowhead identifies a CMV-infected cell whereas the small arrowhead shows the nuclear halo.

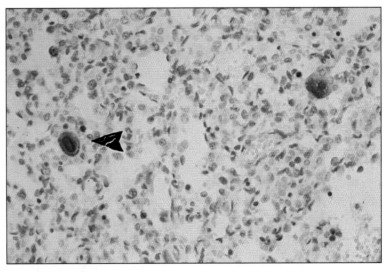

FIGURE 5-13.

An immunoperoxidase stain makes identification of cytomegalovirus (CMV)-infected tissue much easier. The peroxidase stain highlights CMV-infected cells (*arrowhead*), even at early stages of infection when classic cellular changes may not yet be evident.

Radiology

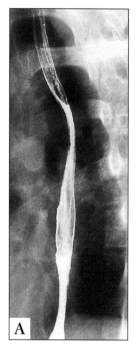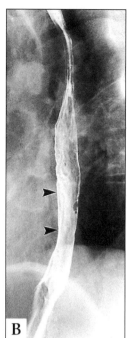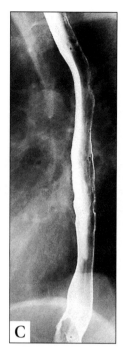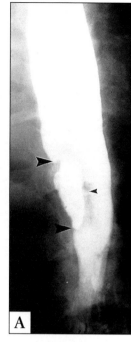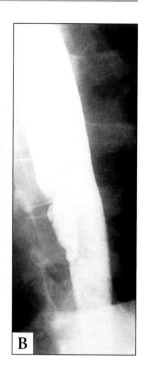

FIGURE 5-14.

A–C, Double-contrast radiographic view of the esophagus shows a large longitudinally-oriented ulcer in the middle to distal two-thirds of the esophagus. The ulcer is shown outlined in double contrast with some barium in the ulcer base. Arrowheads identify the extent of the ulceration. (*Courtesy of* Dr. Arunas E. Gasparitis, Chicago, IL.)

FIGURE 5-15.

A–B, Esophagogram taken during the late phases of infection reveals large deep ulceration (*large arrowhead*) with raised borders secondary to edema. The small arrowhead identifies the edematous border.

Esophagogastroduodenoscopy with biopsy of the ulcer crater is required for diagnosis. Brushings of this area are not helpful. Findings early in the course include mucosal erythema and superficial erosions with geographic, serpiginous, nonraised borders. (*Courtesy of* Dr. Arunas E. Gasparitis, Chicago, IL.)

Endoscopy

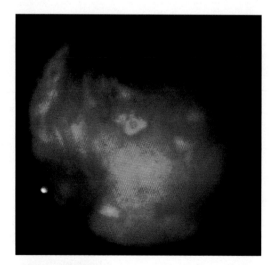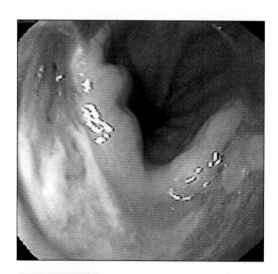

FIGURE 5-16.

This figure shows typical midcourse lesions with shallow ulcers 0.5 to 10 cm in which complete denudation of the esophagus is unusual. These ulcers may be indistinguishable from herpes simplex virus ulceration and biopsy is required. Cytomegalovirus infections of the esophagus is typically most prominent in the mid to distal esophagus.

FIGURE 5-17.

Large ulcerations typical of the late course of infection caused by cytomegalovirus (CMV). These ovoid or elongated ulcers may extend for several centimeters. Herpes simplex virus ulcers are rarely more than several centimeters in length and the presence of one or more giant ulcers is suggestive of CMV esophagitis. Large ulcers may become hemorrhagic.

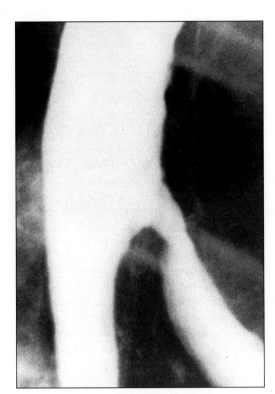

FIGURE 5-18.

The rare complication of formation of a fistula between the esophagus and left main-stem bronchus in a patient with chronic infection caused by cytomegalovirus (CMV). Other complications of CMV include superinfection (viral, bacterial, fungal), stricture, hemorrhage, and perforation (rare). (*From* Fenoglio-Preiser *et al.* [1]; with permission.)

TABLE 5-2. PREVENTION AND TREATMENT OF ESOPHAGITIS CAUSED BY CMV

DRUG FORMULATION	PREVENTION OF CMV INFECTION*	TREATMENT OF ESTABLISHED CMV DISEASE
Acyclovir, for IV use (500 mg/10 mL vial, admixed to final concentration <7 mg/mL)[†]	For seropositive patients[‡] or recipients of organs from seropositive donors: 500 mg/m^2 BSA IV every 8 hours	Not applicable
Ganciclovir, for IV use (500 mg/10 mL vial, admixed to final concentration < 10 mg/mL)[§]	For seropositive patients[‡] or recipients of organs from seropositive donors: 5 mg/kg every 12 hours IV for 5 days, then once daily as maintenance therapy	5 mg/kg every 12 hours IV for 2 weeks,[¶] then once daily for maintenance (if indicated)
Foscarnet, for IV use (12 g/500 mL)	Not applicable	60 mg/kg every 8 hours (or 90 mg/kg every 12 hours) IV for 2 weeks,[¶] then 90–120 mg/kg daily for maintenance (if indicated)
Epidemiologic methods	For seronegative patients: Transfusion of CMV seronegative blood products Organ transplants from CMV seronegative donors Leukofiltration of CMV seropositive blood products	

*For patients at risk.
[†]Adjust dose for renal function.
[‡]Marrow transplantation patients; trials of prophylactic ganciclovir for patients infected with HIV have not been completed.
[§]Use of oral ganciclovir formulations are under current study.
[¶]Induction therapy should be extended if the patient has not completely responded and other etiologies are excluded.

TABLE 5-2.

Therapy for cytomegalovirus (CMV) can be given as prevention of disease in patients known to be immunocompromised or a therapy against established disease proven by tissue biopsy. Current therapy includes ganciclovir and acyclovir for prophylaxis and ganciclovir and foscarnet for treatment of established disease. In AIDS patients with biopsy-proven CMV esophageal ulceration, both ganciclovir and foscarnet therapy have been associated with endoscopically documented ulcer healing in some patients in 2 weeks or less. (*Adapted from* Baehr and McDonald [2].)

Epidemiology

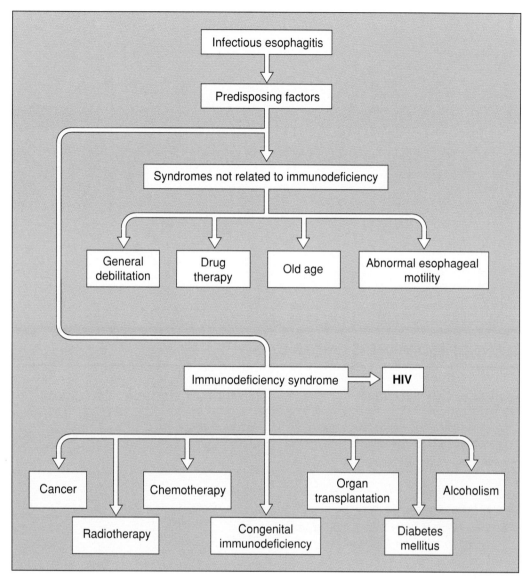

FIGURE 5-19.

Herpes simplex virus is a large, enveloped, double-stranded DNA virus with humans as the only reservoir. Infection occurs most commonly as a reactivation of a silent infection rather than as an exogenous infection. Esophagitis can occur with both HSV type 1 and type 2. The likelihood is that reactivation will occur and then the severity of disease will be inversely related to the immunocompetence of the patient.

Several factors predispose patients to infectious esophagitis. None of these is specific for herpetic infection, but they share a common theme. The common finding is a compromised immune system. At present, with the AIDS epidemic, infectious esophagitis is seen most frequently in these patients; however, because of underreporting of AIDS cases, misdiagnosis of infectious esophagitis and empiric therapy for complications of infectious esophagitis, the actual number of cases per year is not available.

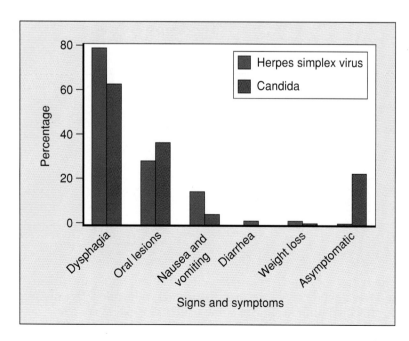

FIGURE 5-20.

Clinical presentation. Eighty percent of patients present with painful or difficult swallowing. Of these, 30% have oral lesions at the time of diagnosis. Unlike esophagitis caused by *Candida*, where 25% of patients will be asymptomatic, virtually all patients with esophagitis caused by herpes simplex virus have symptoms.

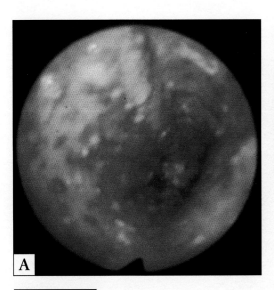

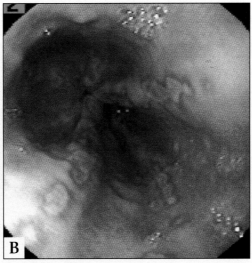

FIGURE 5-21.

Endoscopic findings in esophagitis caused by herpes simplex virus (HSV). Endoscopic findings vary with the severity of the disease and the point at which endoscopy is

performed. Early lesions are vesicular, occurring in the midesophagus, and are rarely seen because few endoscopies are performed at this stage, when the vesicles are fragile and easily ruptured. Midway in the course of the disease sharply demarcated small ulcers with raised margins are noted (**A**). The mucosa surrounding the ulcers is often erythematous and edematous. In the late necrotic phase of the disease process, diffuse esophagitis is noted with confluent esophageal ulcers (**B**).

The location of the biopsy site is essential to accurately diagnose esophagitis caused by HSV accurately. Because the virus is active only in epithelial cells, biopsies should be directed at the ulcer edge and not into the crater, which will only yield necrotic debris. (**A**, *Courtesy of* Dr. S. Kadakia, Brooke Army Medical Center; **B**, *courtesy of* Dr. K. Yamamoto, Madigan Army Medical Center.)

Complications of esophagitis caused by herpes simplex virus

TABLE 5-3. COMPLICATIONS FROM HERPES SIMPLEX VIRUS

Mucosal necrosis	Stricture
Mucosal superinfection	Tracheoesophageal fistula
Hemorrhage	Dissemination

TABLE 5-3.

Herpetic infection of the esophagus in immune compromised patients is generally limited to the mucosa. There can be dramatic complications, such as hemorrhage and fistulization to the trachea. Superinfection can occur with other viruses or bacteria.

Histology

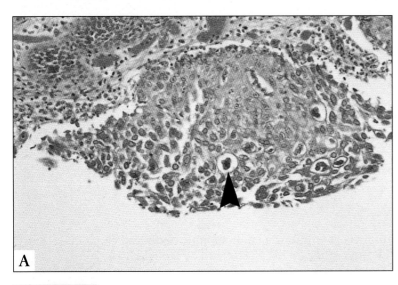

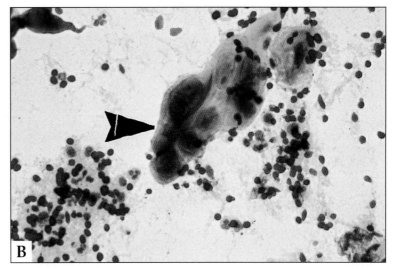

FIGURE 5-22.

Pathologists should be notified that esophagitis caused by herpes simplex virus (HSV) is suspected so that immunohistologic staining can be performed. **A**, HSV invades only the squamous epithelium, causing necrosis of the esophageal mucosa. Findings include multinucleated giant cells and ballooning degeneration of the squamous epithelial cells. Immunohistologic staining clearly identifies cells containing HSV. **B**, Characteristic findings of ballooning degeneration, ground glass nuclei, eosinophilic intranuclear inclusions, and herpetic giant cells (*arrowhead*). Special stains (Papanicolaou's

stain) demonstrate multinucleated cells (*arrowhead*); this makes changes associated with HSV more evident.

Viral culture can be used to augment histopathology in diagnosing herpetic esophagitis. Viral culture is more sensitive than endoscopic inspection and microscopic examination. HSV can be rapidly grown in diploid fibroblasts or rabbit kidney cells. Cytopathic changes in culture occur rapidly and are evident within 24 to 96 hours after inoculation. (**B**, *Courtesy of* Dr. P. McNally, Eisenhower Army Medical Center.)

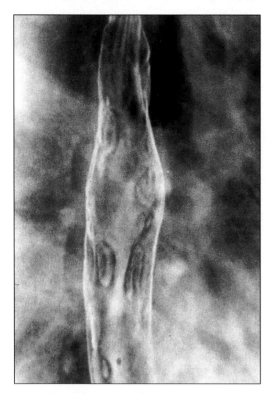

FIGURE 5-23.

Double contrast esophago-gram can be normal or diagnostic. Disease is often midesophageal with discrete, superficial, stellate ulcers. Advanced disease may have plaques, cobblestoning, or even a shaggy ulcerative appearance similar to that seen in infection caused by *Candida.* This figure shows a double-contrast esopha-gogram demonstrating numerous oval mucosal elevations representing a thin, lucent ring of edema surrounding the herpetic ulcers. Note the similarity between the appearance of this radiograph and Figure 5-23A. (*From* Fenoglio-Preiser *et al.* [1]; with permission.)

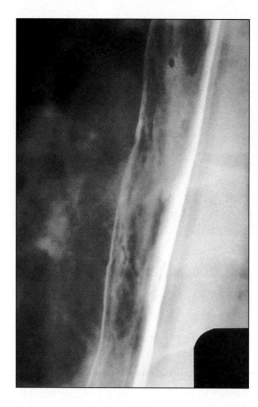

FIGURE 5-24.

Multiple discrete, punctate ulcers are distributed throughout the proximal and middle third of the thoracic esophagus.

TABLE 5-4. PREVENTION AND TREATMENT OF ESOPHAGITIS CAUSED BY HERPES SIMPLEX VIRUS (HSV)

DRUG FORMULATION	PREVENTION OF HSV INFECTION*	TREATMENT OF ESTABLISHED HSV INFECTION
Acyclovir, capsules (200 mg)	200–400 mg orally 4–5 times daily, or 800 mg orally twice daily	200–400 mg orally 5 times daily for 2 weeks
Acyclovir, for IV use (500 mg/10 mL vial, admixed to final concentration <7 mg/mL)	250 mg/m^2 every 12 hours IV	250 mg/m^2 every 8 hours IV for 2 weeks[†]
Foscarnet, for intravenous use (12 g/500 mL)[‡]	Not applicable	60 mg/kg every 8 hours (or 90 mg/kg every 12 hours) IV for 2 weeks, then 90–120 mg/kg daily for maintenance (if indicated)[§]

*For patients at risk.
[†]Intravenous acyclovir therapy can be converted to oral route for completetion of induction therapy in responders.
[‡]For treatment of HSV resistant to acyclovir.
[§]Induction therapy should be extended if the patient has not completely responded and other etiologies are excluded.

TABLE 5-4.

Current therapeutic strategies are based on the severity of disease and immune status of the patient. Clinical decisions must be made to determine if a patient is at significant risk to merit the use of prophylaxis. Options include supportive care, acyclovir or foscarnet. (*Adapted from* Baehr and McDonald [2].)

ESOPHAGITIS CAUSED BY *CANDIDA*

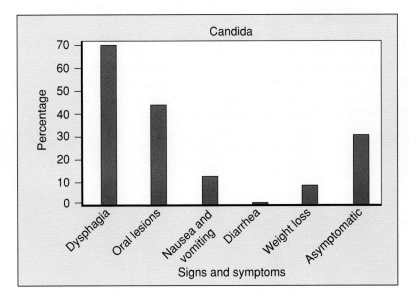

Candida

Percentage / Signs and symptoms

Dysphagia — Oral lesions — Nausea and vomiting — Diarrhea — Weight loss — Asymptomatic

FIGURE 5-25.

Although *Candida* is a normal component of the oral flora, esophageal candidal infection occurs most commonly in the immunocompromised host. Candidiasis is the most common type of infectious esophagitis in patients with HIV involvement, but is also seen in other illnesses, such as progressive systemic sclerosis, diabetes mellitus, following caustic ingestion, after solid-organ or bone-marrow transplantation, esophageal motility disorders, or in esophageal obstruction. Compromise of the host's immune function predisposes the patient to candidal infection. Suppressed lymphocyte function leads to superficial mucosal infection whereas suppressed granulocyte function may permit deep mucosal invasion and disseminated infection. Typical infections progress from colonization to epithelial infection, and then to deeper tissue invasion.

Patients may present with a spectrum of complaints related to the gastrointestinal system. Unlike in esophagitis caused by herpes simplex virus wherein virtually all patients are symptomatic, as many as 25% of patients with esophageal candidiasis are asymptomatic, particularly immunocompetent hosts. Studies indicate that patients with AIDS who have esophageal symptoms and oral candidiasis have a positive predictive value of 71% to 100% for candidal esophagitis.

Diagnosis

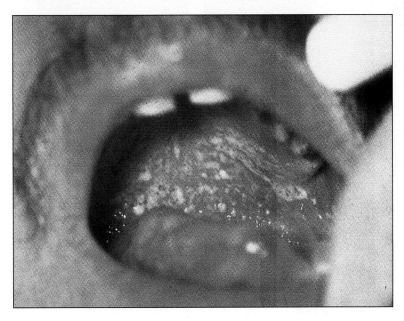

FIGURE 5-26.

The magnitude of the AIDS epidemic and its multiple complications have, to some extent, driven the diagnostic evaluation and management of acute esophageal symptoms in patients with AIDS. Patients presenting with dysphagia or odynophagia and positive results of an oral examination revealing candidiasis should receive empiric treatment with systemic antifungal medication. More invasive diagnostic procedures should be performed in patients who fail to respond to empiric antifungal therapy or have more severe symptoms suggesting an alternative diagnosis. Blind esophageal brushing of the esophagus can be obtained by passing a sheathed brush orally through a nasogastric tube. Sheathed tubes prevent contamination. This technique has a sensitivity of 88% and specificity of nearly 100% when compared with endoscopically obtained specimens. Blind smears can be used but will not diagnose Kaposi's sarcoma, pill-induced injury, esophageal injury caused by gastroesophageal reflux disease or infections caused by human immunodeficiency virus, herpes simplex virus or cytomegalovirus, which can also occur in this setting. (*From* Pounder *et al.* [3]; with permission.)

Pathology

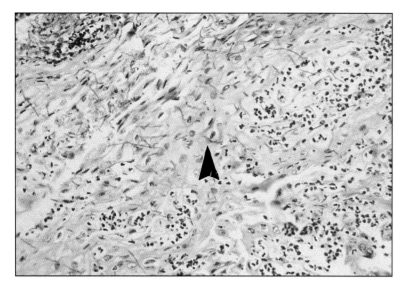

FIGURE 5-27.

Histologic specimen with large numbers of pseudohyphae (*arrowhead*) in the esophageal mucosa on periodic acid-Schiff staining. Specimens can be obtained either from blind esophageal brushing or through endoscopically guided brushings. Silver stain can also be used and may aid in the diagnosis of candidal infection.

Radiologic findings

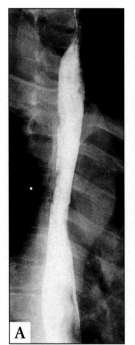 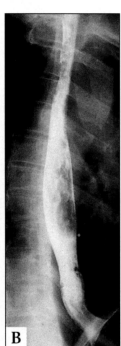 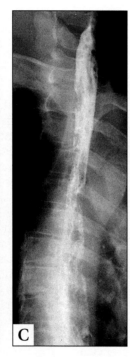 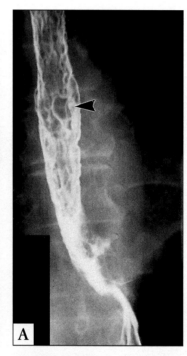 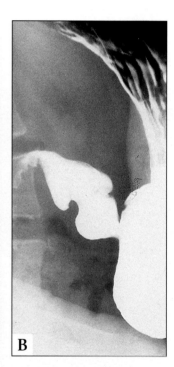

FIGURE 5-28.

Radiologic evaluation of esophagitis caused by *Candida* may be less diagnostic in the early stages because it resembles other causes of esophagitis. **A–C,** Early findings in acute esophagitis caused by *Candida*. Normal or tiny nodular lesions with a granular appearance in the upper half of the esophagus.

FIGURE 5-29.

A–B, Classic findings in acute esophagitis caused by *Candida*. Discrete plaque-like lesions, oriented longitudinally, producing linear or irregular filling defects with distinct margins (*arrowhead*).

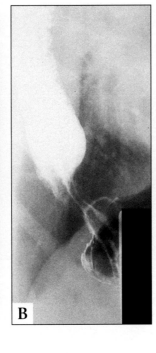

FIGURE 5-30.

A–B, Severe findings in acute esophagitis caused by *Candida* include coalescing plaques. Pseudomembranes may produce a grossly irregular or shaggy pattern.

TABLE 5-5. ENDOSCOPIC GRADING OF ESOPHAGEAL CANDIDIASIS

Grade I

A few small (up to 2 mm) white, raised plaques with hyperemia but with no evidence of ulceration or edema.

Grade II

Multiple raised plaques over 2 mm with edema and hyperemia. No ulcers are noted.

Grade III

Linear and nodular elevated confluent plaques with hyperemia and ulceration.

Grade IV

Grade III plus mucosal friability that may be associated with luminal narrowing.

TABLE 5-5.

Endoscopic grading of esophageal candidiasis. (*Adapted from* Kodsi *et al.* [4].)

Endoscopic Findings

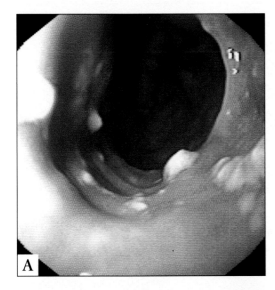

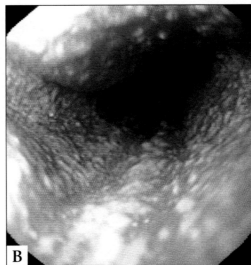

FIGURE 5-31.

Early findings of esophagitis caused by *Candida* with plaques not yet becoming confluent. As the infection worsens, there is associated hyperemia. Brushing and biopsy are diagnostic and help to rule out secondary causes of esophagitis. Generally plaques caused by *Candida* will not wash off. Biopsy should be obtained using hematoxylin and eosin stain as well as stains for fungus (silver and periodic acid-Schiff). **A**, Grade 1; **B**, grade 2. (**A**, *Courtesy of* Dr. A. Tsuchida, Madigan Army Medical Center; **B**, *courtesy of* Dr. K. Yamamoto, Madigan Army Medical Center.)

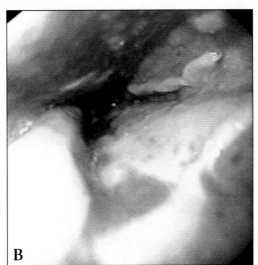

FIGURE 5-32.

Panel A (grade 2-3,) and **panel B** (grade 3-4,) represent the progression of esophageal disease caused by candidiasis. (**B**, *Courtesy of* Dr. M. Lyons, Madigan Army Medical Center.)

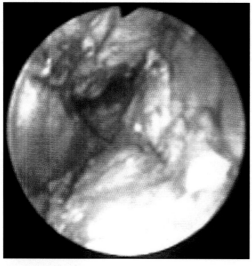

FIGURE 5-33.

Grade 4 esophagitis caused by *Candida* with distal ulceration and hemorrhage. (*Courtesy of* Dr. M. Lyons, Madigan Army Medical Center.)

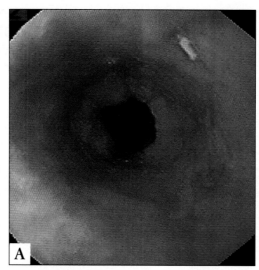

FIGURE 5-34.

A–B, A nearly healed case of severe esophagitis caused by *Candida*, showing a healing ulcer in the foreground.

TABLE 5-6. TREATMENT OF *CANDIDA*-INDUCED ESOPHAGITIS

DRUG FORMULATION	NO OR MINIMAL LYMPHOCYTE DEFECTS AND NORMAL GRANULOCYTES	DECREASED LYMPHOCYTE FUNCTION BUT NORMAL GRANULOCYTES	DECREASED GRANULOCYTE FUNCTION
Oral, nonabsorbable drugs			
Nystatin suspension (1,000,000 units/mL)	1–3 MU orally, 4 times daily	Not applicable	Not applicable
Amphotericin B lozenge (10 mg) or suspension (100 mg/mL)*	1–2 lozenges or 1 mL suspension, 4 times daily	Not applicable	Not applicable
Miconazole oral gel (25 mg/mL)	10 mL orally, 4 times daily	Not applicable	Not applicable
Clotrimazole troches (10 mg)	**10 mg troche, dissolved in mouth 5 times daily**	Not applicable	Not applicable
Clotrimazole vaginal tablets (100 mg)	100 mg tablet, dissolved in mouth 3 times daily	100 mg tablet, dissolved in mouth 3–5 times daily	Not applicable
Oral, absorbable drugs			
Ketoconazole tablets (200 mg)	200 mg orally, once daily	400–800 mg orally, once daily	400–800 mg orally, once daily
Fluconazole capsules (50 or 100 mg)	50 mg orally, once daily	**100 mg orally, once daily**	100–200 mg orally, once daily
Flucytosine capsules (250 or 500 mg)†	Not applicable	Not applicable	50–150 mg kg^{-1} day^{-1}, at 6 hr intervals
Intravenous drugs			
Amphotericin B for IV use (5 mg/mL)	Not applicable	0.3 mg kg^{-1} day^{-1}, intravenously	**0.5 mg kg^{-1} day^{-1}, intravenously**
Fluconazole for IV use (2 mg/mL)‡	100 mg intravenously, once daily	100 mg intravenously, once daily	100–200 mg intravenously, once daily

*Not available in the USA.
†Not for use as a single agent. See text for discussion of the use of this drug.
‡When oral route is not available.
The therapy of choice under each column is given in bold.

TABLE 5-6.

Treatment of esophagitis caused by *Candida*. (*Adapted from* Baehr and McDonald [2].)

Epidemiology and incidence

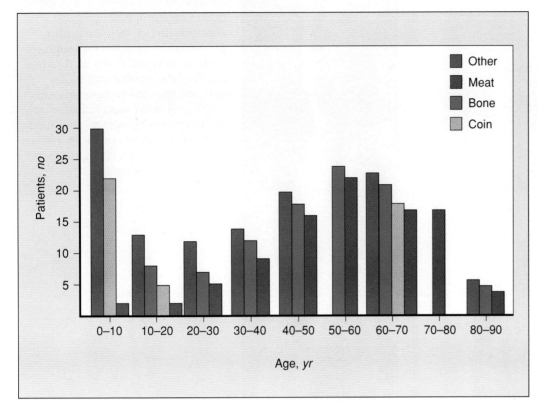

FIGURE 5-35.

Several important factors are related to foreign body impaction. This figure demonstrates the bimodal incidence of impaction with age. Children account for the first peak with impaction of small objects, such as coins, which are easily found and swallowed by curious unsuspecting children. The second peak occurs in the fifth to sixth decade, when patients with pathologic stricture or B-ring cause impaction of common foods at narrowed areas. Poor dentition and the inability to masticate food in elderly patients increases the likelihood of impaction, especially if underlying pathology is present. Other risk factors for impaction include younger than 10 years old and older than 50 years old; underlying disease; ring, web; stricture, tumor; motility disorder; oral disease; poor dentition; dentures; and mental impairment. The magnitude of the problem of foreign body ingestion in the United States remains unclear. Each year 1500 to 2750 persons die from foreign body ingestion. Of the objects that are ingested, 80% to 90% pass into the stomach and do not require therapeutic intervention. (*Adapted from* Giordano *et al.* [5].)

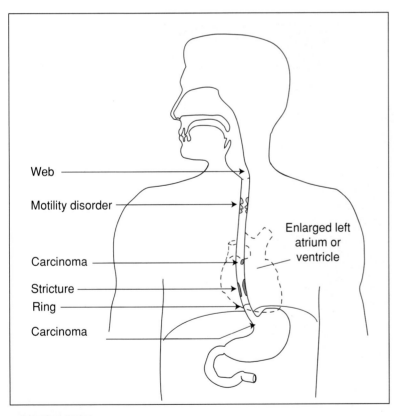

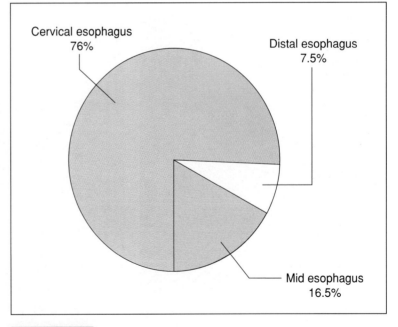

FIGURE 5-37.

Breakdown of impactions by location [6].

FIGURE 5-36.

When considering all age groups, most foreign body impactions occur in patients without attendant esophageal pathology, such as web, ring, or stricture. In the older patient, however, clinicians must consider these lesions and determine if underlying pathology is present. This figure indicates common areas of abnormality at which impactions are likely to occur.

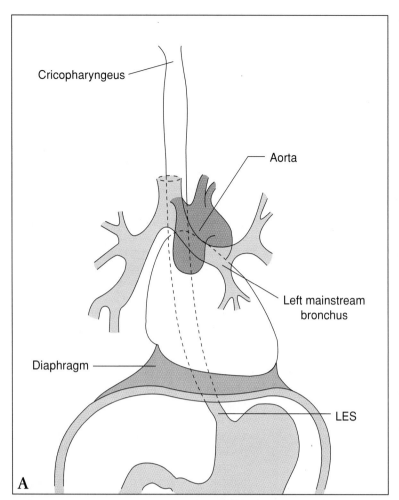

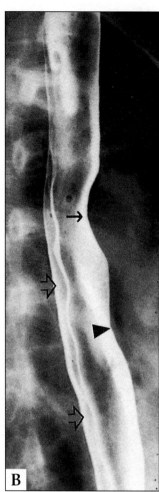

FIGURE 5-38.

A, Locations where normal anatomic structures can cause physiologic narrowing of the esophagus and increase the likelihood of foreign body impaction (the anatomic relationship between the cardiopulmonary system and the esophagus is noted in Figure 5-30). **B,** A radiograph of the normal esophagus demonstrates the compressive effect of the arch of the aorta (*closed arrow*), left mainstem bronchus (*arrowhead*), and spinal processes on the esophagus (*open arrow*). (*From* Fenoglio-Preiser *et al.* [1]; with permission.)

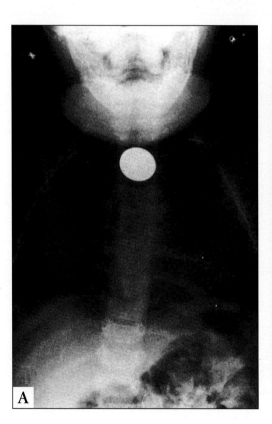

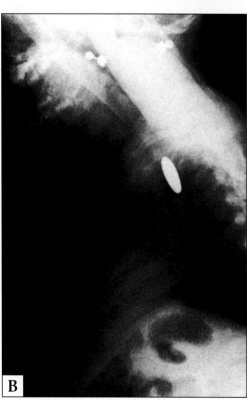

FIGURE 5-39.

Taking plain radiographic films of the neck when evaluating foreign body impaction is important. **Panel A** and **panel B** show a coin in the child's esophagus, with the coin seen head on in the anteroposterior projection. (*From* Yoshida and Peura *et al.* [7]; with permission.)

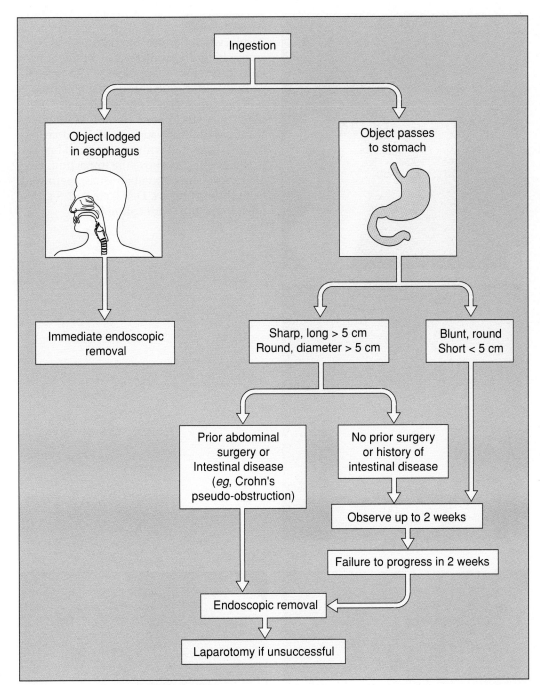

FIGURE 5-40.

Diagnostic evaluation should precede with a complete history and physical examination. The patient is usually able to give specifics concerning the size, consistency, and time of foreign body ingestion. A past history of gastroesophageal reflux disease, dysphagia, loss of teeth, or change in dentures are clues concerning the etiology. Posteroanterior and lateral chest radiographs, as well as neck radiographs with radiographic technique to emphasize soft tissues, are important to assess impaction in the hypopharynx and cervical esophagus as well as airway compromise. Barium swallow is generally not indicated in suspected foreign body impaction because aspiration may occur and the barium may prevent endoscopic visualization. Additionally, other objects should not be swallowed to try to "drive" the impacted object into the stomach.

This figure shows an algorithmic approach to a patient with food impaction. The first consideration when approaching the patient would be the nature of the ingested object. Sharp objects should be considered for removal. Toxic or caustic objects should also be considered for early removal. Location, as determined by radiology studies, is also important. All objects stuck in the esophagus should be considered for removal if adequate resources are available. (*Adapted from* Cotton *et al.* [8].)

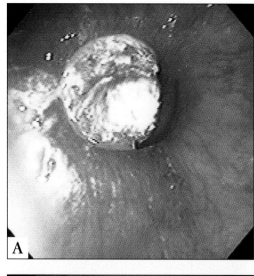
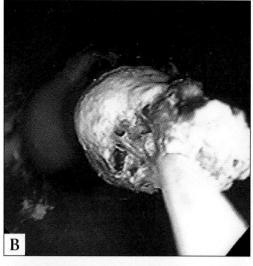

FIGURE 5-41.

Results when barium and barium-soaked cotton balls are swallowed by a patient with food impaction. This patient is a 46-year-old woman with B-ring above a hiatal hernia. **A,** A barium-soaked cotton ball in the midesophagus (a large amount of liquid barium was already suctioned); **B,** extraction of the cotton ball with barium pool below in the esophagus above the impaction; **C,** 4.5 cm × 2 cm cotton ball "mass" removed from the esophagus; **D,** 3.0 cm × 1.5 cm meat impaction with cotton ball.

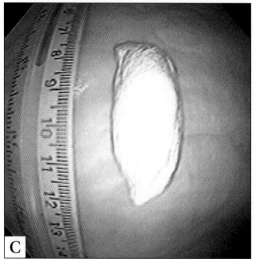
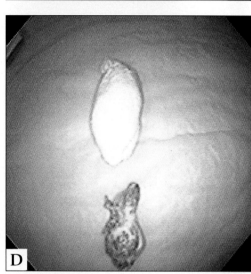

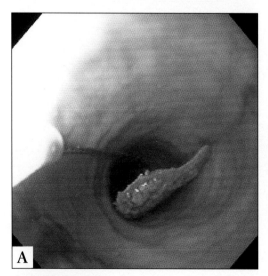
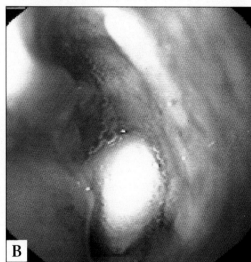
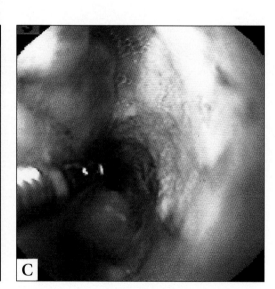

FIGURE 5-42.

Various objects have caused impaction. Food, particularly meat and small pieces of bone, are common. **A,** A chicken bone within the esophageal lumen and mild trauma in the esophagus proximal to the impacted bone. **B,** Squamous cell carcinoma of the esophagus as the underlying abnormality causing narrowing of the esophagus.

C, Subsequent impaction of a theophylline pill that required removal endoscopically with forceps. (**A,** *Courtesy of* Dr. P. McNally, Eisenhower Army Medical Center; **B,** *courtesy of* Dr. K. Yamamoto, Madigan Army Medical Center.)

PILL-INDUCED ESOPHAGITIS

Factors associated with esophageal clearance

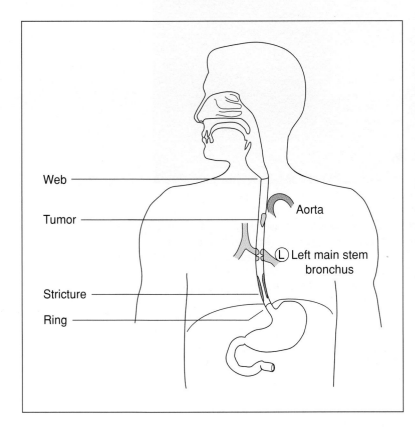

Web

Tumor

Stricture

Ring

Aorta

(L) Left main stem bronchus

FIGURE 5-43.

Location of pill injury. Pill-induced esophageal injury occurs when the caustic contents of pills remain in contact with the esophagus long enough to produce mucosal damage. Anyone who ingests caustic pills is susceptible to pill-induced esophageal injury because the moderate delay in transit through the esophagus is a common event even with normal esophageal motility. Although delays in transit are necessary for pill-induced injury, they alone are not sufficient because the content of the pill must be inherently caustic. Doxycycline and ascorbic acid produce pH levels below 3.0 when dissolved and can cause local burns. Other agents, such as nonsteroidal anti-inflammatory drugs and doxycycline, may produce injury by causing local toxic accumulation within the esophageal mucosa. Risks of pill-induced injury include structural abnormalities, hiatal hernia, stricture, tumor, supine position, old age, abnormal esophageal motility, minimal liquid taken with medications, type of pill, concurrent ingestion of alcohol, and underlying gastroesophageal reflux disease. Factors associated with esophageal clearance include body position during and following pill ingestion (easily modified), saliva production, esophageal motility, structural abnormalities, and volume of water consumed (easily modified).

Clinical presentation

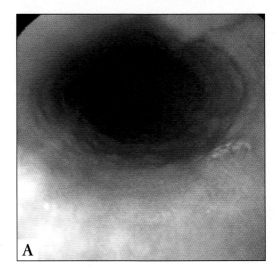

A

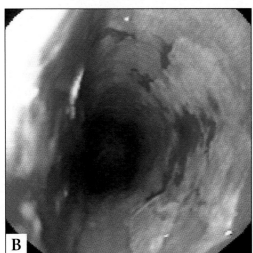

B

FIGURE 5-44.

Patients typically have no prior history of esophageal disease and present with sudden onset of retrosternal pain, exacerbated by swallowing. Pain may be mild or so severe that swallowing may be impossible. Typically, the pain increases over the first 72-hour pill ingestion and gradually subsides. Patients with preexisting esophageal problems, such as gastroesophageal reflux disease (GERD), frequently present with worsening symptoms of heartburn, regurgitation, and dysphagia. In more severe esophageal injury patients may present with odynophagia.

Patients with severe or persistent esophageal symptoms and an appropriate

(continued on next page)

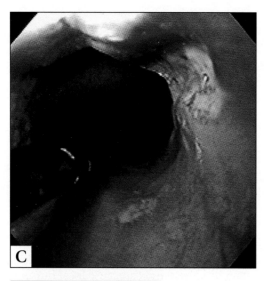

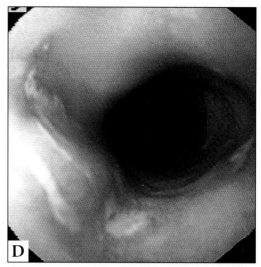

FIGURE 5-44. (*CONTINUED*)

history of pill ingestion should have endoscopy. Findings, often including esophagitis, hiatal hernia, Schatzski's B-ring, or stricture, are all most commonly found in the distal esophagus. Most pill-induced lesions occur in the endoscopically normal esophagus, and are located between the junction of the proximal and middle esophagus. The lesions associated with pill-induced esophageal injury vary with the agent ingested and the duration of injury.

The type of pill and duration of esophageal contact may influence the injury. Punctate ulcers with well-circumscribed borders may be noted with antibiotics, such as doxycycline and erythromycin. A shallow plaque-like ulcer with a thin membrane can also be noted, resulting from lower toxic concentrations or shorter duration of injury. Raised, plaque-like membranes can be seen with quinidine-induced esophageal injury. Pill-induced lesions may be single or multiple, with remnants of pills sometimes noted within the ulcer crater.

A, A discrete tetracycline-induced ulcer with normal surrounding mucosa. **B,** Aggressive plaque-like, membranous ulceration, secondary to doxycycline with adjacent ulcers on each side of the esophagus. Friability and bleeding is noted following intubation of the endoscope. **C,** Large, deep ulcer and smaller more discrete ulceration secondary to erythromycin. **D,** Classic pill-induced "kissing ulcerations." (**A,** *Courtesy of* Dr. T. Peller, Madigan Army Medical Center; **B,** *Courtesy of* Dr. K. Yamamoto, Madigan Army Medical Center.)

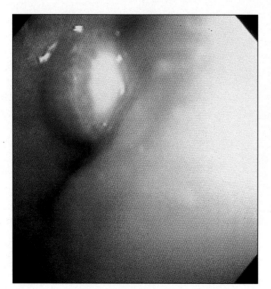

FIGURE 5-45.

Pill fragments may be seen in ulcer bases on endoscopy. In this case, an ibuprofen (Motrin) tablet is seen in the esophagus with adjacent ulceration.

Radiologic findings

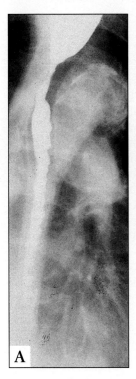
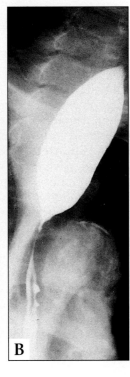

FIGURE 5-46.

A–B, Radiographs demonstrating different cases of quinidine-induced esophageal injury. There is little reason to perform a barium esophagogram in a patient with acute esophageal symptoms and an accepted pill-induced injury. Barium study may play a role in diagnosing underlying pathology, such as gastroesophageal reflux disease, hiatal hernia, stricture, or complications.

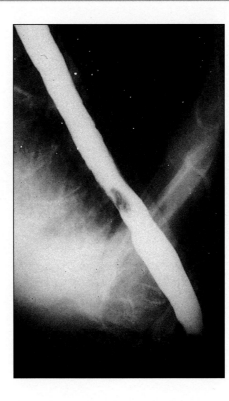

FIGURE 5-47.

A raised membrane in the proximal third of the esophagus. This finding is classic for quinidine-induced esophageal injury, which may be mistaken endoscopically for esophagitis caused by *Candida* because of the whitish membranous plaques. Stricture formation can occur, as shown in Figure 5-40B, which shows a more severe, long-term esophageal injury. This single contrast spot film of the proximal third of the esophagus shows a high-grade smooth stricture at the level of the aortic arch (an area of physiologic narrowing).

Therapy

TABLE 5-7. THERAPY FOR PILL-INDUCED ESOPHAGITIS

Discontinue use of nonsteroidal anti-inflammatory drugs
Acid blockade
Sucralfate
Local analgesia
Supportive care

TABLE 5-7.

Pill-induced esophagitis can cause intense pain, but this is generally short lived (1–3 days). Therapy is supportive with medicine to decrease pain and prevent further injury. A mixture of lidocaine, mylanta, and bendryl in equal parts can decrease pain. Discontinuing injurious agents and decreasing acid, particularly in patients with reflux disease, is also helpful.

Prophylactic interventions

TABLE 5-8. PREVENTION OF PILL-INDUCED INJURY

Taking a large volume of liquid with pills
No pills less than 1 hour before bed
Upright posture during and following pill ingestion
Ingestion of liquid forms of medicines are available

TABLE 5-8.

There are four easily modified actions that will decrease the risk of pill-induced esophageal injury. Esophageal clearance can be improved with simply ingesting more liquid with pills and taking pills in an upright position. These simple measures will generally prevent pill-induced esophageal injury.

ESOPHAGITIS CAUSED BY RADIATION

Pathophysiology

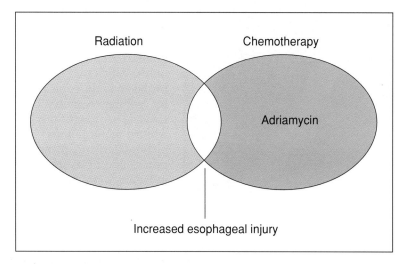

FIGURE 5-48.

The deleterious effect of radiation to the gastrointestinal tract has been reported since 1897. In general, the incidence of radiation-induced injury to the esophagus ranges between 1% to 25%, with serious damage reported in 1% to 5%. This incidence may be increasing because chemotherapeutic agents, such as adriamycin, potentiate radiation damage. Additionally, a recall phenomenon has been observed with adriamycin because subsequent doses without additional radiation produce endoscopic and radiographic findings, which are indistinguishable from those seen with radiation-induced esophagitis.

Incidence and severity of radiation-induced esophageal injury are directly proportional to the radiation dose administered and to the total surface area of esophagus that is irradiated. Radiation acutely damages cells by inhibiting mitosis in the epithelial germinal layer, thus predisposing to esophageal ulceration and sloughing. Endothelial cells of submucosal arterioles are particularly radiosensitive. Although capillary dilation, edema, and leukocyte infiltration are early morphologic changes, with time endothelial proliferation results in ischemia and fibrosis of the submucosa and lamina propria with damage to smooth muscle fibers and neural elements.

Histology

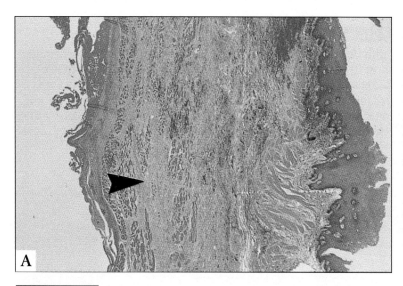

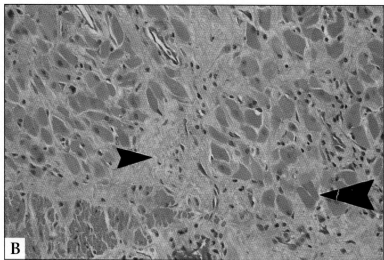

FIGURE 5-49.

Radiation injury to the esophagus. **A,** A patient 10 years after radiation therapy showing epithelial hyperplasia as well as fibrosis (*arrowhead*) throughout the submucosa and esophageal wall. **B,** A higher magnification of the esophageal wall showing extensive fibrosis (*small arrowhead*) interlaced between muscle bundles (*large arrowhead*).

Clinical effects of radiation dose

TABLE 5-9. EFFECT OF RADIATION DOSAGE ON THE ESOPHAGUS

> 30 Gy Nonspecific or none *
> 40 Gy Retrosternal burning and esophagitis
> 50 Gy Severe esophagitis
> 60 Gy Stricture and fistulas

* All can be worsened by chemotherapy.

TABLE 5-9.

The magnitude of injury to the esophagus secondary to radiation therapy is directly proportional to the dose of radiation delivered. At doses less than 30 Gy, little injury is present. As the dose increases esophagitis, stricturing and fistula formation can occur.

Methods to decrease radiation injury

TABLE 5-10. PREVENTING RADIATION-INDUCED ESOPHAGITIS

Specialized ports
Shielding
Dose hyperfragmentation
Alternate day schedule

TABLE 5-10

The esophagus is relatively fixed in location. To minimize radiation injury to the esophagus, radiation oncologists have tried several methods to decrease radiation intensity delivered to the esophagus.

Clinical presentations

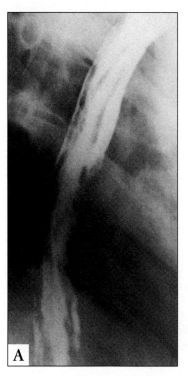
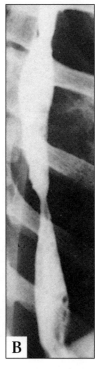
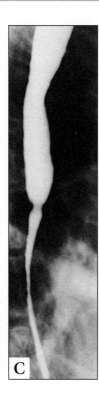

FIGURE 5-50

Esophagitis induced by combined radiation and chemotherapy (doxorubicin). Patients often present to the gastroenterologist during the third to fifth week of radiation therapy, although the natural history of the radiation injury may be altered with the coadministration of chemotherapeutic agents. Retrosternal burning, dysphagia, or odynophagia are typical symptoms that may be persistent and require supportive care to maintain hydration and nutrition. Additionally, patients must be considered for the possibility of superinfection with organisms such as *Candida*. **A,** Barium esophagram performed 10 days after the onset of symptoms demonstrates a dilated esophagus with thickened folds. Peristaltic activity was diminished at fluoroscopy. **B,** Esophagram 16 days after the onset of symptoms demonstrates a narrowed esophagus with markedly irregular mucosa and formation of a stricture in the distal half. No peristalsis was evident at fluoroscopy. **C,** High-grade stenosis involving about 9 cm of the distal esophagus with significant obstruction was found on follow-up examination 2 months after the onset of symptoms. The lumen of the stricture is irregular. The transition from the proximal esophagus, although abrupt, appears benign and is characterized by concentric narrowing. (*From* Boal *et al.* [9]; with permission.)

Complications

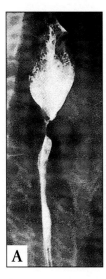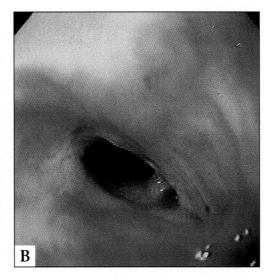

FIGURE 5-51.

At a radiation dose of less than 30 Gy, patients have self-limited, asymptomatic esophagitis. At dosages above 30 Gy, there may be progression to fibrosis and scarring of the esophagus. Strictures are typically smooth and elongated with thickened walls. Neural elements of the esophageal wall are frequently damaged. Esophageal peristalsis may be absent proximal to the stricture. Other complications include ulceration, pseudopolyp formation, mucosal bridging, and fistulization to the tracheal or bronchia apparatus, mediastinum, or aorta. The findings noted at endoscopy vary with the duration of time that the patient has received radiation therapy. The endoscopic findings include a spectrum of injury from acute esophagitis to circumferential ulceration with stricture formation, as demonstrated both radiographically (**A**) and endoscopically (**B**) in this figure. (*From* Wilcox [10]; with permission.)

Therapy

TABLE 5-11. THERAPEUTIC OPTIONS IN RADIATION ESOPHAGITIS

Supportive Care
  Intravenous hydration
  Nutrition support (partial or total parenteral nutrition)
  Narcotic analgesia
  Local anesthetics
Soft or liquid diet
Acid suppression
  Proton pump inhibitors
  H₂ blockers
  Antacids
Prokinetic agents
  Metoclopramide
  Cisapride
Interrupt radiotherapy
  Pursue and treat opportunistic infections
Strictures
    Repetitive dilation
    Steroid injection

TABLE 5-11.

There are many therapeutic options in radiation esophagitis that can markedly improve patients' quality of life. The three that tend to impact the most are acid blockade, prokinetic agents, and repeated dilations. Radiation causes small vessel anteriolitis and nerve damage, which leads to dismotility of the esophagus. Prokinetic agents may improve the function of the esophagus while strong acid blockade can decrease reflux symptoms. Repeated dilations can have very satisfying results, allowing very ill patients to swallow and eat during the last months of their lives.

REFERENCES

1. Fenoglio-Preiser CM, Lantz PE, Listrom MB, *et al.*: *Gastrointestinal Pathology, An Atlas and Text.* New York: Raven Press; 1989:60.

2. Baehr PM, McDonald GB: Esophageal infections: Risk factors, presentation, diagnosis and treatment. *Gastroenterology* 1994, 106:509–532.

3. Pounder RE, Allison MC, Dhillon AP: *A Colour Atlas of the Digestive System.* Chicago: Year Book Medical Publishers; 1989:13.

4. Kodsi BE, Wickremesinghe PC, Kozinn PJ, *et al.*: Candida esophagitis: A prospective Studies of 27 cases. *Gastroenterology* 1976, 71:715–719.

5. Giordano, *et al.*: Current management of esophageal foreign bodies. *Arch Otolaryngol* 1981, 107:249–251.

6. Castell DO: *The Esophagus*, edn 2. Boston: Little, Brown and Company; 1995.

7. Yoshida CM, Peura DA: Foreign bodies. In *The Esophagus*, edn. 2. Edited by Castell DO. Boston: Little, Brown and Company; 1995:379.

8. Cotton PB, Tytgat GNJ, Williams CB: *Annual of Gastrointestinal Endoscopy.* 1988:13.

9. Boal DKB, Newburger PE, Teele RL: Esophagitis induced by combined radiation and adriamycin. *Am J Roentgenol* 1979, 132:567–570.

10. Wilcox CM: *Atlas of Clinical Gastrointestinal Endoscopy.* Philadelphia: WB Saunders; 1995.

Chapter 6

Esophageal Motor Disorders

RAVINDER K. MITTAL

The orderly propulsion of a bolus following its ingestion is caused by a set of coordinated activities in the muscles of the esophagus. This organized motility is caused by a number of complex events that take place in the brain stem, extrinsic and intrinsic nerves, and muscles of the esophagus. From a simplistic point of view, after mastication and organization of the bolus in the mouth, the cheek, tongue, and muscles of the floor of the mouth propel the bolus back into the pharynx. The stimulation of the receptors in the pharynx by the bolus results in afferent impulses that travel along the fifth, seventh, ninth, and tenth cranial nerves into the brain stem. In the medulla oblongata these nerve impulses are coordinated and programmed efferent impulses travel along the vagus nerve and coordinate motor events in the esophagus.

The esophagus in humans is guarded by upper and lower esophageal sphincters. The body of the esophagus is 20 to 25 cm in length and made up of skeletal muscle in the upper one third, a mixture of skeletal and smooth muscle in the middle third, and only smooth muscle in the lower one third. Esophageal enteric nervous system is present in the wall of the esophagus. Efferents from the brain stem connect with the esophageal enteric nervous system and coordinate the motor events in the esophagus. These motor events result in relaxation of the upper and lower esophageal sphincters as well as a peristaltic contraction along the length of the esophagus. Peristaltic contraction in the smooth muscle esophagus and relaxation of the lower esophageal sphincter can also be coordinated by the esophageal enteric nervous system in the absence of central connections.

The motor abnormalities of the esophagus are the result of either systemic disorders affecting the muscles of the esophagus or a loss of central or peripheral control of esophageal peristalsis and its sphincters. A number of systemic diseases, such as scleroderma, diabetes mellitus, dermatomyositis, and the neurologic conditions affecting the brain stem or vagus nerve, can affect the esophageal motility (secondary motor disorders). The etiology of the primary motor disorders of the esophagus is not known; however, the pattern of contraction abnormalities in the esophagus are well described and can be easily identified through the technique of intraluminal pressure measurement (*ie*, manometry). The primary or idiopathic motor disorders of the esophagus are categorized into upper esophageal sphincter dysfunction and Zenker's diverticulum, achalasia of the lower esophageal sphincter and esophagus, diffuse esophageal spasm, nutcracker esophagus or hypertensive esophageal peristalsis, isolated hypertensive lower esophageal sphincter, and gastroesophageal reflux disease.

UPPER ESOPHAGEAL DYSFUNCTION AND ZENKER'S DIVERTICULUM

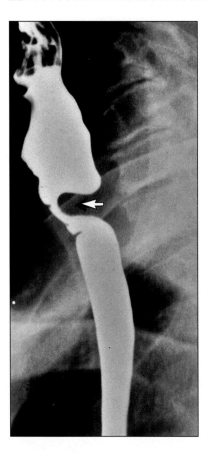

FIGURE 6-1.

Radiologic appearance of cricopharyngeal bar. The indentations (*arrow*) seen in the barium swallow, usually occurring at the level of cervical vertebra 4 or 5, represent either a nonrelaxing or a noncompliant upper esophageal sphincter. The patient usually has oropharyngeal dysphagia; however, asymptomatic individuals can have this radiologic finding.

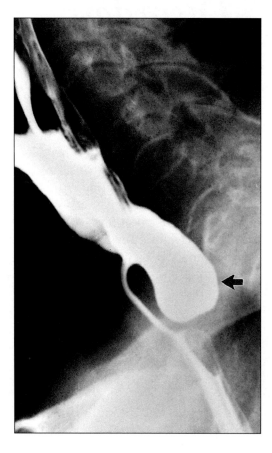

FIGURE 6-2.

Zenker's diverticulum. Radiograph of a 70-year-old patient with oropharyngeal dysphagia, coughing, choking spells, and recurrent pneumonia. Note the outpouching of the pharynx above the level of the cricopharyngeus (*arrow*). This outpouching is located in the posterior wall of the pharynx. Zenker's diverticulum is a true pulsion diverticulum and is the result of increased intrapharyngeal pressures during swallowing as a result of a noncompliant or nonrelaxing upper esophageal sphincter. There may be penetration of the barium into the laryngeal inlet and spilling into the tracheobronchial tree. The treatment of this condition in the setting of severe symptoms is usually cricopharyngeal myotomy.

ACHALASIA OF THE ESOPHAGUS

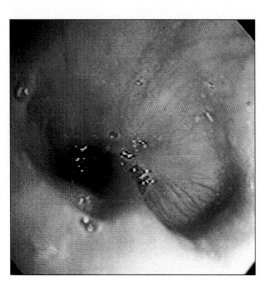

FIGURE 6-3.

Endoscopic view from a patient with achalasia of the lower esophageal sphincter (LES). Note that the region of the LES is tightly closed. Usually a small amount of pressure is needed before the endoscope pops into the stomach. Above the LES there is a wide-mouth diverticulum known as the *epiphrenic diverticulum*.

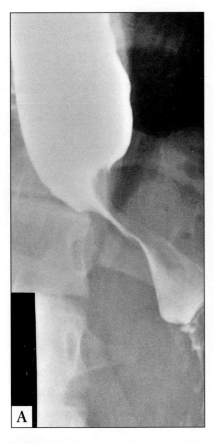
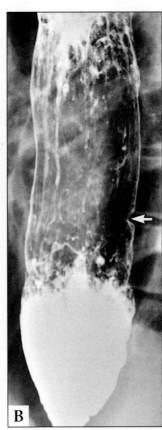

FIGURE 6-4.

Barium swallow in a patient with achalasia of the esophagus. This study shows a dilated esophagus in a patient with achalasia of the lower esophageal sphincter (A). The gastroesophageal junction does not open, resulting in a classical bird's beak appearance at the distal end of the esophagus (B). The serrated margin (*arrow*) in the midesophagus is referred to by radiologists as *tertiary contractions*.

A

B

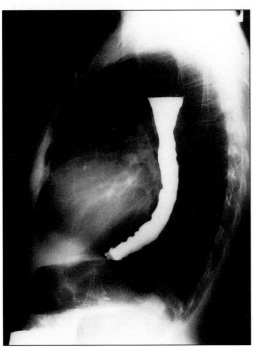
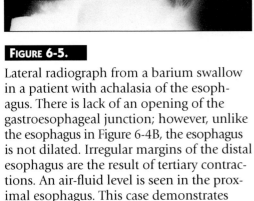
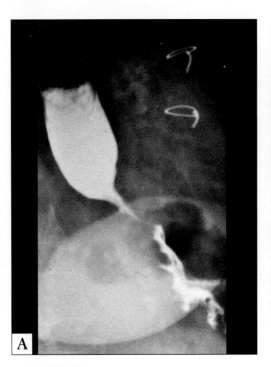

A

B

FIGURE 6-5.

Lateral radiograph from a barium swallow in a patient with achalasia of the esophagus. There is lack of an opening of the gastroesophageal junction; however, unlike the esophagus in Figure 6-4B, the esophagus is not dilated. Irregular margins of the distal esophagus are the result of tertiary contractions. An air-fluid level is seen in the proximal esophagus. This case demonstrates that not all patients with achalasia of the esophagus have dilated, tortuous, and sigmoid esophagus.

FIGURE 6-6.

A–B, Barium swallows of a patient with secondary achalasia. The barium swallows in this figure represent the appearance of the esophagus in a patient with adenocarcinoma of the gastroesophageal junction, which can produce a motility disorder identical to primary or idiopathic achalasia. The gastroesophageal junction shows a bird's beak appearance, and on multiple spot films there was no evidence of an opening of the esophagogastric region. Case reports of metastatic tumor from prostate, breast, lymphoma, lung carcinoma, hepatocellular carcinoma, colon carcinoma, esophageal lymphangioma, and pleural mesothelioma causing secondary achalasia have been described.

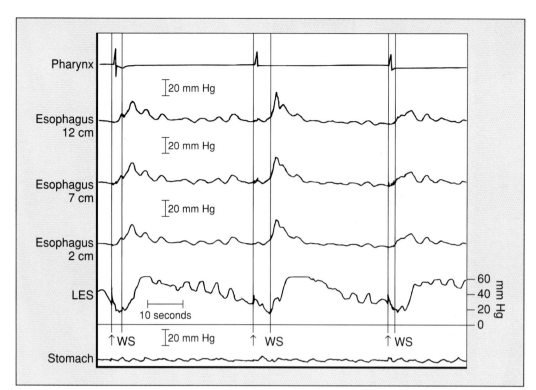

FIGURE 6-7.

Manometric tracing from a patient with achalasia of the esophagus. Simultaneous pressure measurements were made in the stomach, lower esophageal sphincter (LES), at three sites in the distal esophagus (5 cm apart), and at the pharynx. The subject was asked to swallow 5 mL of water for each of the three wet swallows (WS) shown in the tracing. Each swallow results in a pharyngeal contraction followed by a simultaneous pressure wave throughout the distal esophagus. The LES pressure is high (> 40 mm Hg), and there is incomplete relaxation of the LES in response to each of the swallows.

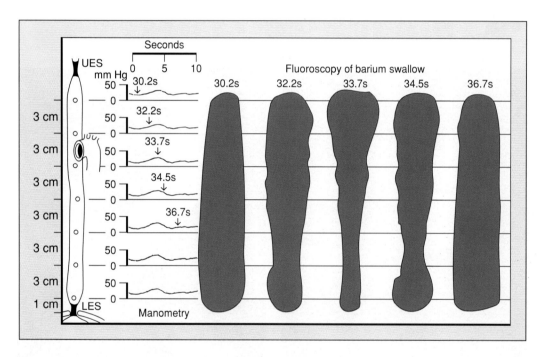

FIGURE 6-8.

Simultaneous pressure recording and fluoroscopy during barium swallow in a patient with achalasia of the esophagus. The esophageal pressures were measured at seven sites spaced 3 cm apart along the length of the esophagus. Note that the swallow resulted in a simultaneous pressure wave throughout the length of the esophagus. This simultaneous pressure wave is not caused by a simultaneous esophageal contraction. Rather, it is caused by an isobaric fluid pressure wave generated between an esophageal contraction at the top end of the esophagus and a closed lower esophageal sphincter region (LES) at the bottom. UES—upper esophageal sphincter. (*Adapted from* Massey *et al.* [5].)

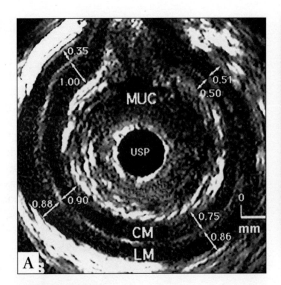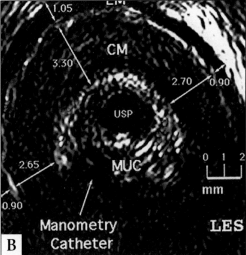

FIGURE 6-9.

Ultrasound images of the lower esophageal sphincter (LES) in a normal subject (A) and in a patient with achalasia of the esophagus (B). These ultrasound images were obtained using a high-frequency intraluminal ultrasound probe (USP). The USP is 6.2 Fr in diameter and contained a 20-MHz transducer. Different layers of the esophagus can be identified using this USP. The ones that are easily identifiable in these figures are the mucosa (MUC), the circular muscle (CM), and the longitudinal muscle (LM). Note excessive thickening of the CM in **panel B**.

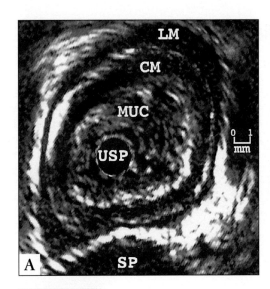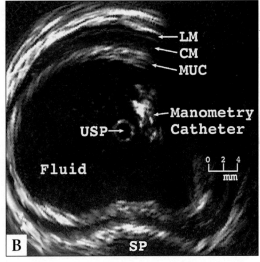

FIGURE 6-10.

Ultrasound images of the esophagus in a normal subject (A) and in a patient with achalasia of the esophagus (B) using a high-frequency intraluminal catheter-based ultrasound probe. The esophagus is 5 cm above the lower esophageal sphincter in the normal subject. The three layers that can be identified include the mucosa (MUC), the circular muscle (CM), and the longitudinal muscle (LM). Note that the mucosa is tightly wrapped around the ultrasound probe (USP) in a normal situation. In the patient with achalasia of the esophagus there is wide separation of the mucosa from the USP. This wide separation is caused by the accumulation of the fluid in an aperistaltic esophagus. SP—spine.

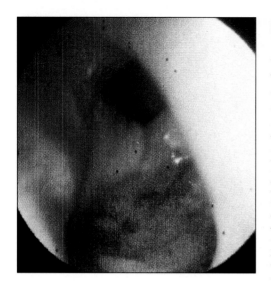

FIGURE 6-11.

Epiphrenic diverticulum in a patient with achalasia of the esophagus. The diverticulum just above the region of the esophagogastric junction can be seen, albeit infrequently, in patients with classical achalasia; it is more common in patients with rigorous achalasia. The latter have hypertensive esophageal peristalsis. The diverticulum is caused by a large increase in the intraesophageal pressure during propulsion of the bolus.

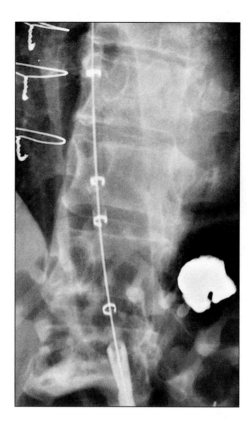

FIGURE 6-12.

Pneumatic dilation of the lower esophageal sphincter using a Rigiflex Balloon (Microvasive, Boston Scientific, Watertown, MA.) in a patient with achalasia of the esophagus. This radiograph was taken at the time of maximal balloon inflation. Note the symmetrical appearance along the whole extent of the balloon and the absence of a waist. A waist on the balloon usually indicates inadequate dilation.

Clinical features and complications of achalasia

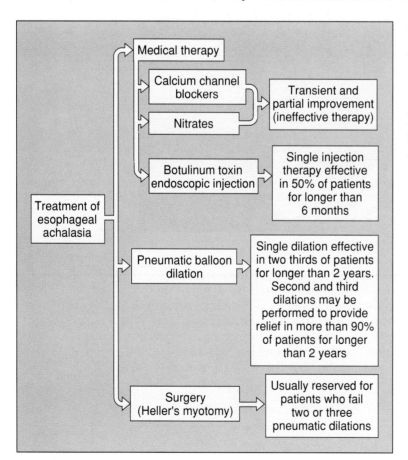

FIGURE 6-13.

Algorithm for treatment of esophageal achalasia. Achalasia of the esophagus can be treated either medically or surgically. Smooth muscle relaxants, nitrate, and calcium channel blockers reduce laser esophageal sphincter pressure and improve dysphagia symptom. Injection of botulinum toxin can also reduce sphincter pressure and improve esophageal emptying; however, standard therapy for achalasia is pneumatic dilation. Patients with recalcitrant symptoms, despite medical therapy, require surgical myotomy.

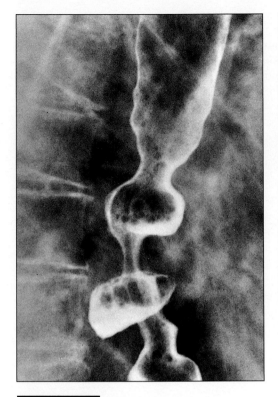

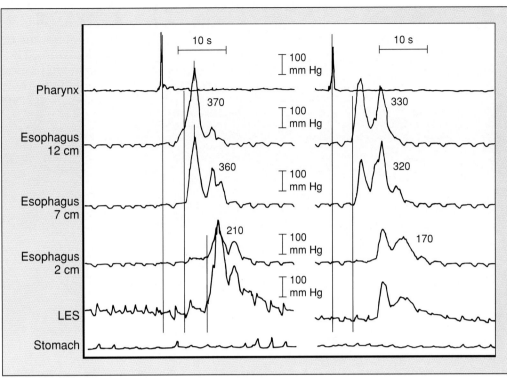

FIGURE 6-14.

Barium swallow study in a patient with diffuse esophageal spasm. Note the corkscrew or rosary-bead appearance along the length of the distal esophagus.

FIGURE 6-15.

Manometric appearance of diffuse esophageal spasm. This manometric tracing is from a patient with diffuse esophageal spasm. Pressure measurements are made simultaneously in the stomach, lower esophageal sphincter (LES), and three sites spaced 5 cm apart in the distal esophagus and pharynx. Two swallows are shown in this trace. Each swallow results in a simultaneous pressure wave between the 7- and 12-cm sites. The esophageal contractions are prolonged and have a double-peaked and triple-peaked appearance. The contraction amplitudes are high. The normal contraction amplitudes are between 50 and 180 mm Hg and duration is less than 6 seconds. In this subject the contraction amplitudes were as high as 370 mm Hg and contraction durations were prolonged.

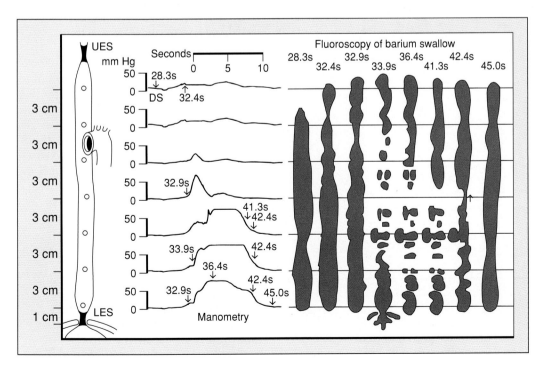

FIGURE 6-16.

Simultaneous manometry and fluoroscopy of barium swallow in a patient with diffuse esophageal spasm. The genesis of simultaneous pressure waves in a patient with diffuse esophageal spasm is different than in a patient with achalasia. The simultaneous pressure waves in a patient with achalasia are the result of fluid pressure built up between a proximal esophageal contraction and a distal closed lower esophageal sphincter (LES). On the other hand, in a patient with diffuse esophageal spasm, true simultaneous contraction does exist in the distal esophagus, which results in compartmentalization of the esophageal lumen. The barium flows in a to-and-fro fashion, resulting in impairment of the esophagus transit. DS—dry swallow; UES—upper esophageal sphincter. (*Adapted from* Massey *et al.* [5].)

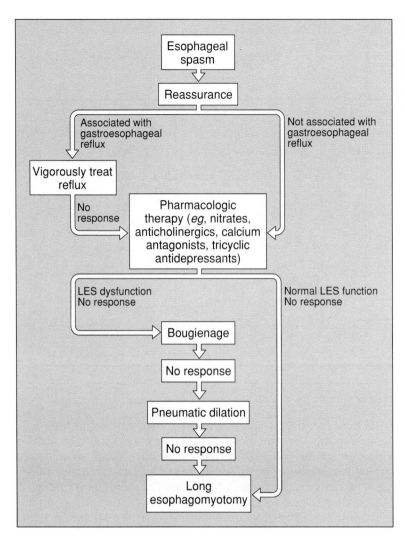

FIGURE 6-17.

Algorithm for the treatment of esophageal spasm. Infrequent symptoms caused by esophageal spasm are best treated by reassurance. Frequent symptoms require medical therapy with antireflux agents or smooth muscle relaxants. Surgical therapy is reserved for most symptomatic patients who are resistant to medical therapy.

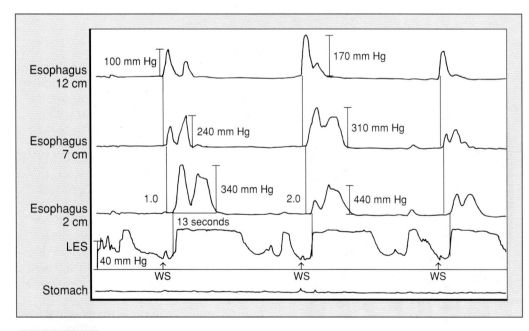

FIGURE 6-18.

Nutcracker esophagus. This manometric tracing was obtained from a patient with noncardiac chest pain. The pressures were measured simultaneously in the stomach, lower esophageal sphincter (LES), and three sites in the distal esophagus, spaced 5 cm apart. Note that the esophageal contractions are high in amplitude and have multiple peaks. Contraction durations are prolonged. In contrast with the diffuse esophageal spasm, these contractions are peristaltic. The LES does not relax completely in response to swallow. In 30% to 50% of patients there is dysfunction of the LES, either in the form of a hypertensive or a partially relaxing LES. Even though a significant number of patients with noncardiac chest pain have this abnormality, there is a lack of temporal association between the chest pain and abnormal esophageal contractions. The prolonged ambulatory motility studies reveal that only 10% to 20% of chest pain events occur in close temporal association with abnormal esophageal contractions in the esophagus. Fifteen percent to 20% of pain events occur in association with acid reflux and the etiology of the remainder remains obscure [9]. Treatment of this disorder with calcium channel blockers and other smooth muscle relaxants results in decreased contraction amplitude without a major improvement in the frequency of chest pain [10]. WS—wet swallow.

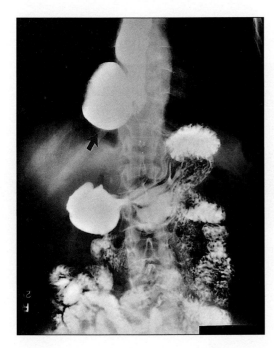

FIGURE 6-19.

Radiograph of esophageal diverticulum. This is an example of an esophageal pulsion diverticulum (*arrow*). The pulsion diverticulum is seen in the setting of esophageal motility disorders, such as hypertensive esophageal peristalsis, diffuse esophageal spasm, or achalasia of the esophagus.

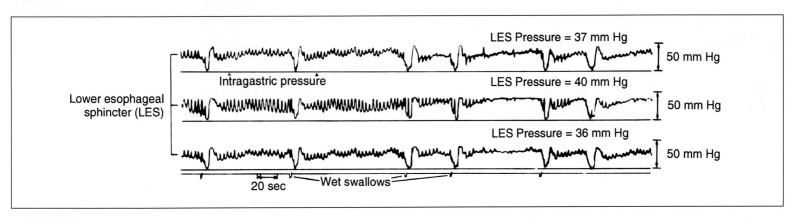

FIGURE 6-20.

Esophageal manometric tracing of a patient with hypertensive lower esophageal sphincter (LES) pressure. Normally the LES pressure is less than 35 mm of mercury. This patient complained of symptoms of moderate dysphagia for solids and liquids for longer than 5 years. The LES pressures were greater than 35 mm of mercury. Complete relaxation of the LES pressure in response to swallowing was present. The mechanism of dysphagia in a patient with complete relaxation of the LES is not clear. It is, however, most likely related to the poor compliance or opening mechanism of the region of the LES, resulting in poor transit.

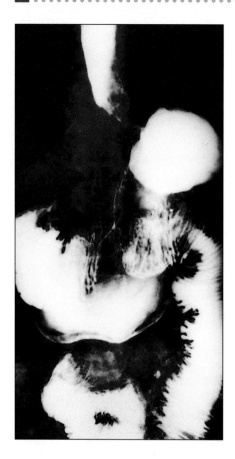

FIGURE 6-21.

Radiographic view of scleroderma of the esophagus, stomach, and duodenum. This picture was taken one-half hour after patient swallowed barium. Note that barium is still present in the esophagus. There is also retained barium in the stomach. The duodenum is enlarged and the small intestine is dilated. Scleroderma is a connective tissue disorder characterized by replacement of the smooth muscles with fibrous tissue. There is loss of peristalsis and dilation of the esophagus. The lower esophageal sphincter is usually very weak, which can result in severe reflux disease and reflux-related esophageal stricture.

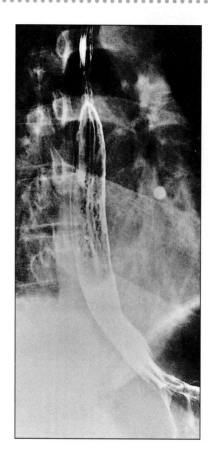

FIGURE 6-22.

Radiographic view of scleroderma of the esophagus. In addition, the patient has esophagitis caused by candidal infection.

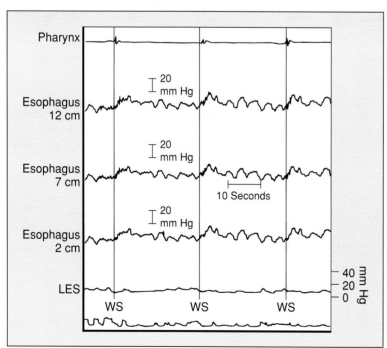

FIGURE 6-23.

Manometric tracing from a patient with severe involvement of scleroderma. The pressures are measured simultaneously in the stomach, lower esophageal sphincter (LES), and three sites in the esophagus and pharynx spaced 5 cm apart. Three wet swallows (WS) are shown on this tracing. Note that the LES pressures are low (5–7 mm Hg). In response to WS there is a small-amplitude, simultaneous pressure wave along the entire length of the distal esophagus. These pressure waves most likely represent the isobaric pressure wave, as described in achalasia of the esophagus.

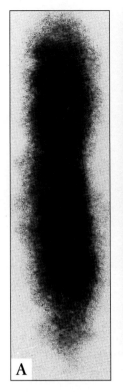

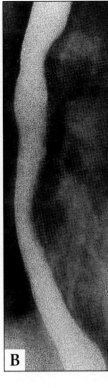

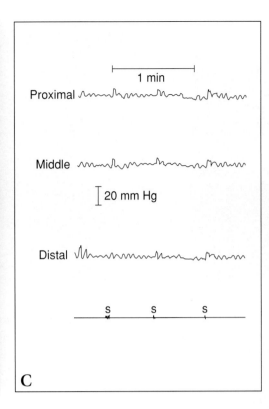

FIGURE 6-24.

Illustration of esophageal function in a woman with scleroderma and severe esophageal motor impairment. The esophageal motor function was assessed by three separate techniques: radionuclide scintigraphy (**A**), barium swallow (**B**), and esophagography (**C**). There was complete retention of the radionuclide material in the esophagus after four swallows. The fluoroscopic study showed similar retention of the barium associated with absent peristalsis, and the manometric study showed absence of peristalsis and esophageal contractions in the distal esophagus. The sensitivity and specificity of the three tests used to assess esophageal motor function are similar. (*From* Klein *et al.* [11]; with permission.)

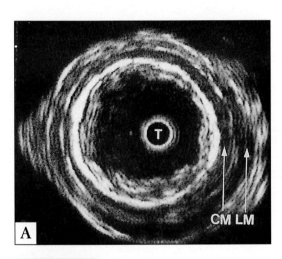

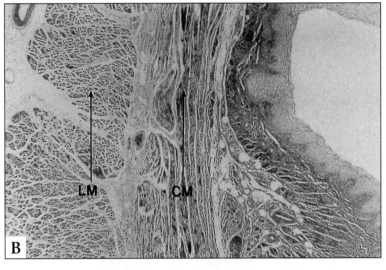

FIGURE 6-25.

Ultrasound images of the normal distal esophagus using high-frequency intraluminal ultrasonography. These images were obtained using an IVUS system (Diasonic, Milpitas, California). This catheter is 6.2 Fr in diameter and contains a 20-MHz transducer. The transducer rotates 360 degrees and provides images of the seven different layers of the esophagus. This figure represents the image of a distal esophagus obtained in a normal subject showing the correlation of the different layers with the ultrasonographic images. Seven different layers of the esophagus (mucosa, submucosa, muscularis mucosa, circular muscle [CM], septum, longitudinal muscle [LM], and adventia) can be seen on these images. There is excellent correlation between different ultrasonographic images (A) to the histologic images obtained on an autopsy specimen (**B**). The muscularis propria (CM and LM layers) appear darker than the mucosa and submucosa on these images. T—transducer. (*From* Miller *et al.* [12]; with permission.)

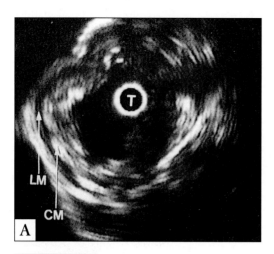
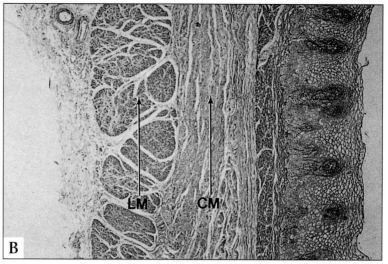

FIGURE 6-26.

Ultrasonographic and histologic images in a patient with scleroderma. Note the increase in the echogenicity of the circular muscle (CM) as well as longitudinal muscle (LM) layers compared to the normal esophagus. There appears to be an excellent direct correlation between the increase in the echogenicity and the extent of fibrous matter in scleroderma. CM is usually more involved than LM. In addition to histologic correlation, there was also direct correlation between the 24 pH scores and the severity of abnormality detected by the ultrasonographic technique. T—transducer. (*From* Miller *et al.* [12]; with permission.)

ANTIREFLUX MECHANISMS

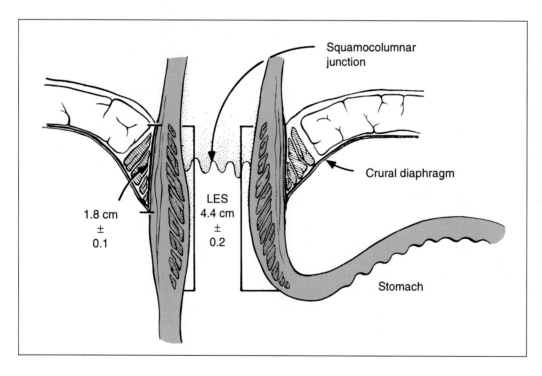

FIGURE 6-27.

Anatomy of the two lower esophageal sphincters. Anatomic relationship between the lower esophageal sphincter (LES) and crural diaphragm based on electrophysiologic measurements. The length of the LES is approximately 4.4 cm and of the crural diaphragm is 1.8 cm. The crural diaphragm encircles the proximal half of the LES. Approximately 2.5 cm of the lower esophageal sphincter is intra-abdominal in location. The squamocolumnar junction is usually located either in the middle or at the proximal end at the LES. (*Adapted from* Heine [13].)

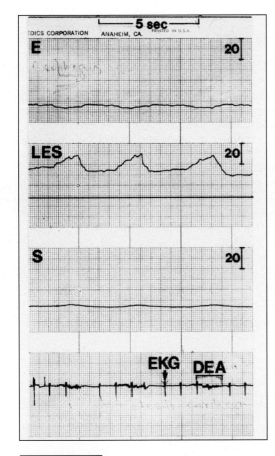

FIGURE 6-28

An esophageal manometric pressure tracing shows the contribution of lower esophageal sphincter (LES) and crural diaphragm to the esophagogastric junction pressure. A tonic component measures as end-expiratory pressure is due to the contraction of the smooth muscles of the LES. With each inspiration there is an increase in LES pressure, which is due to contraction of the crural diaphragm. E—esophagus; S—stomach; DEA—diaphragm electrical activity; EKG—electrocardiogram.

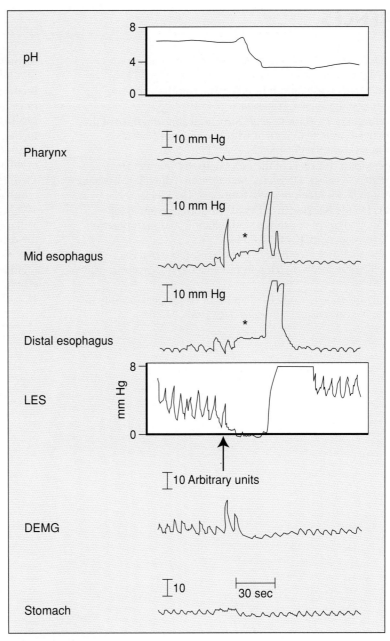

FIGURE 6-29.

A spontaneous, transient, lower esophageal sphincter (LES) relaxation. The onset of relaxation is indicated by the arrow. Relaxation occurred in the absence of swallow as manifested by the absence of pharyngeal pressure wave. The LES relaxation is complete to the level of intragastric pressure (indicated by the horizontal line) and is sustained for longer than 20 seconds. Transient LES relaxation is associated with inhibition of the crural diaphragm as indicated by the loss of inspiratory increase in LES pressure and diaphragmatic electromyography (DEMG). Note the esophageal contractions at the onset of LES relaxation. Reflux (drop in esophageal pH) occurs after complete LES relaxation has been achieved, and is associated with an increase in intraesophageal pressure (common cavity, marked by an asterisk). A secondary peristaltic clearance response can be seen at the end of LES relaxation. Transient LES relaxation is the major mechanism of gastroesophageal reflux in normal controls as well as patients with reflux disease. Transient LES relaxation is a neural reflex that is controlled through the brain stem and is mediated through the vagus nerve. (*see* Chapter 4 for further discussion of gastroesophageal reflux.)

REFERENCES

1. Dantas RO, Cook IJ, Dodds WJ, *et al.*: Biomechanics of cricopharyngeal bars. *Gastroenterology* 1990, 99:1269–1274.

2. Cruse JP, Edwards DAW, Smith JF, *et al.*: The pathology of cricopharyngeal dysphagia. *Histopathology* 1979, 3:223.

3. Cook IJ, Blumberg ST, Cash K, *et al.*: Structural abnormalities of the cricopharyngeus muscle in patient with pharyngeal (Zenker's) diverticulum. *Gastroenterol Hepatol* 1992, 7:556–562.

4. Clouse RE: Motor disorders of the esophagus. In *Gastrointestinal Diseases: Pathophysiology, Diagnoses, Management.* Edited by Sleisenger MH, Fordtran JS. Philadelphia: WB Saunders; 1993:341–371.

5. Massey BT, Dodds WJ, Hogan WJ, *et al.*: Abnormal esophageal motility: An analysis of concurrent radiographic and manometric finding. *Gastroenterology* 1991, 101:344.

6. Becker DJ, Castell DO: Acute airway obstruction in achalasia: Possible role for defective belch reflex [review]. *Gastroenterology* 1989, 97:1323–1326.

7. Cremer B, Donoghue E, Code CF: Pattern of esophageal motility in diffuse esophageal spasm. *Gastroenterology* 1958, 34:782.

8. Richter JE, Castell DO: Diffuse esophageal spasm, a reappraisal. *Ann Intern Med* 1984, 100:242.

9. Breumelhof R, Nadorp JHSM, Akkermans LMA, *et al.*: Analysis of 24 hr esophageal pressure and pH data in unselected patients with non-cardiac chest pain. *Gastroenterology* 1990, 99:1257.

10. Richter JE, Dalton CB, Bradley LA, *et al.*: Oral nifedipine in the treatment of non-cardiac chest pain in patients with nutcracker esophagus. *Gastroenterology* 1987, 93:21.

11. Klein HA, Wald A, Graham TO, *et al.*: Comparative studies of esophageal function in systemic sclerosis. *Gastroenterology* 1992, 102:1551–1556.

12. Miller LS, Liu JB, Klenn BJ, *et al.*: Intraluminal ultrasonography of the distal esophagus in systemic sclerosis. *Gastroenterology* 1993, 105:31–39.

13. Klein HA, Wald A, Graham TO, *et al.*: Comparative studies of esophageal function in systemic sclerosis. *Gastroenterology* 1992, 102:1551–1556.

Chapter 7

The Pharynx

WILLIAM J. RAVICH
BRONWYN JONES

Although the average gastroenterologist passes through the pharynx hundreds of times a year while performing routine endoscopy, the average gastroenterologist is remarkably unfamiliar with this region. Until recently, gastroenterology textbooks barely referred to it. The pharynx has been generally considered the domain of the otolaryngologist. In a schematic drawing illustrating endoscopic anatomy of the esophagus, one well-known atlas of endoscopy, showed in great detail the relationship of the esophagus to mediastinal structures, but used two parallel broken lines to portray the pharynx.

The pharynx is the avenue to the esophagus. Without it the esophagus would be as useless as the appendix. Moreover, esophageal peristalsis is actually only a continuum of the pharynx's response to swallowing. It is not always easy to distinguish between pharyngeal and esophageal causes of dysphagia on the basis of symptoms alone, and evaluation of swallowing disorders is often best directed by someone familiar with the pharynx as well as the esophagus. Therefore, a gastroenterologist should have some knowledge of pharyngeal function and dysfunction. This chapter offers a brief introduction to the pharynx, using methods often used by the gastroenterologist in evaluating esophageal disease. By looking up at the pharynx and knowing what to look for, the gastroenterologist should be able to recognize and either direct or redirect evaluation to those who might best help the patient.

This chapter also concentrates on three methodologies—radiology, manometry, and endoscopy—to illustrate what these techniques demonstrate about pharyngeal physiology and disease. The intent is not to provide a comprehensive atlas, as might be appropriate for an otolaryngologist's use, but rather to offer an introduction to an area that gastroenterologists must deal with regularly, but about which they know surprisingly little.

Note: *To avoid excessive cross references, certain figures in the chapter are repeated for comparisons of different disease states against a normal finding. It is hoped that this information helps to prevent any confusion on the reader's part regarding the individual images.*

Even more than in esophageal disease, radiographic studies are a key diagnostic technique in the evaluation of dysphagia. Routine barium radiography, however, depending on fluoroscopy and spot films to detect abnormalities, is inadequate for the evaluation of the pharynx and can miss (or misinterpret) both functional and structural abnormalities. Dynamic imaging using video recordings is essential, allowing the repeated and slow-motion playback often required to understand the motor events involved with swallowing and to detect subtle (and occasionally not so subtle) structural lesions. Because of its central role in the evaluation of the pharynx, the majority of the images in this chapter are taken from videoradiographic studies. It should be recalled, however, that slides are often a poor means of illustrating dynamic function. The interested gastroenterologist is encouraged to review the videoradiographic studies performed on their own patients with an experienced videoradiologist.

Although esophageal manometry is a standard part of gastroenterology, application of manometry to evaluation of the pharynx is only rarely used in clinical practice. In part, this reflects the focus of gastroenterology in general. It also reflects the limitations of pharyngeal manometry as currently performed, making accurate assessment of pharyngeal function problematic. The figures explain some of the technical issues that influence the accuracy and interpretation of pharyngeal manometry. There are few published studies using acceptable technology in disease states and a consequent dearth of information about the sensitivity and specificity of pharyngeal manometry for the diagnosis of pharyngeal motor dysfunction. Even when it demonstrates abnormal function, it is unclear how much pharyngeal manometry adds to the information provided by videoradiography; however, there have been important advances in the understanding and technique of pharyngeal manometry that require the attention of the gastroenterologist, especially in the use of this methodology to confirm the presence of dysfunction of the upper esophageal sphincter.

Although endoscopy of the pharynx has been predominantly the preserve of the otolaryngologist, the gastroenterologist also performs pharyngoscopy regularly during the course of intubation and extubation of the pharynx. All too often, gastroenterologists seem to close their eyes (figuratively, if not literally) during passage through the pharynx, and endoscopy notes rarely even mention the pharynx. Although the endoscopes used for upper endoscopy may not be optimal for careful examination of the pharynx, and although few gastroenterologists have a great deal of expertise in pharyngeal pathology, it is worthwhile to have at least passing familiarity with the pharynx, if only so that the patient can be appropriately referred when further evaluation is warranted.

Anatomy

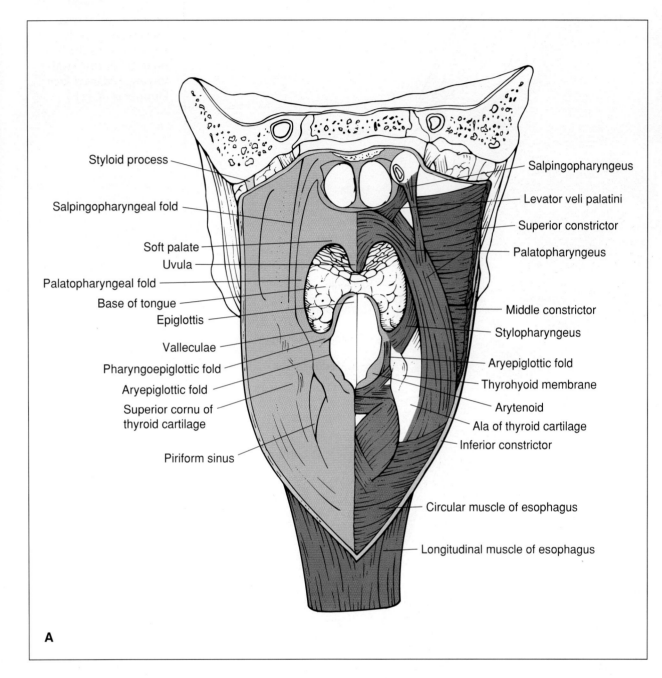

Styloid process

Salpingopharyngeal fold

Soft palate

Uvula

Palatopharyngeal fold

Base of tongue

Epiglottis

Valleculae

Pharyngoepiglottic fold

Aryepiglottic fold

Superior cornu of thyroid cartilage

Piriform sinus

Salpingopharyngeus

Levator veli palatini

Superior constrictor

Palatopharyngeus

Middle constrictor

Stylopharyngeus

Aryepiglottic fold

Thyrohyoid membrane

Arytenoid

Ala of thyroid cartilage

Inferior constrictor

Circular muscle of esophagus

Longitudinal muscle of esophagus

A

FIGURE 7-1.

Schematic drawings of the pharynx from posterior (**A**) and lateral (**B**) perspectives. Note the relationships of the valleculae and piriform sinuses to the base of tongue, epiglottis, and larynx.

(*continued on next page*)

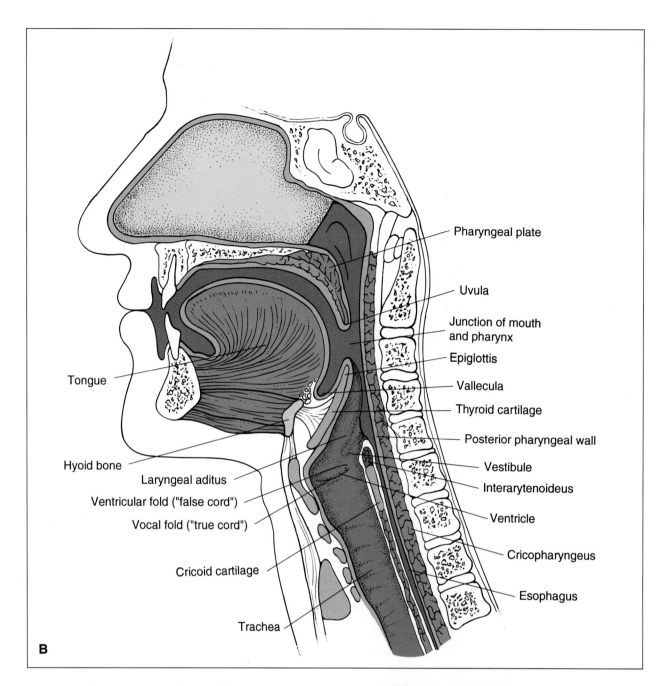

FIGURE 7-1. (CONTINUED)
Because the pharynx is part of both the respiratory and alimentary tracts, both the nasopharynx and larynx must be effectively isolated from the pharynx during swallowing. (*Adapted from* Donner *et al.* [1].)

Pharyngeal plate

Uvula

Junction of mouth and pharynx

Epiglottis

Vallecula

Thyroid cartilage

Posterior pharyngeal wall

Vestibule

Interarytenoideus

Ventricle

Cricopharyngeus

Esophagus

Tongue

Hyoid bone

Laryngeal aditus

Ventricular fold ("false cord")

Vocal fold ("true cord")

Cricoid cartilage

Trachea

B

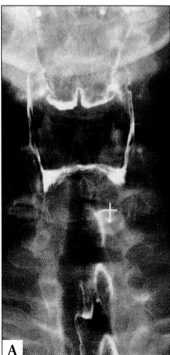

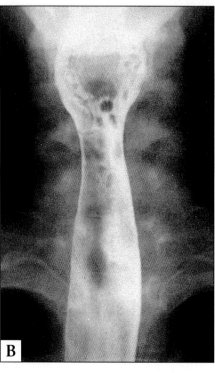

FIGURE 7-2.

A, Radiograph demonstrates the structures of the pharynx at rest in an anteroposterior view, coated with a contrast medium. The paired valleculae lie proximally just below the angle of the mandible and the paired piriform sinuses inferiorly, just above the level of the vocal cords (seen as an indentation of the midline air column). Minimal contrast is retained in the valleculae and piriform sinuses, which is not unusual with high-density barium. **B**, A film of the distended pharynx during transit of a barium bolus demonstrates the oval appearance during the act of swallowing when the normal landmarks have been obliterated. (**A**, *From* Jones and Donner [2]; with permission. **B**, *From* Jones *et al.* [3]; with permission.)

A

B

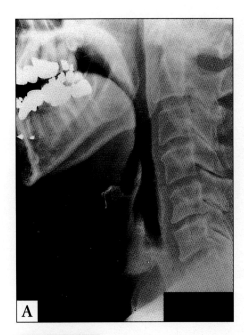
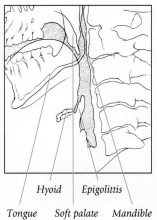

Hyoid   Epigolittis

Tongue   Soft palate   Mandible

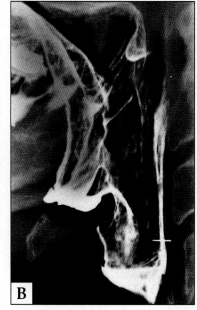
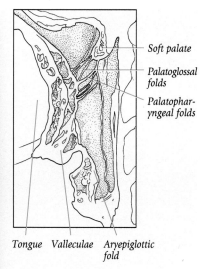

Soft palate

Palatoglossal
folds

Palatophar-
yngeal folds

Tongue   Valleculae   Aryepiglottic
fold

A   **B**

FIGURE 7-3.

Pharynx in the lateral position. **A,** A soft-tissue–density view in the lateral position of the air-filled mouth, nasopharynx, pharynx, and larynx. Note that the soft palate rests against the back of the tongue, the hyoid is parallel to the mandible, and the epiglottis is upright. **B,** During phonation the soft palate elevates to a right angle and the tongue moves forward, opening up the valleculae and the entire anteroposterior diameter. As a result, a number of pharyngeal structures have been exposed, including the vertical palatopharyngeal fold, the aryepiglottic fold, and paired palatoglossal folds. The valleculae and piriform sinus have been pulled open; minimal retention exists in the valleculae and piriform sinuses. This degree of retention is within normal limits. (**A,** *From* Jones *et al.* [4]; with permission. **B,** *From* Rubessin *et al.* [5]; with permission.)

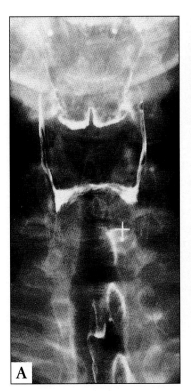
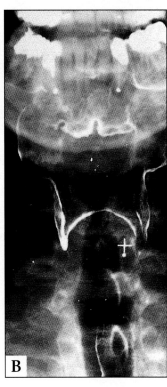

A   **B**

FIGURE 7-4.

Effect of insufflation. Anteroposterior view of the pharynx at rest (**A**) and during insufflation produced by a Valsalva maneuver (**B**) [2]. The normal pharynx distends symmetrically, but there is greater distention above the valleculae, where the pharynx is supported only by the thyrohyoid membrane than inferiorly where distention is limited by the rigid thyroid cartilage. Loss of distensibility can occur from inflammation, fibrosis, or infiltrative disease. In horn players the pouches can reach an enormous size from chronic pressure produced by blowing into their instruments. (*From* Jones *et al.* [2]; with permission.)

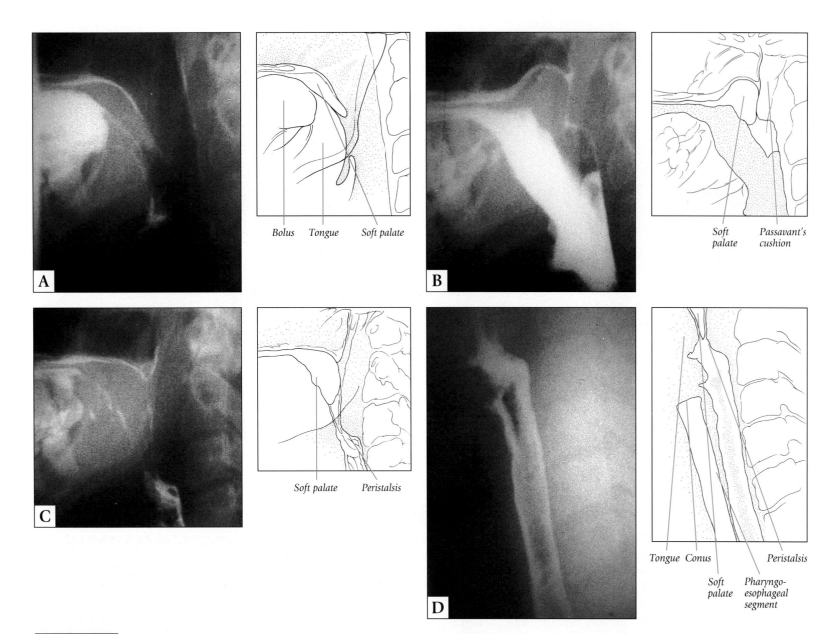

FIGURE 7-5.

Normal swallow. Stop frames from a cinepharyngoesophagogram. **A**, Bolus is retained in the mouth by apposition of the superoposterior portion of the tongue and the soft palate. Some contrast has been introduced through the nose; therefore, the nasal surfaces of the free edge of the soft palate are coated with contrast. **B**, Tongue thrust propels the bolus into the pharynx as the soft palate elevates to a right angle to oppose a converging segment of the superior pharyngeal wall (Passavant's cushion). **C**, The contact tongue, soft palate, and posterior pharyngeal wall completely occlude the

pharyngeal cavity behind the bolus. The posterior indentation at the top of the advancing barium bolus represents the pharyngeal propagative (peristaltic) wave. **D**, The epiglottis is completely inverted and the larynx is completely elevated and closed resulting in the appearance of the "conus", the squared off superior aspect of the closed airway. Note the posterior pharyngeal propagative wave and that the lumen at the level of the pharyngoesophageal segment is completely open. (**A**, **C–D**, *From* Jones *et al.* [6]; with permission. **B**, *From* Jones and Donner [4]; with permission.)

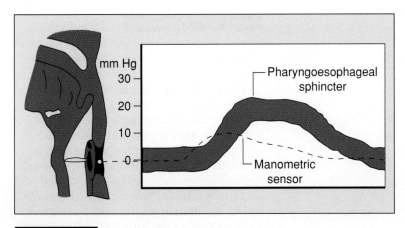

mm Hg
30
20
10
-0
Pharyngoesophageal sphincter
Manometric sensor

FIGURE 7-6.

Movement of upper esophageal sphincter (UES) during swallowing. A critical problem in the application of manometric technique to the pharynx is the mobility of the larynx and pharynx. As

illustrated, both the sensor and UES move orad during swallowing, but the movement is asynchronous. The sensor moves first, probably as a result of elevation of the soft palate. It reaches a maximum orad excursion of approximately 1 cm. The UES segment then begins to rise, reaching a maximum excursion of 2 cm, passing the sensor as the latter descends back to its resting position. Elevation of the UES is caused by laryngeal elevation, which may also be a factor, along with UES relaxation and pharyngeal propulsive force in opening the pharyngoesophageal segment. This asynchronous movement makes positioning of the manometric sensor difficult. Traditional placement in the center of the high-pressure zone results in a period in which the sensor actually descends (relative to UES position) into the cervical esophagus, causing an artifactually prolonged relaxation. An alternative approach to the problem of sphincter segment motion is the use of a water-perfused sleeve catheter assembly, which records the highest pressure along the sleeve's length. The sleeve ensures that axial movement does not result in displacement of the sphincter segment off the recording sensor. (*Adapted from* Dodds *et al.* [7].)

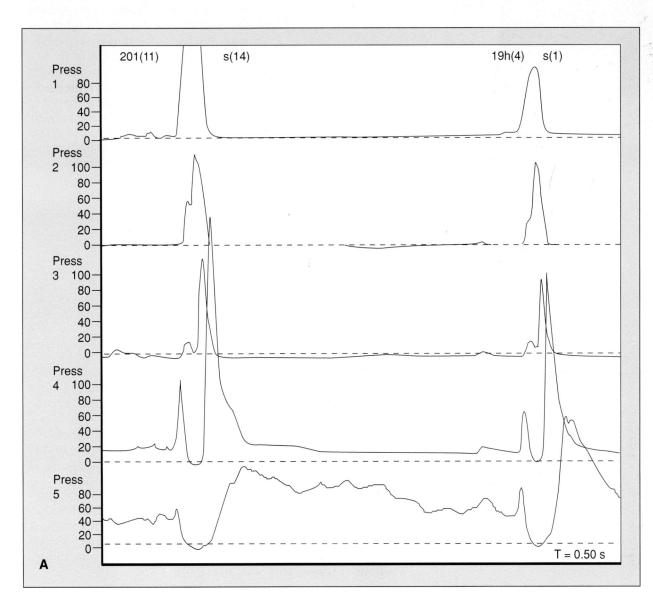

FIGURE 7-7.

A and **B,** Normal pharyngeal manometry. These figures demonstrates normal pharyngeal–upper esophageal sphincter (UES) pressure response using a solid-state manometric catheter with a 4-mm diameter and with sensors placed at 2-cm intervals. The distal sensor (channel 5) is positioned in the mid-portion of the resting UES. Channels 1 and 2 show a prolonged pressure wave representing a combination of intrabolus pressure and compression of the base of tongue against the upper pharynx. The relative height of the pressure of the two components of this wave differs substantially among individuals and depends on placement of the sensor. An attenuated wave of intrabolus pressure is also noted in channel 3, which, as would be expected, is simultaneous with the

(*continued on next page*)

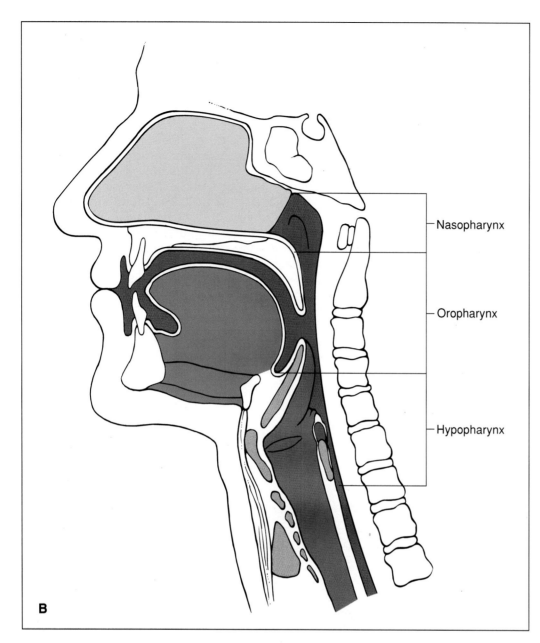

Nasopharynx

Oropharynx

Hypopharynx

B

FIGURE 7-7. (CONTINUED)

first component of channels 1 and 2. Channel 3 shows a contractile wave, beginning somewhat after those in channels 1 and 2, and representing the propagation wave (pharyngeal peristalsis). The sensor recording pressures in channel 5, located in the traditional position used to record UES relaxation, reveals an apparent prolonged relaxation. Based on information about UES movement during swallowing (*see* Fig. 7-6), Castell and co-workers [8] have suggested that the proper location measuring UES relaxation is the proximal end of the UES, as confirmed by the "M" configuration seen in channel 4, a pattern produced by the initial rise of pressure resulting from the sphincter's rising over the sensor, followed by actual sphincter relaxation, and then propagation of the peristaltic wave through the sphincter segment. The relaxation thus observed is substantially shorter than that seen in channel 5. Although physiologically sound, it remains to be established that this placement modification reliably compensates for sensor and sphincteric movement. Note the negative pressure at the nadir of UES relaxation (pressure = -7), a normal finding in pharyngeal manometry. The dotted line indicates intrapharyngeal baseline. (**B**, *Adapted from* Donner *et al.* [1].)

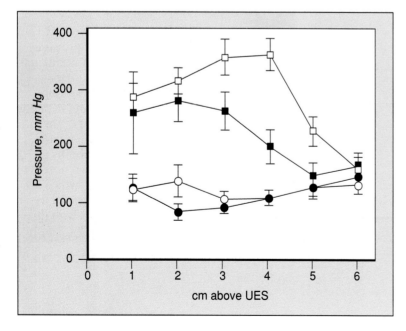

FIGURE 7-8.

Normal asymmetric pharyngeal contractile pressure. The pressures noted during pharyngeal contractions may be asymmetric. In this study by Sears and associates [10], mean pharyngeal contraction pressures in the anterior (*open square*), posterior (*closed square*), right lateral (*open circle*), and left lateral (*closed circle*) orientations at different levels above the manometrically recorded upper esophageal sphincter are displayed. The pressures recorded on the anterior and posterior axes are significantly higher in the anterior and posterior directions than in the lateral direction. The differences tend to diminish as the sensor is located more proximally. A recent study by Olsson and coworkers [9] suggests that the highest pressures may relate, at least in part, to compression by the tilting epiglottis. (*Adapted from* Sears *et al.* [10].)

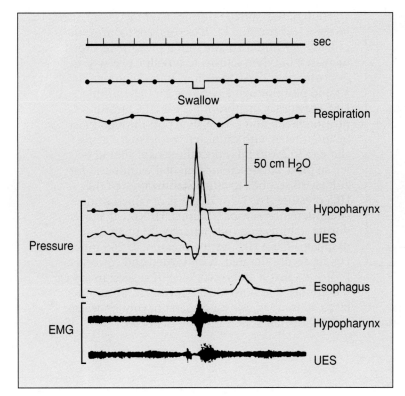

FIGURE 7-9.

Initiation of upper esophageal sphincter (UES) relaxation. This study demonstrates the response of the pharynx and UES to swallowing in terms of both motility and electrical activity. The manometric tracing is shown on the upper two channels whereas the electromyographic (EMG) recording is shown in the lower two channels. Resting UES tone results from tonic electrical stimulation while there is little or no electrical activity in the pharynx at rest. Swallowing generates a crescendo-decrescendo pattern of electrical activity in the superior constrictor, causing contraction of the pharyngeal constrictors. At the same time, there is an abrupt termination of electrical activity in the UES, which is temporally associated with UES relaxation. (*Adapted from* van Overbeck [11].)

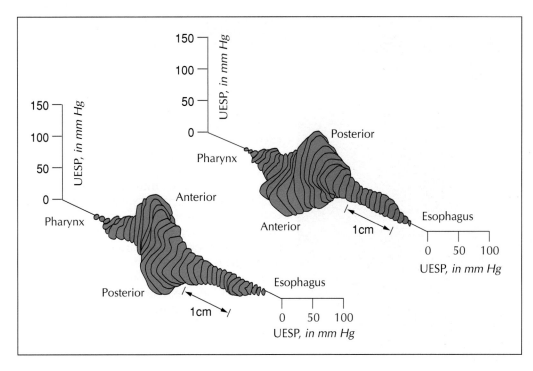

FIGURE 7-10.

Normal asymmetry of the upper esophageal sphincter (UES). The radial asymmetry of UES pressures has been recognized for many years. Pressures recorded in the anterior and posterior directions are far higher than those from the right or left lateral direction. This figure shows a pressure profile of the normal UES as measured by an 8-lumen water-perfusion catheter system. The figure at the lower left shows the same data as the one at the upper right, rotated 180 degrees. Note that there is some degree of axial asymmetry in addition to the more dramatic radial asymmetry. This has made it difficult to establish accurate normal values for UES pressures using a small number of radially arrayed side-port sensors. Recently, a circumferential solid-state sensor has been used to circumvent this problem. (*Adapted from* Welch *et al.* [12].)

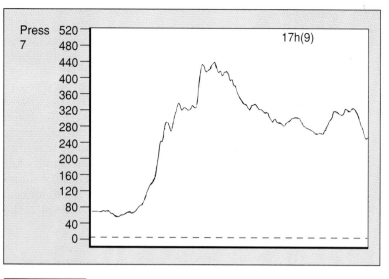

FIGURE 7-11.

Changes in upper esophageal sphincter (UES) pressure during catheter stimulation. The UES reacts to various types of stimulation.

Traction of the catheter during manometry can also increase UES pressure for 10 seconds or more. As the catheter is withdrawn, the initial pressure recorded increases, but then returns to baseline over a 4- to 5-second period. As a result of this phenomenon, a rapid pull-through technique for determining UES pressure is inappropriate for UES pressure measurement, and even a slow pull-through must be interpreted with caution to avoid this reactive change. To avoid this effect the sensor should be left in place after each incremental withdrawal for at least 20 seconds to allow stabilization of the UES pressure. The recording was obtained using a circumferential sensor (channel 5). Note that even during stabilization this patient with pharyngeal dysphagia has a UES resting pressure of 265 mm Hg, markedly elevated. Both Castell and coworkers [13] and Olsson and coworkers [9] suggest in separate studies that normal UES pressures are about 80 to 90 mm Hg using a catheter of similar design, but slightly larger (4.5 mm) in diameter.

PATHOLOGIC FINDINGS

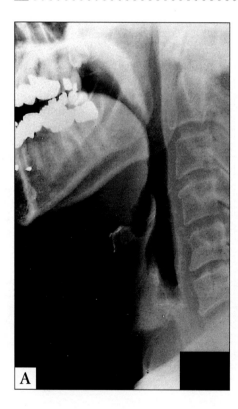
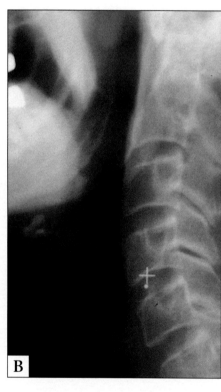

FIGURE 7-12.

Prevertebral atrophy. **A,** Normal study. A soft-tissue view in the lateral position of the air-filled mouth, nasopharynx, and larynx demonstrating that the prevertebral soft tissue is of normal thickness. **B,** Prevertebral atrophy. A lateral plain film of the neck in a patient with neurogenic dysphagia demonstrates almost complete loss of the prevertebral soft tissue, indicating muscle atrophy or weakness. The patient had suffered with poliomyelitis as a child. Dysphagia was a common occurrence in acute bulbar polio. Late recurrence or onset of dysphagia is a feature of the post-polio syndrome, a condition thought to be caused by long-term compensatory overuse of the remaining unaffected neurons [14]. (**A,** *From* Jones *et al.* [4]; with permission.)

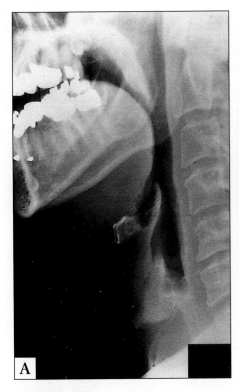

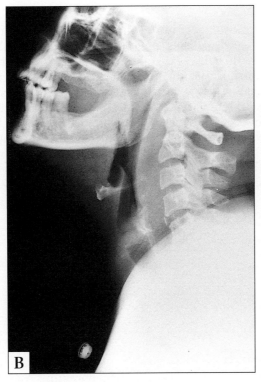

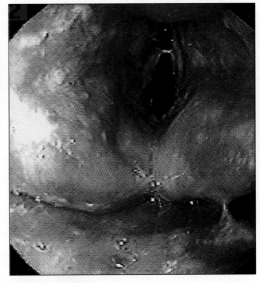

FIGURE 7-13.

Superior vena caval syndrome. **A,** Normal lateral view compared with **panel B,** in which diffuse soft-tissue swelling of the prevertebral soft tissues is present. The patient had superior vena caval syndrome and the edema was caused by venous engorgement. The patient complained of dysphagia, a result of increased turgidity of the pharyngeal soft tissues. Dysphagia may occur during conditions that affect the pharyngeal soft tissue. Dysphagia is common during pharyngitis, although odynophagia tends to dominate the clinical picture and patients are rarely studied radiographically because the diagnosis is obvious. Patients with a history of radiation therapy for head and neck malignancy may develop dysphagia resulting from peripharyngeal soft-tissue injury. In postradiation injury, the videoradiographic findings may be similar to those seen in neurogenic dysphagia. (**A,** *From* Jones *et al.* [4]; with permission.)

FIGURE 7-14.

Mucositis after radiation treatment. Severe edema with diffuse exudate of larynx and hypopharynx in a patient recently treated with radiation for squamous cell carcinoma of the larynx. The patient had severe dysphagia. The larynx is also edematous and somewhat shaggy-looking, representing similar effects. Radiographic studies may show impaired motor function, reflecting soft-tissue inflammation. (*Courtesy of* David Kafonek, Baltimore, MD.)

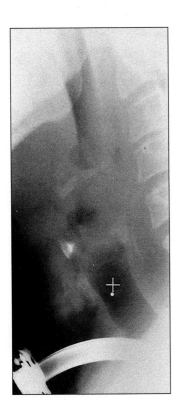

FIGURE 7-15.

Neck abscess. Radiographic view of a lateral film of the neck shows soft-tissue swelling of the prevertebral soft tissues and air in the soft tissues in the prevertebral area and also anteriorly in the neck. The patient previously had a tracheostomy. Note that the soft tissue has a fuzzy appearance compared with the relative homogeneity seen in the normal soft tissue of the neck (*see* normal soft tissue in Fig. 7-2A, for comparison).

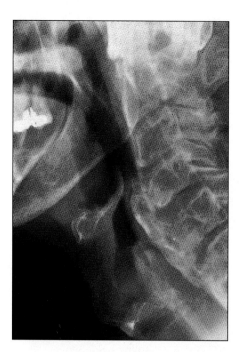

FIGURE 7-16.

Cervical osteophytes causing obstruction. Cervical osteophytes are commonly seen in middle-aged and elderly patients. They are usually an incidental finding. Even in patients with swallowing disorders, osteophytes are rarely responsible for dysphagia. Symptoms can occur by one of two basic mechanisms: either through narrowing by direct compression or by the impairment of pharyngeal wall movement in the area of osteophytes. Plain film and shows bony excrescences along the anterior aspect of many of the cervical spine vertebral bodies consistent with diffuse idiopathic skeletal hyperostosis (Forestier's arthritis). Note the proximity of the epiglottis to the upper border of the bony mass. Unless videoradiographic study demonstrates greater than 50% narrowing of the lumen, both liquid barium and a barium-impregnated solid bolus usually pass without delay in the absence of some other abnormalities. (*From* Jones *et al.* [4]; with permission.)

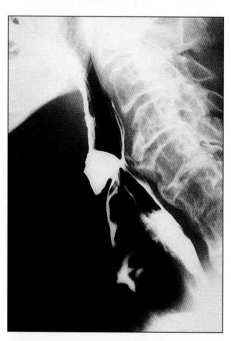

FIGURE 7-17.

Cervical osteophytes causing impaired motility. Aside from compromising swallowing by luminal obstruction, osteophytes may cause dysphagia by affecting the motor function of the pharynx. Radiograph from a frame of a video study demonstrates retention in the valleculae and piriform sinuses and some contrast in the larynx. The videoradiographic study demonstrated a pharyngeal propagative wave that stopped abruptly at the level of the osteophyte and that the epiglottis did not tilt fully as it hit the osteophyte posteriorly. The lumen, however, appeared to open adequately during bolus passage. The interrupted peristaltic wave may be caused by fixation of the soft tissue overlying the osteophyte. (*From* Jones *et al.* [4]; with permission.)

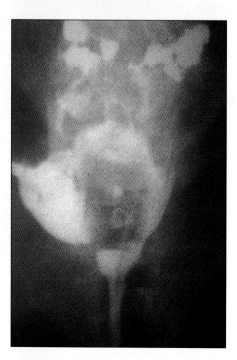

FIGURE 7-18.

Unilateral paresis. Radiograph from a frame of a video study of a patient with unilateral paresis. During swallowing there is asymmetric bulging of the pharynx, with that on the right bulging much farther than that on the left, a sign of right-side weakness. Unilateral dysfunction most often occurs in a patient with dysfunction of the central nervous system that causes asymmetric injury, such as a cerebrovascular attack, brain tumor, or head trauma. Brainstem injury is more likely to cause pharyngeal dysfunction than cerebral injury. It can also result from local soft tissue or neural injury resulting from accidental or surgical neck trauma. (*From* Jones *et al.* [15]; with permission.)

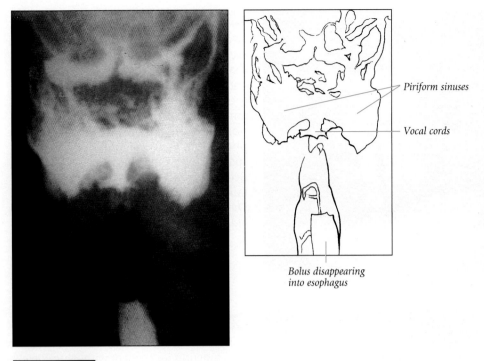

Piriform sinuses

Vocal cords

Bolus disappearing into esophagus

FIGURE 7-19.

Bilateral paresis. In this radiograph from a frame of a video study there is bilateral symmetric bulging of the pharynx with marked retention in the piriform sinuses consistent with paresis. Barium has entered the larynx, penetrating to, and just

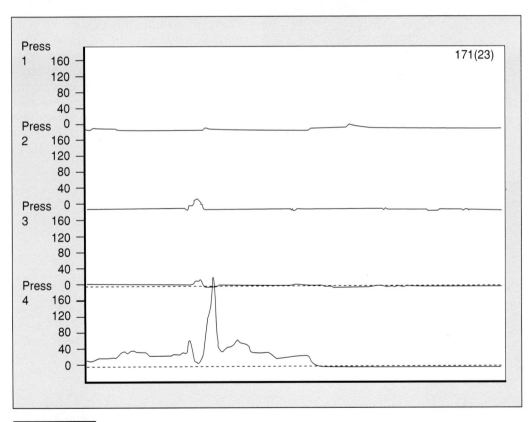

FIGURE 7-20.

Pharyngeal manometry in pharyngeal paresis. Neurologic disorders can affect pharyngeal function, usually producing paresis that may be focal or diffuse. This figure illustrates the manometric findings in a patient with diffuse paresis involving the tongue and pharynx. The catheter used for the study has four sensors at variable intervals along its length (channels 1 and 2 are 5 cm apart; channels 2 and 3 are 2 cm apart; sensors 3 and 4 are 3 cm apart). There is no pressure response at the back of the tongue (channel 1), and those seen in the mid-pharynx (channels 4 and 5) are low (10 and 20 mm Hg, respectively), reflecting profound weakness, and simultaneous caused by failure of the contraction to occlude the lumen. Although upper esophageal sphincter (UES) pressure is low, the presence of a normal "M-spike" configuration of UES elevation, relaxation, and high amplitude contraction is remarkable, suggesting preservation of muscle function at this level. The nadir of relaxation is 6 mm Hg above intrapharyngeal baseline, normal according to the study of Olsson *et al.* [9]. The PE segment normally is opened by videoradiography. Segmental preservation of contractile activity of this type is not uncommon. Whether manometric findings can help to establish a specific diagnosis has not been adequately studied. The most common causes of neurogenic dysphagia are cerebrovascular disease, head trauma, brain tumor, and amyotrophic lateral sclerosis. A substantial number of patients presenting with neurogenic dysphagia to a multidisciplinary swallowing disorders center (The Johns Hopkins Swallowing Center, The Johns Hopkins Medical Institutions, Baltimore, MD) have neurogenic dysphagia visible on videoradiography without other findings to suggest a specific diagnosis. (*Adapted from* Olsson *et al.* [9].)

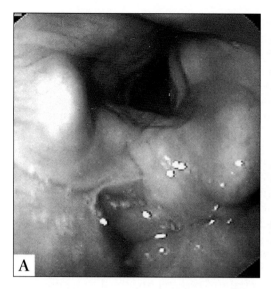

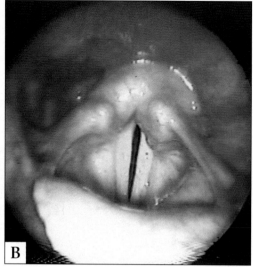

FIGURE 7-21.

Normal vocal cord motion. **A**, The larynx is seen with the vocal folds open at rest. Note that at rest the arytenoid processes and vocal folds are symmetric and that the former are widely separated. The small amount of clear secretions present, a normal finding in the pharynx. **B**, During phonation, the vocal folds close and the space between the arytenoid processes decreases; however, symmetry is maintained. (**A**, *Courtesy of* Gillian Zeldin and David Kafonek, Baltimore, MD. **B**, *Courtesy of* Laura Purcell, Baltimore, MD.)

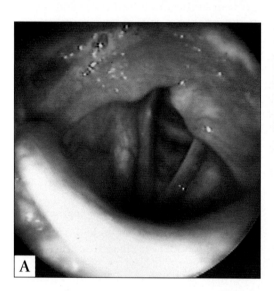

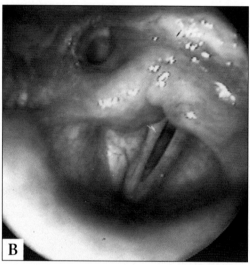

FIGURE 7-22.

Abnormal vocal cord motion. Abnormal vocal cord function in a patient with neurologic dysfunction. **A**, The larynx, as seen through the laryngoscope, is asymmetric at rest. Notice that the left arytenoid process appears to lie forward of right and that the contour of the left arytenoid and aryepiglottic fold is different than that of the right. **B**, These abnormalities are brought out during phonation. Although right arytenoid moves forward and to the left, the left arytenoid has not changed position. The left vocal fold is fixed whereas the right vocal fold actually crossed the midline in an effort to compensate for the left's deficiencies. Note the increased retained secretions in the piriform sinuses, reflecting associated pharyngeal paresis and retention. (*Courtesy of* Laura Purcell, Baltimore, MD.)

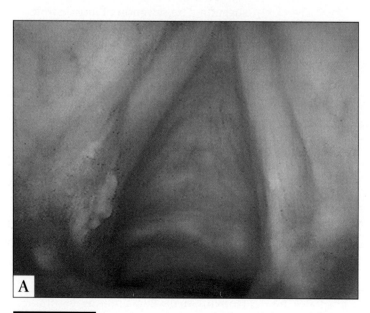

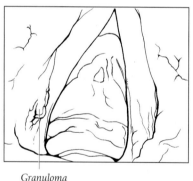

Granuloma

FIGURE 7-23.

Granuloma of the larynx. Granulomata may vary in size from barely perceptible nodules to large masses. The condition usually results from chronic irritation. The most common cause is voice abuse. They may also result from trauma, smoking, chronic coughing, and reflux disease. **A**, Small bilateral granulomas located in the typical position on the medial aspect of the vocal fold, about two thirds of the way from the anterior end. This is the location of the tip of the vocal process of the arytenoids. **B**, A large granuloma of unknown origin

(*continued on next page*)

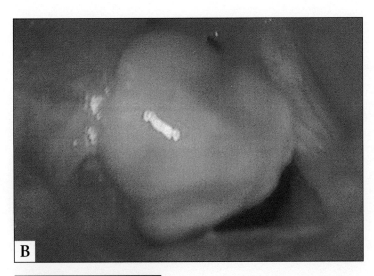

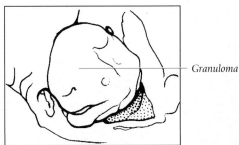

Granuloma

FIGURE 7-23. (CONTINUED)

involving the left vocal fold. The granuloma almost obliterates the view of the right vocal fold, even though vocal folds are open. If the cause is treatable, such as voice abuse or gastroesophageal

reflux disease, treatment can lead to rapid regression of the lesion. (*Courtesy of* Haskins Kashima, Baltimore, MD.)

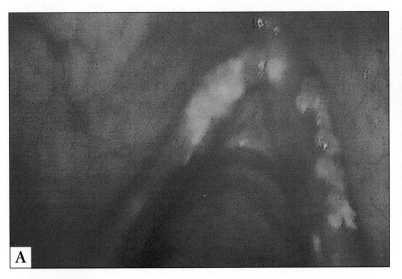

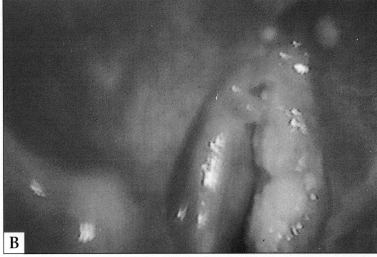

FIGURE 7-24.

Leukoplakia and carcinoma in situ. Leukoplakia describes white, plaque-like lesions. It may result from chronic inflammation or represent a malignancy. **A,** Benign leukoplakia of both vocal cords in a patient presenting with hoarseness. It is typically flat and located on the upper margin of the vocal folds. Even benign disease has a premalignant potential. The biopsies demonstrated epithelial atypia.

B, Leukoplakia of the right vocal cord, in a patient with hoarseness. The lesions are more elevated and nodular in appearance than those in **panel A.** There is also a small red nodule on the left vocal fold. Biopsies revealed bilateral carcinoma-in-situ and areas of invasive carcinoma on the right side. (*Courtesy of* Haskins Kashima, Baltimore, MD.)

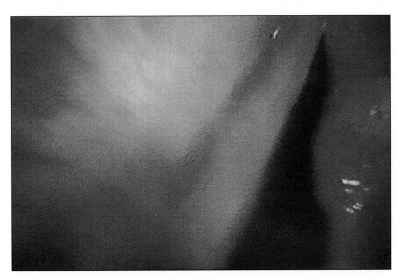

FIGURE 7-25.

Cancer of the larynx. Cancer of the right vocal fold, appearing as a distinct nodular thickening. The entire right vocal fold looks redder than the left, although a white patch on the nodule is evident. Cancer of the larynx can be colored white, red, or (as in this patient) variegated, depending on the degree of keratosis present in a given area. (*Courtesy of* Haskins Kashima, Baltimore, MD.)

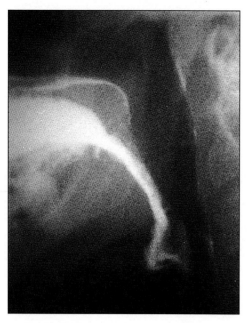

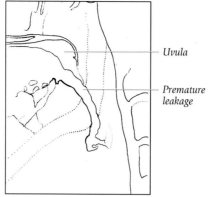

Uvula

Premature
leakage

FIGURE 7-26.

Premature leakage. Radiograph of a patient with neurogenic dysphagia. There is premature leakage from the mouth into the valleculae along the back of the tongue consistent with impaired tongue function or an inability to maintain the seal between the oral cavity and pharynx. Note that the soft palate is not elevated, indicating that the patient has not yet begun to swallow. Some contrast has been placed in through the nasopharynx, coating the nasal and free edge of the uvula. (*From* Jones *et al.* [4]; with permission.)

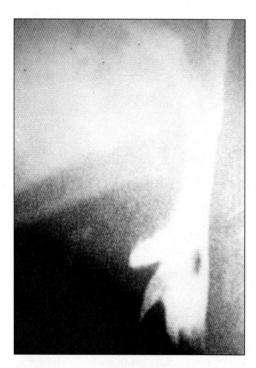

FIGURE 7-27.

Nasopharyngeal regurgitation. Radiograph of a patient with neurogenic dysphagia. The lateral stop-frame print from a cinepharyngoesophagogram shows nasopharyngeal regurgitation behind an incompletely elevated soft palate. Normal elevation of the soft palate and contraction of the posterior nasopharyngeal wall seals the nasopharynx, preventing nasopharyngeal regurgitation. Regurgitation during swallow most often implies neurogenic dysfunction. Note that the epiglottis is upright and there is laryngeal penetration into the open larynx. (*From* Jones *et al.* [3]; with permission.)

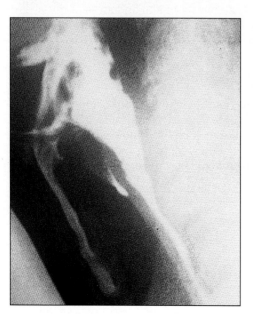

FIGURE 7-28.

Laryngeal penetration. Radiograph of the pharynx in a patient with amyotrophic lateral sclerosis. There is laryngeal penetration with subglottic extension of barium into the trachea. The epiglottis has remained upright, one factor in the failure to protect the airway. Epiglottic tilt, laryngeal elevation, and vocal cord approximation are all important in the prevention of airway penetration. The loss of any one of these defenses does not necessarily result in penetration; however, in neurogenic dysphagia, impairment of multiple factors is not uncommon. Note the degenerative joint disease in the cervical spine. (*From* Jones and Donner [4]; with permission.)

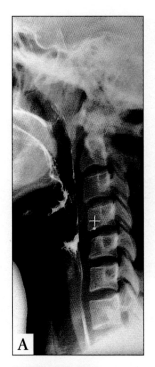
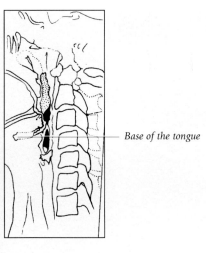

Base of the tongue

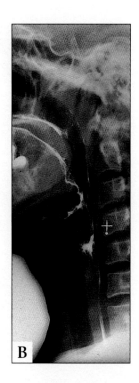

A **B**

FIGURE 7-29.

Lingual tonsil. **A–B,** Radiographs demonstrating a small rounded mass at the base of the tongue. Although this finding could represent cancer, it actually is due to an enlarged lingual tonsil. This finding is more common in younger individuals. Although it can cause dysphagia, it is limited to patients with extremely bulky lesions. It can be treated with laser therapy to reduce the amount of tissue; however, treatment is rarely indicated. In this patient, the enlarged lingual tonsil was an incidental finding.

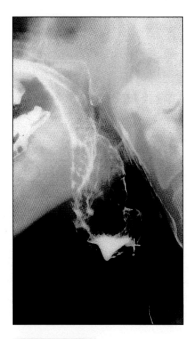

FIGURE 7-30.

Cancer of the tongue base. Radiograph of a patient with a cancer of the base of the tongue. There is an extremely large, bulky tumor of the whole of the base of the tongue consistent with cancer. Note that this interferes with the function of the tongue and the epiglottis, which appears somewhat thickened and may be involved. There is retention in the valleculae. (*From* Jones *et al.* [4]; with permission.)

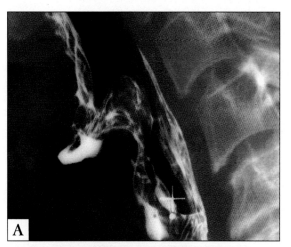

A

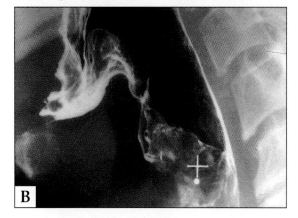

B

FIGURE 7-31.

Carcinoma of the epiglottis. **A,** Radiograph shows obvious thickening of the epiglottis, and the tongue base appears nodular. The extent of tumor involvement is unclear. **B,** With insufflation by means of phonation, and by coning in on the area of the epiglottis, it is now clear that the valleculae are involved by small nodular masses and that the aryepiglottic folds appear nodular. Oblique views with insufflation help determine whether involvement is unilateral or bilateral. Without insufflation the extent of tumor involvement may be underestimated, as seen in this example, or the tumor may not be evident at all. (*From* Rubessin *et al.* [16]; with permission.)

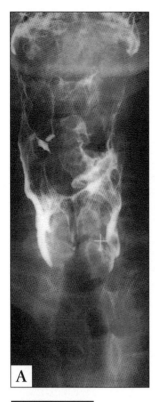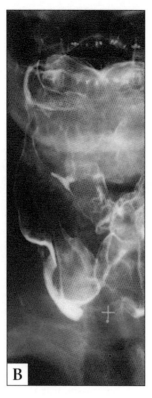

A   **B**

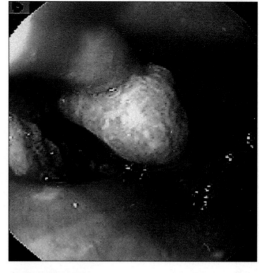

FIGURE 7-33.

Cancer of the pharynx. Endoscopic view of a large mass involving the left pharynx. Notice the mass with a granular mucosal surface protruding from the left aryepiglottic fold as well as the left wall of the pharynx. The white erosion posterior to the mass is the site of a recent biopsy. Note that the left arytenoid process deviated to the right as a result of pressure from the mass. The patient presented with a 6-cm mass on the left side of the neck, representing an involved lymph node. The patient had a long history of esophageal dysphagia and a tight stricture in the distal esophagus that had required dilatation 1 year before he presented with the neck mass. The last esophagoscopy 8 months before had not detected a pharyngeal abnormality.

FIGURE 7-34.

Retention cyst. Radiograph of frontal (**A**) and slightly oblique (**B**) views of the pharynx during insufflation shows a round ring shadow in the right piriform sinus consistent with a benign lesion, such as a retention cyst. The findings should be confirmed by pharyngoscopy. The asymmetry in **panel B** is caused by the oblique angle at which the image is obtained.

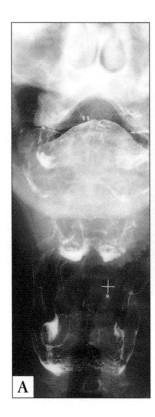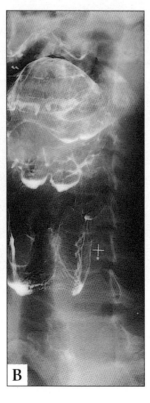

A   **B**

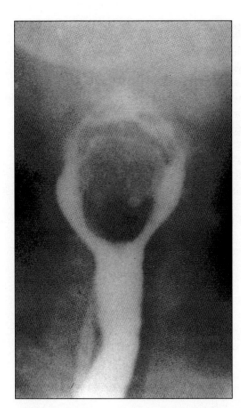

FIGURE 7-35.

Epiglottic pseudomass. Radiograph demonstrating an apparent large midline filling defect. Although superficially resembling a tumor, it actually represents the completely symmetrically inverted epiglottis and associated flow phenomenon. The flow defect is created when the epiglottis deflects the liquid (and food) into the lateral food channels of the piriform sinuses. Flow phenomena may dramatically alter the appearance of pharyngeal and pharyngoesophageal (PE) segment findings; a small mass can appear larger and a web or tight PE segment can look like a long stricture.

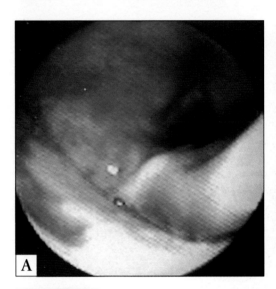

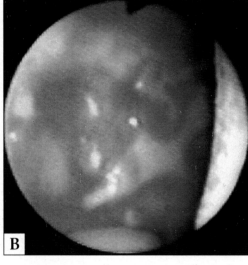

FIGURE 7-36.

Pharyngeal ulcerations in cicatricial (bullous) pemphigoid. **A,** Severe ulceration of the hypopharynx. A large confluent ulcer is present on the posterior pharynx. In addition, there is a small ulcer of the overlying the right arytenoid. **B,** Well-demarcated elongated and stellate ulcerations of the oropharynx (the back of the tongue is seen to the right). The presence of gingivitis and conjunctivitis in the patient suggests cicatricial pemphigoid. Although classically thought of as a skin disease, only about 50% of patients with cicatricial pemphigoid actually have skin involvement. Of interest is that the patient presented with dysphagia and videoradiographic studies suggesting pharyngeal paresis. Inflammatory changes can cause pharyngeal weakness that can appear neurogenic in origin. Whether the motor abnormalities seen represent a direct effect of edema or an effect of associated myositis or neural injury is uncertain.

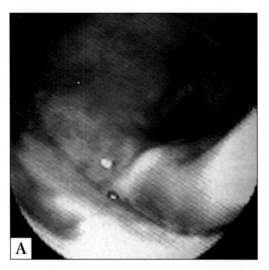

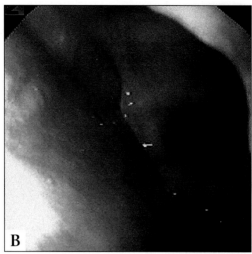

A **B**

FIGURE 7-37.

Cicatricial pemphigoid before and after treatment. The same patient as seen in Figure 7-36 before (**A**) and after (**B**) treatment with steroids and cyclophosphamide for 5 months. Although the post-therapy image is from a slightly more cephalad perspective, the views of the two images cover the same area. Note that the large ulceration of the posterior hypopharynx has completely resolved and the right arytenoid looks normal. Some ulceration of the posterior aspect of the epiglottis remained, but this could not be photographed satisfactorily. The videoradiographic study also improved.

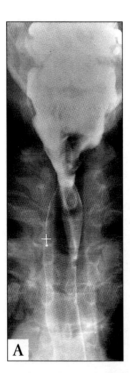

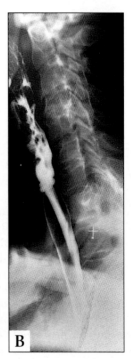

A **B**

FIGURE 7-38.

Benign mucosal pemphigoid. Frontal (**A**) and lateral (**B**) radiographs of the pharynx during swallowing demonstrate multiple concentric narrowings consistent with multiple webs. Although occasionally of congenital origin, multiple webs may be a sequela of earlier inflammation. The patient had benign mucosal pemphigoid. (**A**, *From* Jones [2]; with permission. **B**, *From* Jones *et al.* [3]; with permission.)

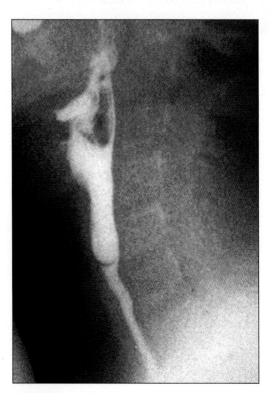

FIGURE 7-39.

Cervical esophageal web. Isolated webs of the hypopharynx, pharyngoesophageal (PE) segment, and cervical esophagus are relatively common causes of dysphagia. In this lateral radiograph taken during barium transit, a horizontal band is seen on the anterior wall of the pharynx at the junction of the pharynx and cervical esophagus with the apparent luminal narrowing below, representing a flow phenomenon caused by the jet effect of the web. Unlike similar short band-like constricting lesions commonly found at esophagogastric junction (*ie*, Schatzki's rings), which are generally circumferential, rings of the pharynx and cervical esophagus are usually asymmetric, indenting the lumen from a single wall. Solitary webs suggest the possibility of sideropenic dysphagia (Plummer-Vinson syndrome); however, sideropenic dysphagia is rare in the United States and most webs are not associated with iron deficiency.

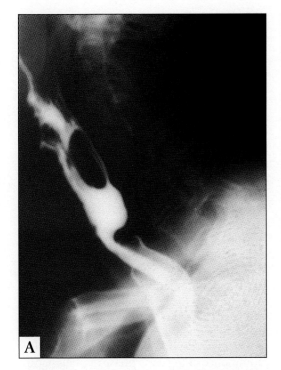

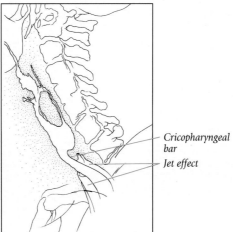

Cricopharyngeal bar
Jet effect

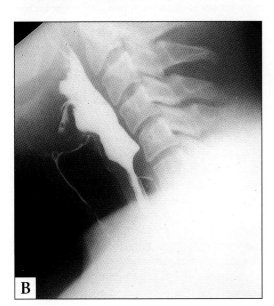

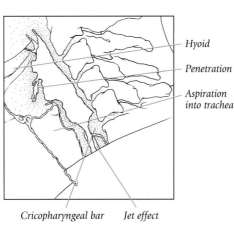

Hyoid

Penetration

Aspiration into trachea

Cricopharyngeal bar   Jet effect

FIGURE 7-40.

Hypopharyngeal (cricopharyngeal) bar. **A,** Lateral radiograph in a patient with hypopharyngeal bar. There is a prominent horizontal bar protruding from the posterior wall of the pharynx at the level of cervical vertebral bodies 5 and 6. There is a flow phenomenon (jet effect) in the cervical esophagus, produced by the barium "squirting" through the narrowed pharyngoesophageal (PE) segment. **B,** Pharyngeal paresis with a prominent cricopharyngeus resulting from lack of "push" with a jet phenomenon indicating luminal narrowing. There is also laryngeal penetration during swallowing and subglottic extension into the trachea. As in **panel A,** there is a hypopharyngeal bar; however, the presence of marked laryngeal penetration suggests that there is pharyngeal dysfunction as well; an impression confirmed on review of the videoradiography, which demonstrated marked pharyngeal paresis. Hypopharyngeal bars are common and often associated with other pharyngeal and esophageal abnormalities. In most patients, the bar is a secondary phenomenon and does not appear to contribute significantly to the patient's symptoms. The bar in this patient narrows the lumen by about 50% (when compared with the normal esophagus). This is sufficiently tight to cause symptoms without other contributing factors. Whether the hypopharyngeal bar is a significant factor in the production of dysphagia in patients with a neurogenic pharynx may be difficult to determine. It appears that opening of the PE segment is not caused only by relaxation of the upper esophageal sphincter. The PE segment is also "pulled" open by the elevating larynx and "pushed" open by the advancing bolus. Defects in any of these components may produce the radiographic finding of a hypopharyngeal bar. A myotomy may be inappropriate, or at least less likely to be effective, if upper esophageal sphincter relaxation is normal. (*From* Jones *et al.* [6]; with permission.)

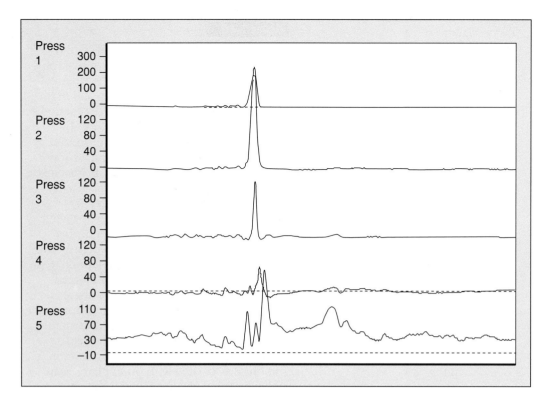

FIGURE 7-41.

Pharyngeal manometry in upper esophageal sphincter (UES) dysfunction. Pharyngeal manometry in a patient with dysphagia, predominantly with solids. On videoradiography, there was a prominent hypopharyngeal bar with a good pharyngeal contractile wave. This manometry study demonstrates failure of UES relaxation (channel 5) with a nadir of pressure at 22 mm Hg above the intrapharyngeal baseline and residual pressure of 50 to 60 mm Hg at the onset of contraction detected in the sensor located 2 cm (channel 4), the usual timing of the nadir of relaxation. The triphasic appearance of the UES during swallowing is simultaneous with the early slow phase of pharyngeal contraction and may be a manifestation of increased pressure, as the bolus is forced through a narrowed sphincter segment. Pharyngeal strength is maintained and pharyngeal contraction is propagative. A subtle change is the unusual prominence of the early phase of pharyngeal contraction at the sensor just above the UES.

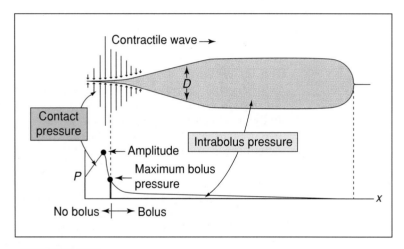

FIGURE 7-42.

Concept of intrabolus pressure. Although manometrists tend to focus on pressure amplitude and coordination, consideration of the relationship between bolus movement and the contractile wave suggests that the absolute pressure amplitude may be less important than usually assumed. The biomechanical concept of intrabolus pressure, as applied by Brasseur and Dodds [18], is an important concept in interpreting manometric data. This figure demonstrates the concept of intrabolus pressure. In the upper schematic, the bolus is showed as the torpedo-shaped object being propelled from the left to right. Its tail is being compressed by the radial force of the muscular wall contraction. The manometric pressure response is shown below. Notice the gradual build-up of pressure within this area in advance of the contractile wave, the slow, early phase of the actual pharyngeal contraction, and the fast, late phase of the contraction wave. The middle phase is temporarily associated with the compression of the bolus at the tail of the bolus, whereas the late phase represents direct contact pressure of the wall against the pressure sensor. Partial downstream obstruction results in increased intrabolus pressure, increased height and area of the middle phase of contraction, and delayed complete expulsion of the bolus, which would occur at a higher pressure. In an extreme situation, the pressure required to push the bolus through the obstruction may exceed the amplitude of the pressure wave, resulting in retrograde bolus flow through the nonoccluded proximal lumen. (*Adapted from* Brasseur *et al.* [18].)

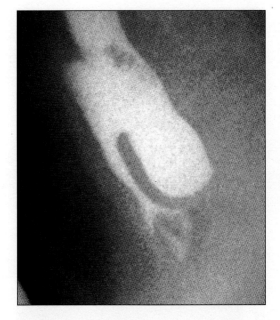
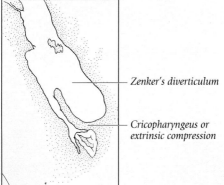

Zenker's diverticulum

Cricopharyngeus or extrinsic compression

FIGURE 7-43.

Zenker's diverticulum. A lateral radiograph (taken from a cinepharyngoesophagogram) shows a large posterior Zenker's diverticulum extending from just above the cricopharyngeus. There is a hypopharyngeal bar, representing either abnormal upper esophageal sphincter function or, alternatively, an effect of direct compression of the pouch itself on the pharyngoesophageal segment. For years, based on the radiographic findings, it was assumed that the diverticulum represented an effect of downstream obstruction caused by cricopharyngeal dysfunction. Surgeons have generally favored performing a cricopharyngeal myotomy at the time of diverticulectomy or diverticulopexy.

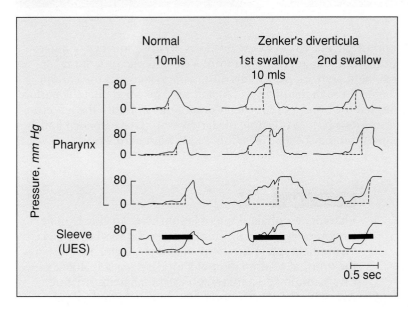

FIGURE 7-44.

Abnormal upper esophageal sphincter (UES) opening in Zenker's diverticulum. It has been assumed for many years, based on the radiographic appearance of the pharyngoesophageal segment, that Zenker's diverticula result from increased pharyngeal pressure due to UES dysfunction. Although early manometric studies using high-compliance water-perfusion systems appeared to confirm this impression, later studies using improved low-compliance technology failed to confirm sphincter dysfunction. Sensor displacement may explain the results of these studies. The figure shows the effect of bolus volume on intrabolus pressure and UES relaxation. Increased intrabolus pressure and failure of UES relaxation is a volume-related phenomenon seen in patients with Zenker's diverticula, and not in normal volunteers. These findings are felt to support the role of UES dysfunction in the pathogenesis of Zenker's diverticula. (*Adapted from* Cook *et al.* [19].)

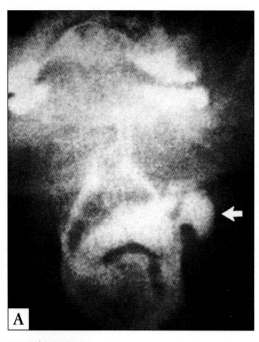 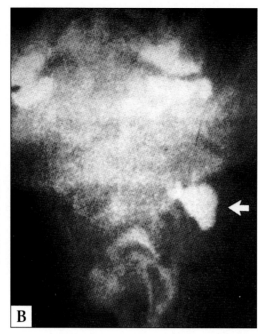 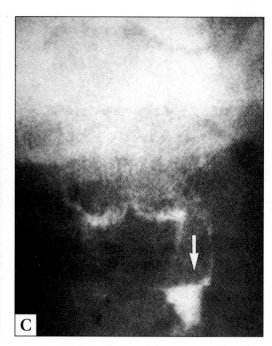

FIGURE 7-45.

Lateral pharyngeal pouches (*arrows*). Zenker's diverticula are not the only pouches that occur in the pharynx. Lateral pharyngeal pouches at the level of the valleculae are relatively common findings that may increase in older patients. In general, they do not appear to cause symptoms and most appear only during bolus transit as a result of transient expansion under increased pharyngeal pressure. Pouches that remain filled at the completion of a swallow may produce symptoms of aspiration by spilling their contents back into the unprotected larynx between swallows. In this sequence of antero-posterior radiographs (taken from a cineradiographic study), a lateral pharyngeal pouch fills during the swallow as the barium passes through the pharynx (**A**) and remains filled after the barium has left the pharynx (**B**). Then the contents spill into the left piri-form sinus (**C**). At this time the larynx would have opened and aspiration may occur. (*From* Jones [20]; with permission.)

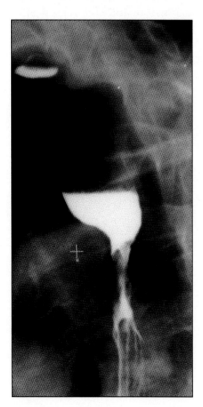 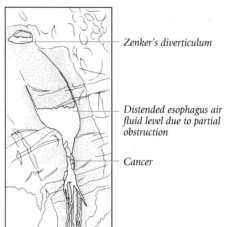

Zenker's diverticulum

Distended esophagus air fluid level due to partial obstruction

Cancer

FIGURE 7-46.

Pharyngoesophageal interrelationships. An elderly male patient presenting with chronic and solid food dysphagia. The radiograph (taken from an oblique angle) demonstrates the unusual combination of a moderate-sized Zenker's diverticulum and a midesophageal malignant stricture. Although the specific combination is rare, multiple ab-normalities of pharyngeal function or structure is more generally appreciated. At the least, this poses difficulty in determining the contribution of the specific abnormalities to clinical presentation. In this patient, laser therapy of the esophageal cancer successfully eradicated his dysphagia, but the coughing was unaffected and presumably was caused by the diverticulum. The possibility that combined abnormali-ties of the pharynx and esophagus may be causal relation-ship should also be considered.

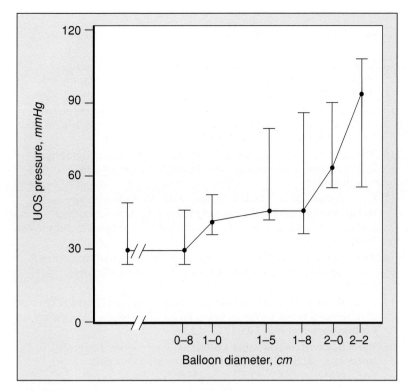

FIGURE 7-47.

Changes in upper esophageal sphincter (UES) pressure during esophageal stimulation. The UES reacts to various types of stimulation. In this study by Andreollo and coworkers [21], balloon distention within the proximal esophagus produces an increase in UES pressure. The increase is directly related to the amount of distention. This observation may account for the frequent findings of a prominent hypopharyngeal bar in patients with esophageal dysmotility or obstructing lesions. (*Adapted from* Andreollo [21].)

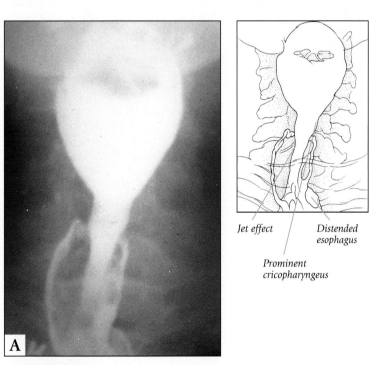

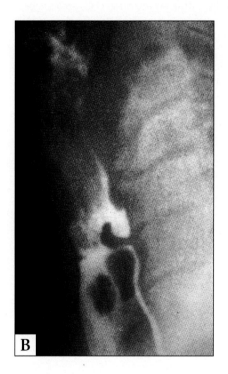

Jet effect   Distended esophagus

Prominent cricopharyngeus

FIGURE 7-48.

Pharyngoesophageal interrelationships. **A,** A spot film during swallowing demonstrates a patient with achalasia with a distended esophagus up to a very prominent cricopharyngeus. There is luminal narrowing at the pharyngoesophageal segment and a jet effect consistent with the luminal narrowing, but one also contributed to by the large caliber of the cervical esophagus. The patient presented with pharyngeal dysphagia rather than regurgitation or esophageal symptoms. **B,** Another patient with achalasia demonstrates a distended esophagus and a small Zenker's diverticulum with a prominent cricopharyngeus. The jet effect is again noted. There is degenerative change in the cervical spine. (**A,** *From* Jones and Donner [15]; with permission. **B,** *From* Jones [22]; with permission.)

REFERENCES

1. Donner MW, Basoma F, Robertson DL: Anatomy and physiology of the pharynx. *Gastrointestinal Radiol* 1985, 10:196–212.

2. Jones B, Donner MW: Examination of the patient with dysphagia. *Radiology* 1988, 167:319–326.

3. Jones B, Gayler BW, Donner MW: Pharynx and cervical esophagus. In *Radiology of the Esophagus*. Edited by Levine MS. Philadelphia: WB Saunders; 1989:311–336.

4. Jones B, Donner MW: Interpreting the study. In *Normal and Abnormal Swallowing: Imaging in Diagnosis and Therapy*. Edited by Jones B and Donner MW. New York: Springer-Verlag, 1991; 51–75.

5. Rubessin SE, Jessurun J, Robertson D, *et al.*: Lines of the pharynx. *Radiographics* 1987, 7:212–237.

6. Jones B, Kramer SS, Donner MW: Dynamic imaging of the pharynx. *Gastrointest Radiol* 1985, 10:213–224.

7. Dodds WJ, Kahrilas PJ: Pharyngeal manometry. *Dysphagia* 1987, 1:209–214.

8. Castell JA, Dalton CB, Castell DO: Pharyngeal and upper esophageal manometry in humans. *Am J Physiol* 1990, 258:G173–G178.

9. Olsson R, Nilsson H, Ekberg O: Simultaneous videoradiography and pharyngeal solid state manometry (videomanometry) in 25 non-dysphagic volunteers. *Dysphagia* 1995, 10:36–41.

10. Sears VW, Castell JA, Castell DO: Radial and longitudinal asymmetry of human pharyngeal pressures during swallowing. *Gastroenterology* 1991, 191:1559–1563.

11. van Overbeck JJM: Upper esophageal sphincterotomy. *Dysphagia* 1991, 6:228–234.

12. Welch RW, Luckmann K, Ricks PM, *et al.*: Manometry of the normal esophageal sphincter and its alteration in laryngectomy. *J Clin Invest* 1979, 63:1036–1041.

13. Castell JA, Dalton CB, Castell DO: Effect of body position and bolus consistency on the manometric parameters and coordination of the upper esophageal sphincter and pharynx. *Dysphagia* 1990, 5:179–186.

14. Jones B, Bucholz DW, Ravich WJ, Donner MW: Swallowing dysfunction in the post-polio syndrome: a cinefluorographic study. *Am J Roentgenol* 1992, 158:283–286.

15. Jones B, Donner MW: Abnormalities in pharyngeal function. In *Textbook of Gastrointestinal Radiology*. Edited by Gore RM, Levine MS, Laufer I. Philadelphia: WB Saunders; 1994:226–243.

16. Rubessin SE, Jones B, Donner MW: Contrast pharyngography: The importance of phonation. *AJR Am J Roentgenol* 1987, 148:269–272.

17. Cunningham ET Jr, Jones B, Donner MW: Normal anatomy and techniques of examination of the pharynx. In *Alimentary Tract Radiology*. Edited by Freeny PC, Stevenson GW. St Louis: Mosby–Year Book; 1994:94–130.

18. Brasseur JG, Dodds WJ: Interpretation of intraluminal manometric measurements in terms of swallowing mechanics. *Dysphagia* 1991, 6:100–119.

19. Cook IJ, Gabb M, Panagopoulos V, *et al.*: Pharyngeal (Zenker's) diverticulum is a disorder of upper esophageal sphincter opening. *Gastroenterology* 1992, 103:1229–1235.

20. Jones B, Ravich WJ, Donner MW, *et al.*: Pharyngoesophageal interrelationships: Observations and working concepts. *Gastrointestinal Radiol* 1985, 10:225–233.

21. Andreollo NA, Thompson DG, Kendall CPN, Earlam RJ: Functional relationships between cricopharyngeal sphincter and oesophageal body in response to graded intraluminal distention. *Gut* 1988, 29:161–166.

22. Jones B: Pharyngeal findings in 21 patients with achalasia of the esophagus. *Dysphagia* 1987, 2:87–92.

Chapter 8

Tumors of the Esophagus

SALIMA HAQUE

Tumors of the esophagus may be broadly classified as either benign or malignant. Benign neoplasms are uncommon and are rarely of any clinical significance. They are usually found incidentally and are symptomatic only when large. Leiomyomas are the most frequently occurring type of benign neoplasm, followed by fibrovascular polyps. Squamous papillomas, granular cell tumors, lipomas, neurofibromas, and inflammatory fibroid polyps are all uncommon types. In the United States, esophageal carcinomas account for about 4% of all malignant tumors [1]. At least 90% of these tumors are squamous cell carcinomas; however, 6% to 10% are adenocarcinomas, and the incidence appears to be increasing. They occur more often in males and are associated with smoking and high alcohol intake levels. Clinically, in its early stages, the disease may be difficult to diagnose; however, in more advanced stages, it may present with progressive dysphagia, anorexia, and weight loss. As a result the prognosis is poor; 30% to 40% of patients have advanced disease at the time of initial presentation. The most important factors for prognosis are depth of infiltration into the esophageal wall, lymph node involvement, and tumor size.

EPITHELIAL NEOPLASMS

Benign tumor

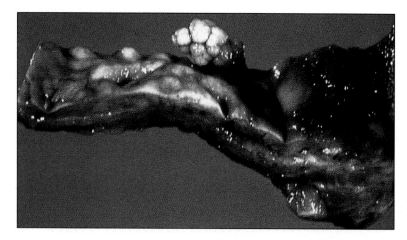

FIGURE 8-1.

Squamous papillomas are rarely found in the esophagus. They are usually identified incidentally, the most common site being the mid-esophagus. Some of them may be associated with human papillomavirus (HPV) infection. Macroscopic appearance varies from single to multiple sessile nodules or polyps. In this illustration, multiple nodules can be seen on the mucosal surface of the esophagus in a patient with papillomatosis. Squamous papillomatosis is usually seen in young children and may be numerous. (*From* Lewin *et al.* [2]; with permission.)

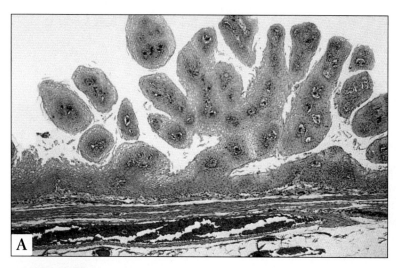

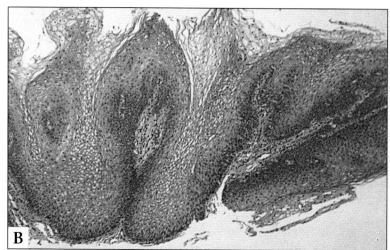

FIGURE 8-2.

A, Microscopic appearance of squamous papilloma. The mucosal surface is irregular, with hyperplasia and hyperkeratosis of squamous epithelium. It is associated with upward elongation of papillae (connective tissue core), thus giving the mucosa a papillary configuration. **B,** Higher magnification of the squamous papilloma showing a thickened epithelium thrown up into papillary folds containing a central fibrovascular core. (**A,** *From* Oota and Sobin [3]; with permission; **B,** *From* Lewin *et al.* [2]; with permission.)

TABLE 8-1. MALIGNANT TUMORS OF THE ESOPHAGUS

Squamous cell carcinoma >90%

Special types
Verrucous carcinoma
Basaloid carcinoma
Spindle cell variant
Small cell carcinoma
Adenosquamous carcinoma

Adenocarcinoma 6%

Mucoepidermoid carcinoma
Choriocarcinoma
Adenoidcystic carcinoma

Leiomyosarcoma (rare)
Malignant melanoma
Malignant lymphoma and plasmacytoma
Metastatic tumors
Rare sarcomas

TABLE 8-1.

Malignant tumors of the esophagus. The great majority of malignant tumors of the esophagus are carcinomas. Among these, squamous cell carcinoma is the most common primary neoplasm, followed by adenocarcinoma. Other malignant tumors are uncommon. Primary lymphoma is very rare in the esophagus but several cases have been reported in the AIDS setting. Kaposi's sarcoma has also been reported in patients with AIDS. Tumor metastatic to the esophagus is infrequent. More commonly, the esophagus is involved by direct spread from tumors arising in contiguous organs, such as lung, stomach, thyroid, and larynx.

SQUAMOUS CELL CARCINOMA

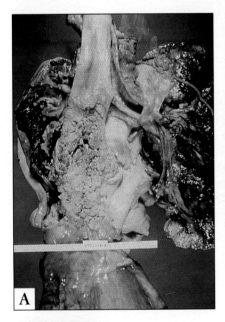 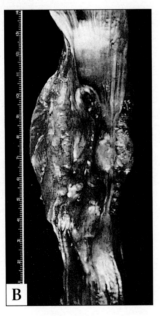 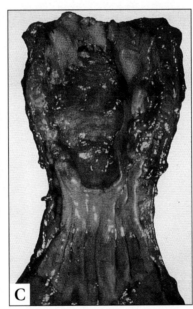 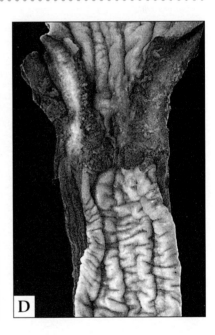

FIGURE 8-3.

Squamous cell carcinoma is the most common malignant neoplasm of the esophagus and constitutes 90% to 95% of all esophageal carcinomas. It commonly affects males, with the peak age of onset between 50 and 70 years. Smoking tobacco and excessive alcohol consumption are the two most important risk factors. Human papillomavirus infection and a variety of dietary triggers have also been suggested as risk factors. Among the predisposing conditions and attendant associations are celiac sprue, prior irradiation, tylosis palmaris et plantaris, Plummer-Vinson syndrome, achalasia, and stricture resulting from the ingestion of lye. Squamous cell carcinoma may occur anywhere in the esophagus but is most commonly found in the middle, and secondly, in the lower third portions. Macroscopic appearance of advanced esophageal carcinomas vary from exophytic mass to ulcerated, infiltrating lesion, to a combination of all these. **A,** In this figure the squamous cell carcinoma is shown to be grossly exophytic, fungating, and partially ulcerated, involving the distal esophagus. The tumor had extensively involved the esophageal wall, spreading into the periesophageal soft tissue. **B,** An exophytic and infiltrating squamous cell carcinoma causing annular constriction of the esophagus. The tumor showed massive circumferential infiltration of the esophageal wall, resulting in obstruction of the lumen. **C,** Squamous cell carcinoma may also present as a large excavating esophageal ulcer, as seen in this figure. The carcinoma had infiltrated into the periesophageal soft tissue. Note the tumor nodules in the surrounding periesophageal soft tissue. The esophagus has a rich lymphatic supply, which accounts for the frequent lymphatic spread to surrounding lymph nodes. Metastasis to distant organs is also common, especially to the liver, lungs, pleura, and adrenals. Occasionally the tumor extends directly into the mediastinum. **D,** The infiltrating squamous carcinoma showed only focal surface ulceration, although the tumor had extensively spread along the submucosa underneath of the intact esophageal mucosa. This type of submucosal extension is common in all types of esophageal carcinoma. The tumor may also spread into the submucosa of the stomach through the submucosal lymphatics. (**B,** *Courtesy of* Beth Israel Hospital, Boston; **C** and **D,** *From* Ming [4].)

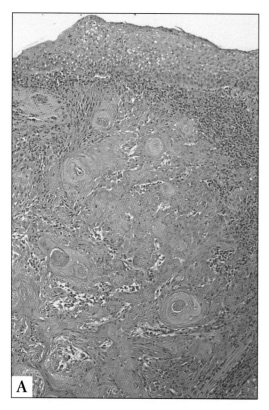

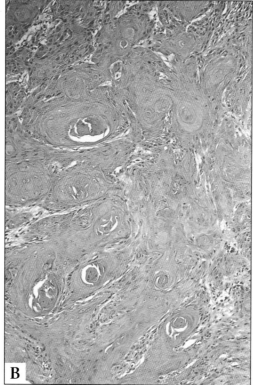

FIGURE 8-4.

Microscopic features of esophageal squamous cell carcinoma range from well-differentiated to poorly differentiated squamous cell carcinomas. The well-differentiated tumors contain squamous nests, pearls, intercellular bridges, and individual cell keratinization. Moderately differentiated squamous cell tumors have features such that they may be considered to be between well- and poorly differentiated carcinomas. Undifferentiated squamous cell carcinomas have no special differentiating features and do not make keratin. The tumor cells may have pleomorphic nuclei and scanty cytoplasm with many mitotic figures. **A,** Histologic appearance of well-differentiated squamous cell carcinoma of the esophagus infiltrating the submucosa. The tumor is producing abundant keratin, manifested in the form of squamous pearls, and is evoking an intense inflammatory reaction around itself. Note the dysplastic squamous epithelium on the surface. **B,** Higher magnification of the tumor shown in **panel A,** showing keratin nests and pearls in greater detail.

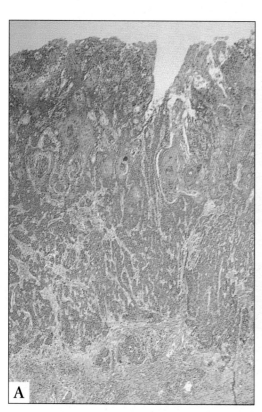

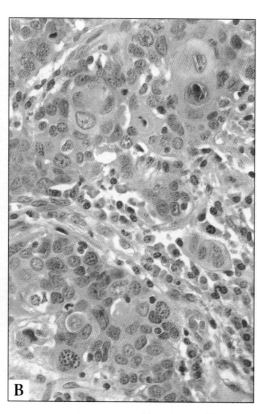

FIGURE 8-5.

A, Histologic appearance of invasive, moderately differentiated squamous cell carcinoma of the esophagus. Note the presence of keratin pearls in the superficial portion of the tumor and the less well-differentiated nonkeratinizing squamous cells at the lower infiltrating margin. **B,** Higher magnification of an island of a moderately differentiated squamous cell carcinoma from the view in **panel A,** showing individual cell keratinization. Note the presence of inflammatory cells in the background.

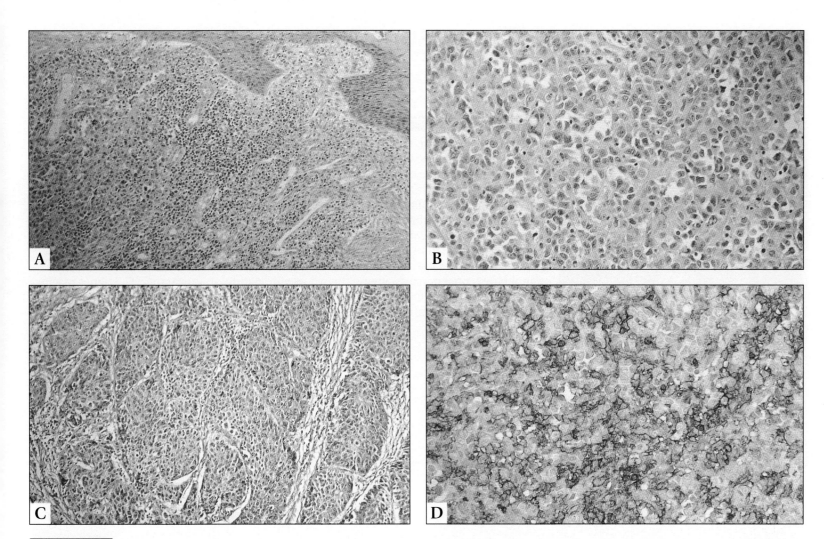

FIGURE 8-6.

FIGURE 8-6.

A, Histologic appearance of undifferentiated squamous cell carcinoma diffusely infiltrating the esophagus. **B,** The tumor has no differentiating features and is composed of sheets of single, large cells with pleomorphic nuclei and scanty cytoplasm. The overlying squamous epithelium had a focus of in situ carcinoma making the diagnosis easier. **C,** A few islands of poorly differentiated squamous cell carcinoma. Immunohistochemical stains such as cytokeratin, vimentin, or leukocyte common antigen may be necessary to identify undifferentiated carcinoma from lymphoma and sarcoma. **D,** The sheets of undifferentiated carcinoma cells showing strong positive staining for cytokeratin.

TABLE 8-2. ESOPHAGEAL TNM PATHOLOGIC STAGING

Classification
Primary tumor (T) class

Tis	Carcinoma in situ
T1	Invades lamina propria or submucosa
T2	Invades muscularis propria
T3	Invades adventitia
T4	Invades adjacent structures

Nodal (N) class

N0	No regional node metastases
N1	Regional node metastases

Distant metastases (M) class

M0	No distant metastases
M1	Distant metastases

Stage grouping

0	Tis N0 M0
I	T1 N0 M0
IIA	T2–T3, N0 M0
IIB	T1–T2, N1 M0
III	T3 or T4 N1 M0
IV	AnyT AnyN M1

TABLE 8-2.

Accurate staging of esophageal cancer is important for therapeutic management and evaluation of treatment. This table illustrates the staging scheme developed by the American Joint Committee on Cancer in Cooperation with the TNM Committee of the International Union Against Cancer. The classification given here applies to all esophageal carcinomas. The pathologic stage is based on examination of the resected esophagectomy specimen. The clinical staging is based on clinical examination before treatment is given and includes physical examination, endoscopy, imaging, and endoscopic ultrasonography. Computed tomography and endoscopic ultrasound scanning are particularly useful in the evaluation of the depth of invasion and of the status of the lymph nodes. (*Adapted from* American Joint Committee on Cancer [1].)

■ SPECIAL TYPES OF SQUAMOUS CELL CARCINOMA

Basaloid carcinoma

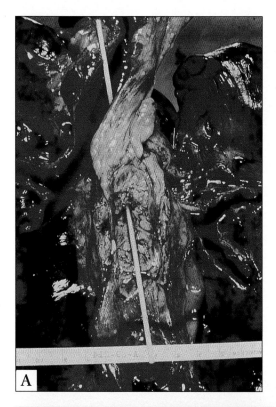

FIGURE 8-7.

A, Basaloid carcinoma, or basaloid variant of squamous cell carcinoma, arising in the distal portion of the esophagus as an infiltrating, annular, constricting neoplasm. The tumor had infiltrated through the esophageal wall into the main bronchus, resulting in the production of an esophagobronchial fistula. The cotton swab is going through the tract of the fistula. This is a rare, highly malignant, esophageal tumor usually occurring in the distal part of the esophagus. Note that the macroscopic appearance is similar to that of conventional squamous cell carcinoma of the esophagus. **B,** Microscopically, it presents as islands of infiltrating, poorly differentiated carcinoma, often exhibiting differentiation toward pseudoglandular structures resembling adenoid cystic carcinoma. Many of the infiltrating islands of tumor have central necrosis, giving them a pseudoglandular appearance. **C,** Higher magnification of basaloid carcinoma to show the comedocarcinoma-like central necrosis and characteristic peripheral palisading.

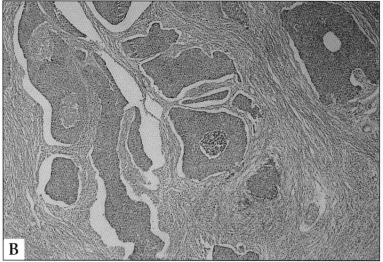

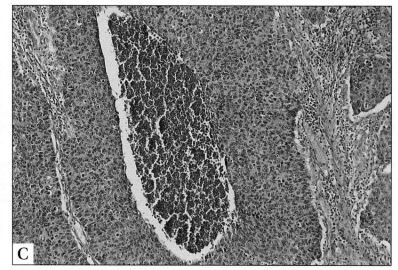

Verrucous carcinoma

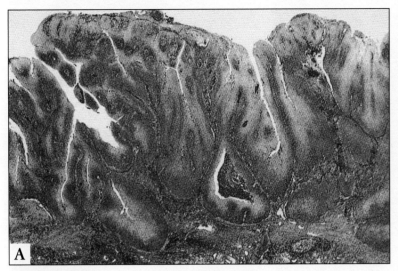

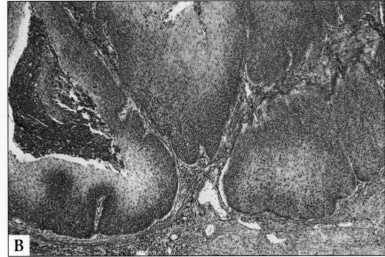

A, Verrucous carcinoma showing papillary architecture. This appearance is similar to that of verrucous carcinoma in other organs. Each papillary frond is made up of well-differentiated squamous cells surrounding a delicate fibrovascular core. Marked acanthosis and parakeratosis are present with blunt pegs extend into the submucosa of the esophagus. **B**, Higher magnification of the deeper end of tumor showing broad blunt pegs of squamous epithelium with central necrosis. Dysplasia is minimal and is confined to the basal layer. Macroscopic appearance is either that of a polypoid or an exophytic papillary mass. Verrucous carcinoma is a rare tumor, which grows slowly. It is less aggressive than the usual squamous cell carcinoma and does not appear to metastasize. The tumor may invade locally. (*From* Oota and Sobin [3]; with permission.)

Spindle cell variant (carcinosarcoma) of squamous cell carcinoma

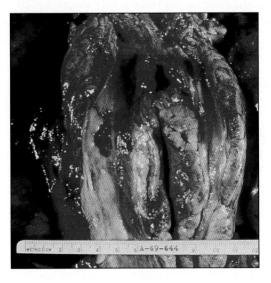

FIGURE 8-9.

Spindle cell carcinoma in the lower esophagus, presenting as a large polypoid mass. The surface of the tumor is partially ulcerated and necrotic. The tumor did not have a well-defined pedicle and showed extensive infiltration of the submucosa. This is a rare neoplasm, which usually presents as a large polypoid mass occurring in the middle and distal portions of the esophagus.

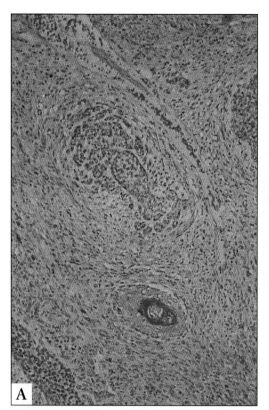 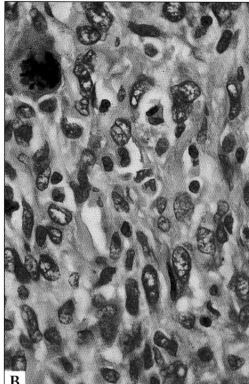 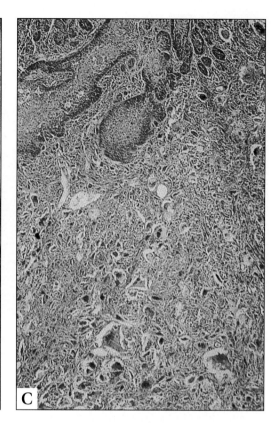

FIGURE 8-10.

A, Microscopic appearance of the spindle cell variant of squamous cell carcinoma, showing small foci of squamous cell carcinoma and large interlacing bundles of malignant spindle cells. B, Higher magnified view of the spindle cell component, showing sarcoma-like cells and mitosis. C, Spindle cell carcinoma composed of large pleomorphic elongated cells and bizarre giant cells, which resemble malignant fibrous histiocytoma. Superficially invasive squamous cell carcinoma is present in the upper portion of the picture. The epithelial component of this neoplasm may be meager, confined only to a few in situ and superficially invasive areas. Mesenchymal differentiation toward bone, cartilage, or muscle may be present in the tumor. (*From* Lewin *et al.* [2]; with permission.)

Small cell carcinoma

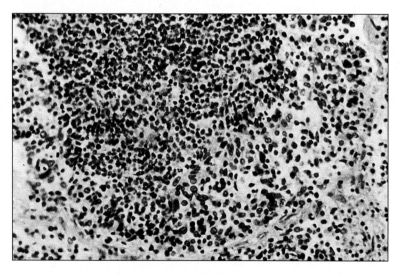

FIGURE 8-11.

Small cell carcinoma of the esophagus growing in a diffuse infiltrative pattern. This very rare, very aggressive neoplasm is composed of small cells with scanty cytoplasm and hyperchromatic nuclei. It has a predominance among women, in whom it usually occurs in the lower and then in the mid-esophagus. Histologically, such neoplasms are identical to small cell undifferentiated (oat cell) carcinoma of the lung. Macroscopically, the tumor usually presents as an exophytic, fungating mass and rarely may occur in multiple foci. Histologically, the tumor has a diffuse growth pattern; it is made up of anaplastic small cells with round to oval hyperchromatic nuclei and scanty cytoplasm. The tumor cells may form rosettes and glands. Squamous pearls and, at times, foci of squamous carcinoma, may also be present. This tumor may be associated with production of ectopic hormones, such as calcitonin and adrenocorticotropic hormone.

ADENOCARCINOMA

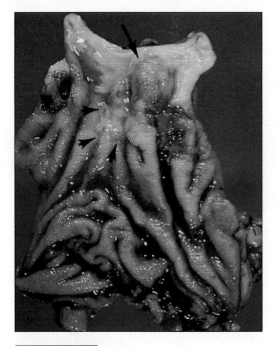

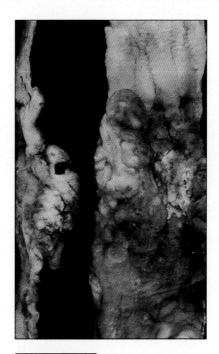

FIGURE 8-12.

Adenocarcinomas of the esophagus usually involve the lower third of the esophagus, but more rarely may be seen in the mid- or upper esophagus. They commonly arise from metaplastic columnar epithelium (*ie*, Barrett's esophagus), as shown in this illustration. Note the irregular gastroesophageal junction (*small arrows*) and the nodular tumor mass (*large arrow*). Adenocarcinomas may also arise from heterotopic gastric mucosa or from the submucosal glands. It is one of the most significant complications of Barrett's esophagus of the "specialized cell" type (columnar with goblet cells). In Barrett's esophagus, the normal squamous epithelium of the esophagus is replaced by glandular-type epithelium as a consequence of long-standing gastroesophageal reflux disease. It is usually seen in men between the ages of 40 and 60, but also has been reported in children. The incidence appears to be increasing. (*From* Lewin *et al.* [2]; with permission.)

FIGURE 8-13.

An exophytic, ulcerated adenocarcinoma arising in Barrett's esophagus. The gross appearance of adenocarcinomas is very similar to that of squamous cell carcinomas of the esophagus, varying from plaques to large, fungating, ulcerated masses. When arising in Barrett's epithelium, these tumors may be multiple. Endoscopically and grossly, they may be flat or may resemble an ulcerated Barrett's mucosa, which is not easily recognizable as a tumor; however, they may also appear as a large exophytic, fungating mass. (*From* Lewin *et al.* [2]; with permission.)

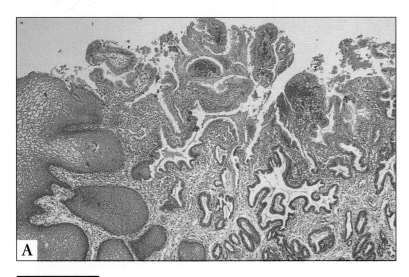

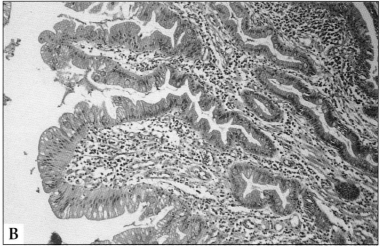

FIGURE 8-14.

A, Histologic appearance of Barrett's esophagus with dysplasia. Note the hyperplastic squamous epithelium on the side. B, High-power view, showing the characteristic goblet cells intermixed with columnar cells as seen in metaplastic Barrett's esophagus. Adenocarcinoma arising in Barrett's esophagus is always preceded or accompanied by dysplasia. In the literature the presence of high

grade dysplasia seen in association with adenocarcinoma has been reported from 68% to 100% of cases.

The histologic appearance of adenocarcinoma varies widely from the well-differentiated intestinal type to diffuse, poorly differentiated carcinoma, to carcinomas with signet-ring cell features. The spectrum of histologic features seen in adenocarcinoma arising in Barrett's esophagus.

(*continued on next page*)

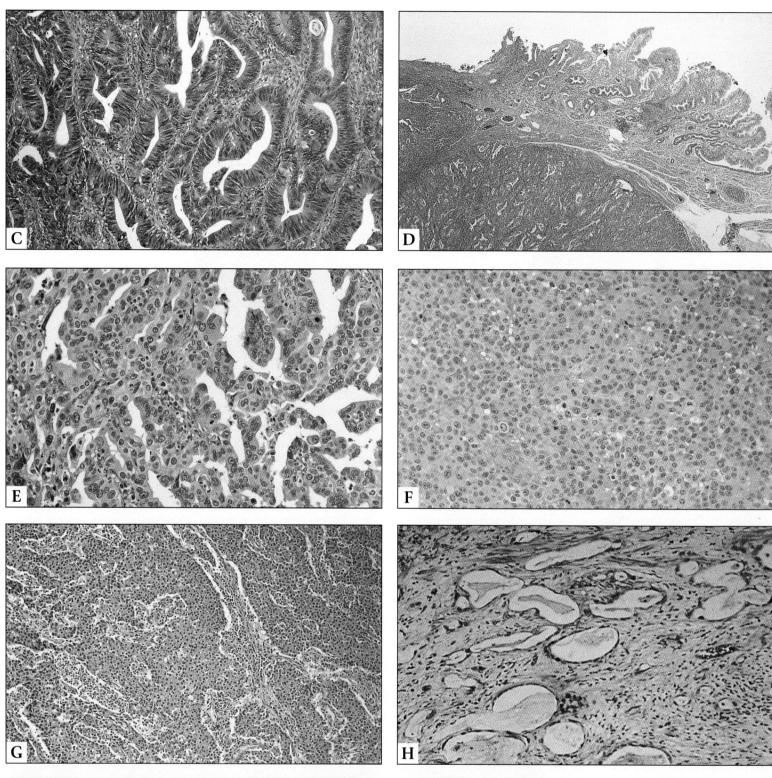

FIGURE 8-14. (CONTINUED)

C, Well-differentiated adenocarcinoma, intestinal type; D, moderately differentiated adenocarcinoma showing extensive intramural spread. The metaplastic columnar epithelium on the surface had many foci of high grade dysplasia; E, higher magnification of the view of the carcinoma seen in **panel D**; F–G, poorly differentiated adenocarcinoma with some cells containing mucin vacuoles; H, mucinous carcinoma; I, signet-ring cell carcinoma. The histologic appearance and tumor grade do not appear to correlate with survival rates. These carcinomas are all very similar to squamous cell carcinomas in their biologic behavior and prognosis. (H and I, *From* Lewin *et al.* [2]; with permission.)

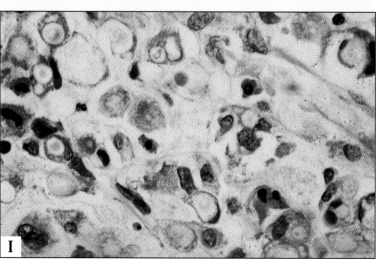

TABLE 8-3. DYSPLASIA IN BARRETT'S ESOPHAGUS: HISTOLOGIC CRITERIA

HIGH-GRADE DYSPLASIA	LOW-GRADE DYSPLASIA
Crypt architecture	Crypt architecture is preserved
Distorted, marked branching	
Lateral budding	
Back-to-back glands	
Nuclei	Nuclei
Stratified to apical surface	Stratified near base, not the apex
Loss of polarity	Enlarged
Hyperchromatic	Hyperchromatic
Variable size and shape	Crowded
Abnormality extends to mucosal surface	Abnormality extends to mucosal surface

TABLE 8-3.

Dysplasia in Barrett's esophagus: histologic criteria. Barrett's esophagus is associated with an increased risk of adenocarcinoma. Dysplasia usually precedes adenocarcinoma, but may also be associated with adenocarcinoma. Thus, it can be used as a marker for detecting patients at high risk for developing carcinoma. Dysplasia is usually classified as high grade, low grade, and indefinite for dysplasia. The diagnosis of dysplasia is based on both architectural and cytological abnormalities, as shown in this table. The diagnosis may be made difficult by inflammatory/reactive changes as well as interobserver variation. Ancillary techniques for better detection of dysplasia are being researched. Among these, DNA content flow cytometry may come to play an important role.

Malignant melanomas

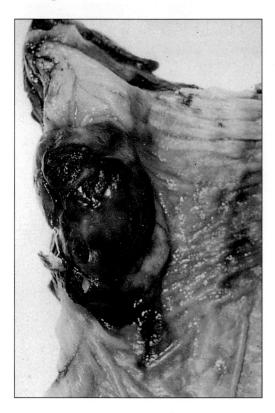

FIGURE 8-15.

Primary malignant melanoma of the esophagus presenting as a large, polypoid mass. A few cases of primary malignant melanoma of the esophagus have been reported. It is important to document the intraepithelial component of the neoplasm in the adjacent squamous mucosa in order to exclude it from metastatic melanoma. Primary tumors may also be associated with pigmentation (melanosis) of the uninvolved mucosa. Although primary melanomas can involve any part of the esophagus, they tend to occur more commonly in the lower third. Prognosis for the patient with this finding is extremely poor (*From* Morson and Dawson [5]; with permission.)

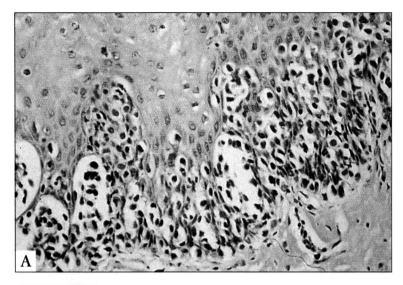

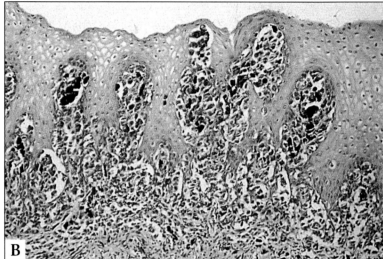

Microscopic appearance of the intraepithelial component (junctional activity) necessary for diagnosis of primary malignant melanoma, as seen in the esophageal mucosa adjacent to the focus of the malignant melanoma. **A,** Proliferation of melanocytes in the basal layer of the squamous mucosa. **B,** The melanocytes are pigmented and extend upward, toward the surface of the mucosa. (*From* Lewin *et al.* [2]; with permission.)

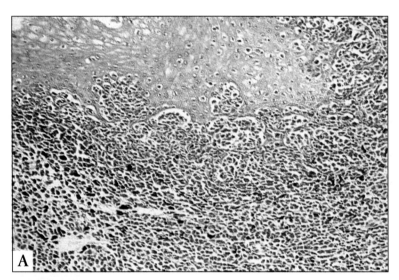

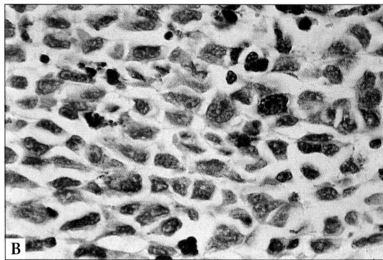

A, Malignant melanoma arising in the esophageal mucosa and infiltrating deep into the submucosa. The tumor is composed of large, malignant, epithelioid cells with prominent nuclei and nucleoli. Note the presence of melanocytic nests in the squamous mucosa. Immunohistochemical staining with S-100 protein, vimentin, and monoclonal antibody such as HMB-45 are helpful in confirming diagnosis. HMB-45 is a more specific, but less sensitive, marker. **B,** Higher magnification of **panel A** showing the tumor cells to be large with increased nuclear-cytoplasmic ratio, pleomorphic nuclei, and prominent nucleoli. Many pigment-laden macrophages are also present. (*From* Lewin *et al.* [2]; with permission.)

■ MESENCHYMAL NEOPLASMS

Fibrovascular polyps

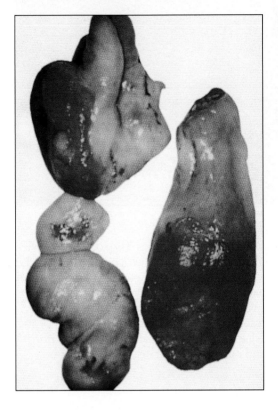

FIGURE 8-18.

Fibrovascular polyps are fairly common benign tumors; they are found more often in men, in whom they typically appear in the upper third portion of the esophagus. Endoscopically, they may present as sessile or pedunculated masses. They do, however, often grow to a much larger size and have long stalks. As shown in this figure, the fibrovascular polyp has assumed a large sausage-shaped configuration, causing nearly complete obstruction. (*From* Ming [4].)

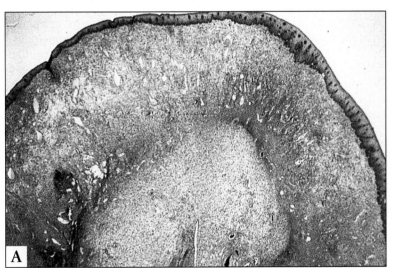

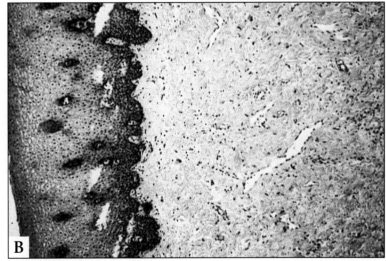

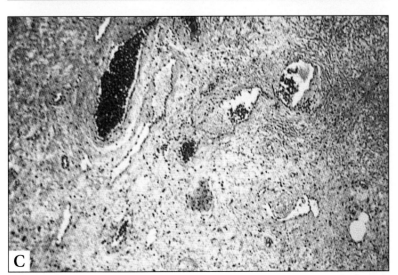

FIGURE 8-19.

A, Microscopic examination has shown these tumors to be mainly submucosal and covered by normal, surface squamous epithelium. **B** and **C,** The bulk of the tumor is made up of loose, edematous, and at times, myxoid connective tissue with dilated blood vessels and scattered mononuclear cells. Strands of spindle cells and islands of adipose tissue may also be present. (*Courtesy of* R. E. Petras, MD.)

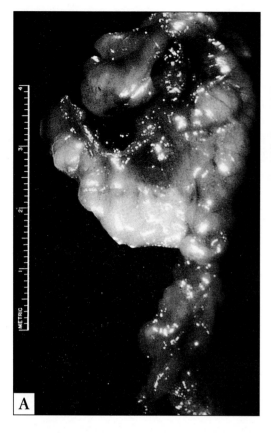
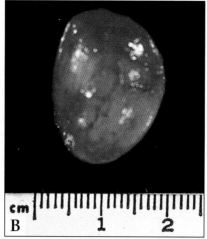
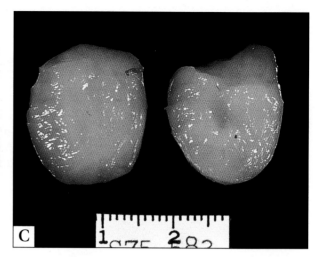

FIGURE 8-20.

Leiomyomas are the most commonly seen benign tumors of the esophagus. They occur more often in men. Although they can be found anywhere in the esophagus, they have a predilection for the lower third portion. Most leiomyomas are found incidentally and are asymptomatic. Larger tumors may cause dysphagia. **A,** Large, multinodular esophageal leiomyoma. The lesion is submucosal with an intact surface epithelium. Larger leiomyomas tend to be multilobular and may have surface ulceration. **B–C,** Nodular leiomyoma with a smooth outer surface. Cut surface appears to be grayish-tan and whorled. Macroscopically, the leiomyoma appears as a well-circumscribed rubbery mass. Most leiomyomas are intraluminal and intramural but, rarely, may present as a mediastinal mass. (**A,** *From* Ming [4].)

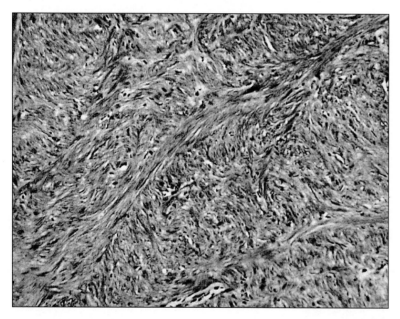

FIGURE 8-21.

Esophageal leiomyoma with smooth muscle cells arranged in interlacing bundles. Note the lack of mitosis and bland appearance of the neoplasm. Microscopic features of leiomyoma include spindle-shaped smooth muscle cells with cigar-shaped nuclei arranged in varying patterns, such as herringbone, storiform, or palisading with rare or no mitosis. Its malignant counterpart, leiomyosarcoma, is rare in the esophagus. It grossly resembles the leiomyoma. Leiomyosarcomas also tend to occur in older men and have a poor prognosis. Histologically, the tumor is made of stromal cells, similar to those seen in the benign leiomyoma. The tumor is, however, markedly hypercellular with numerous mitotic figures. (*From* Ming [4].)

REFERENCES

1. American Joint Committee on Cancer: *Manual for Staging of Cancer,* edn. 4. Philadelphia: JB Lippincott Company; 1992.

2. Lewin KJ, Riddell RH, Weinstein WM: *Gastrointestinal Pathology and Its Clinical Implications.* New York: Igaku-Shoin; 1992.

3. Oota K, Sobin LH: *Histological Typing of Gastric and Oesophageal Tumors.* Geneva: World Health Organization; 1977.

4. Ming S-C: *Atlas of Tumor Pathology, series 2—Fascicle: Tumors of the Esophagus and Stomach.* Bethesda, MD: Armed Forces Institute of Pathology; 1973.

5. Morson BC, Dawson IMP, Day DW, *et al.*: *Morson and Dawson's Gastrointestinal Pathology,* edn 3. Oxford: Blackwell Scientific; 1990.

6. Fenoglio-Preiser C, Lautz PE, Listrom MB, *et al.*: *Gastrointestinal Pathology: An Atlas and Text.* New York: Raven Press; 1992.

Chapter 9

Esophageal Causes of Noncardiac Chest Pain

RICHARD I. ROTHSTEIN

Noncardiac chest pain (NCCP) is a common and important clinical problem. The most common esophageal cause of NCCP is gastroesophageal reflux disease (GERD); other esophageal etiologies include abnormal esophageal motility, altered nociception, or an "irritable esophagus". With many similarities in the presenting symptoms of cardiac and noncardiac chest pain, certain historical features may suggest an esophageal cause; however, it is important first to determine a possible cardiac cause. If results of studies are negative for a cardiac cause of pain, the diagnostic work-up should be directed at identification of obvious upper gastrointestinal disease (tumor, infection, injury) with endoscopy with or without barium radiography. If this is unrevealing of a source, specific testing for GERD (acid-perfusion test, ambulatory pH monitoring) or esophageal motor disorders (esophageal manometry, ambulatory manometry) should be undertaken. Specialized provocative testing for altered esophageal sensitivity (edrophonium, balloon distention) may reveal the esophagus to be involved in the production of an individual's symptom of chest pain.

▮ BACKGROUND AND EPIDEMIOLOGY

As many as 30% of coronary arteriograms performed in the evaluation of chest pain demonstrate normal or insignificant coronary anatomy to explain the symptoms, suggesting alternative noncoronary causes. These patients with NCCP with normal coronary anatomy have an excellent prognosis, with follow-up in studies of up to 10 years demonstrating a less than 1% death rate from cardiac disease [1–3]. Despite reasonable exclusion of coronary artery disease and explanation to the patient of this, patients with NCCP continue to have chest pain that compromises their lifestyle, with a possible inability to work; they persist with visits to physicians' offices and emergency departments for further evaluation of their chest pain symptoms [4–6].

The sources for chest pain symptoms in these patients include noncoronary cardiac disease, pulmonary disease, musculoskeletal disorders, panic disorder, and disorders of the esophagus or other gastrointestinal organs. Studies of patients with angina-like pain, excluding those with evidence of cardiac disease, revealed esophageal causes for symptoms in 50% [7–14]. Thus, esophageal disease is a common cause for production of symptoms in patients with NCCP; gastroenterologists are often responsible for the evaluation of this group of patients.

CHARACTERISTICS OF ESOPHAGEAL CHEST PAIN

Patients with NCCP may present with the same angina-like symptoms as patients found to have coronary artery disease. Patients presenting to emergency departments are often anxious about possible cardiac disease, and may share with those patients who are found to have coronary ischemic pain symptoms of fear and autonomic discharge (diaphoresis, pallor, dizziness, tremor). In NCCP patients referred to an esophageal laboratory after cardiac disease has been excluded, symptoms of heartburn and regurgitation were seen in the majority, while almost half had experienced dysphagia along with their chest pain symptoms, and only 11% had no esophageal symptoms other than their chest pain [15]. However, these esophageal symptoms are not isolated to patients with chest pain in whom cardiac disease is ruled out, for they were found to be present in about half of chest pain patients with proven coronary disease [16]. Although certain characteristics of the pain history may prompt investigation into possible esophageal causes, it is reasonably necessary to exclude cardiac disease as the first evaluation.

MECHANISMS OF ESOPHAGEAL CHEST PAIN

The specific mechanisms producing esophageal chest pain are not well understood. Acid reflux may stimulate chemoreceptors and trigger the sensation of heartburn or chest pain, but data from patients with abnormal total reflux time and esophagitis suggest that only about 20% of reflux events produce symptoms [17].

Esophageal motor disorders may cause myoischemia [18] or distention and result in symptom production. Ingestion of cold liquids, stimulating thermoreceptors, may induce aperistalsis with esophageal distention and resultant chest discomfort [19]. Dysfunction of the belch reflex may also result in acute esophageal distention and discomfort [20]. Studies of esophageal balloon distention as a provocative test show that smaller inflation volumes produce chest pain sensations in patients with NCCP, compared with controls, suggesting abnormal sensory perception of distention as a mechanism for pain production [21,22]. This hypersensitivity, along with the discovery that in some patients identical pain symptoms are triggered by acid reflux events, motor abnormalities, and provocative tests, has led to the concept of the "irritable esophagus" [23].

Investigations have found a high degree of anxiety disorders, depression, and somatization among patients with NCCP, similar to patients with irritable bowel syndrome [24]. Panic disorder is a common condition and probably afflicts at least one third of patients with NCCP, has a psychophysiologic and cognitive etiology, and needs to be considered in the evaluation of patients with unexplained angina-like chest pain [25].

GERD, ESOPHAGEAL MOTILITY DISORDERS, AND CHEST PAIN

In patients with NCCP, 24-hour pH monitoring shows abnormal reflux in about half [7,15,26,27]. GERD may also produce symptoms in patients with proven obstructive coronary disease, and combined ambulatory Holter and pH monitoring can help to elucidate the cause. In one such study, abnormal reflux parameters were identified in 39% of patients, with half experiencing chest pain coinciding with identifiable reflux events [28].

Although upper gastrointestinal endoscopy and biopsy may identify patients with reflux esophagitis, the majority of symptomatic patients with NCCP have normal findings. Barium radiography and esophageal scintigraphy may demonstrate gastroesophageal reflux to be present in a given patient, but do not necessarily correlate to symptoms. The acid-perfusion (Bernstein) test has good specificity, but a poor sensitivity; it has been supplanted in most centers by ambulatory pH monitoring. Prolonged pH monitoring has excellent sensitivity and specificity and permits the correlation between chest pain and acid reflux episodes, even when total reflux exposure may not be excessive [15,29].

Recent studies suggest a role for empiric acid inhibition to identify and treat reflux-related chest pain, with test characteristics as good as or better than the Bernstein test [30,31]; further studies will be needed to compare empiric acid-suppressive therapy with other standard evaluations. Treatment of acid-related symptoms with omeprazole in patients with proven obstructive coronary artery disease being optimally managed with antianginal therapy was similarly effective in relieving chest pain symptoms, improving 65% of those who had at least some of their symptoms related to GERD [32].

Historically, esophageal spasm was described in association with noncardiac chest pain. The disorder called *nutcracker esophagus*, consisting of high-amplitude peristaltic contractions which may be of prolonged duration, was subsequently identified to be the most common esophageal motility disorder (EMD) identified in patients with NCCP, accounting for about half of EMDs when present [9,33]. Although some of the motor disorders may directly relate to causation of pain, through mechanisms of spasm or distention (*eg*, achalasia, diffuse spasm), most investigators now consider the EMDs to be an epiphenomenon found in chronic patients with chest pain or as a response to stress [34,35].

Prolonged ambulatory esophageal testing and provocative testing

The esophagus is likely the source of a patient's chest pain if the usual discomfort is shown to occur during an abnormal esophageal event that could cause the pain, such as acid reflux, abnormal motility, or both. Comparison of stationary and ambulatory esophageal studies in patients with NCCP shows that patients with acid-related chest pain most often have normal baseline esophageal manometry, whereas abnormal baseline manometry is more likely associated with an abnormal motility episode during spontaneous pain [11,12]. In patients undergoing combined 24-hour pH and motility testing, an esophageal cause for NCCP symptoms is found in 10% to 47% [36]. Gastroesophageal reflux accounts for the majority (about 70%) of these symptoms, whereas abnormal motility events account for the minority.

Esophageal provocative testing has evolved as a method to reproduce esophageal chest pain while patients are in the esophageal laboratory; the procedure is similar to performing cardiac stress tests to bring out symptoms or findings of ischemic heart disease. Historically, ergonovine maleate and bethanechol had been used as esophageal provocative tests; however, they are nonspecific stimulants and may produce chest pain from coronary artery disease and are limited in their use by significant side effects (*eg*, coronary spasm, headache, nausea, pain at injection site, sweating) [37,38].

The most frequently used esophageal provocative test is administration of the cholinesterase inhibitor edrophonium. The test is believed specific for the esophagus, has few side effects, and provokes chest pain in only 20% to 30% of patients with NCCP [39,40].

Intraesophageal balloon distention often reproduces chest pain in patients with NCCP (60%) but produces chest discomfort in only 20% of asymptomatic volunteers; patients are found to have their pain stimulated by lower inflation volumes of esophageal distention (21,22).

The addition of balloon distention to acid-perfusion and edrophonium testing provides an increased identification of the esophagus as the likely source of the NCCP [41,42]. Although helpful in the search for an esophageal cause of chest pain, prolonged esophageal ambulatory studies and provocative tests are limited by variable diagnostic yield, the lack of standard criteria, and the intermittent nature of chest pain.

Evaluation of patients with NCCP

Following a search for a coronary ischemic cause of chest pain, a thoughtful review of its differential diagnosis and a stepwise evaluation should be undertaken. The differential diagnosis includes, but is not limited to, cardiac causes (*eg*, mitral valve prolapse, microvascular angina, pericarditis), pulmonary causes (*eg*, pleurisy, parenchymal diseases), musculoskeletal causes (*eg*, costochondritis, myofascial syndromes), gastrointestinal diseases (*eg*, peptic ulcer disease, gallbladder disease, esophageal tumor or infection), panic disorder, and the esophageal disorders of reflux, dysmotility, and abnormal nociception. In many patients with NCCP, cardiac, esophageal, musculoskeletal, and psychiatric problems may overlap, suggesting a common abnormality, such as a smooth muscle disorder or abnormal visceral nociception, but much remains to be determined in the study of the interrelationships of these disorders [43–45].

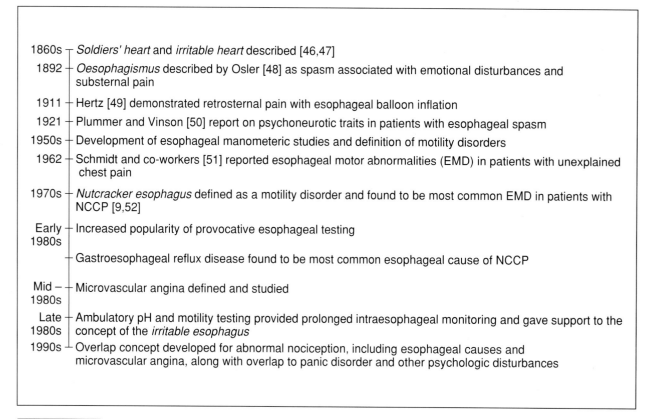

1860s — *Soldiers' heart* and *irritable heart* described [46,47]

1892 — *Oesophagismus* described by Osler [48] as spasm associated with emotional disturbances and substernal pain

1911 — Hertz [49] demonstrated retrosternal pain with esophageal balloon inflation

1921 — Plummer and Vinson [50] report on psychoneurotic traits in patients with esophageal spasm

1950s — Development of esophageal manometeric studies and definition of motility disorders

1962 — Schmidt and co-workers [51] reported esophageal motor abnormalities (EMD) in patients with unexplained chest pain

1970s — *Nutcracker esophagus* defined as a motility disorder and found to be most common EMD in patients with NCCP [9,52]

Early 1980s — Increased popularity of provocative esophageal testing

— Gastroesophageal reflux disease found to be most common esophageal cause of NCCP

Mid – 1980s — Microvascular angina defined and studied

Late 1980s — Ambulatory pH and motility testing provided prolonged intraesophageal monitoring and gave support to the concept of the *irritable esophagus*

1990s — Overlap concept developed for abnormal nociception, including esophageal causes and microvascular angina, along with overlap to panic disorder and other psychologic disturbances

FIGURE 9-1.

Major developments in the history of noncardiac chest pain (NCCP). The early descriptions of patients with chest pain refer to the interplay of emotional issues or possible altered pain perception with disordered function of the esophagus [46–50]. Following the development of esophageal manometric recording, esophageal motor disorders were specifically defined and found in association with symptoms in patients with NCCP [9,51,52]. Studies using provocative or prolonged ambulatory esophageal events permitted a correlation of symptoms with defined esophageal events. More recently, an overlap concept has emerged, linking the "irritable esophagus" with "sensitive heart" (microvascular angina) and panic disorder, as associated causes of chronic chest pain.

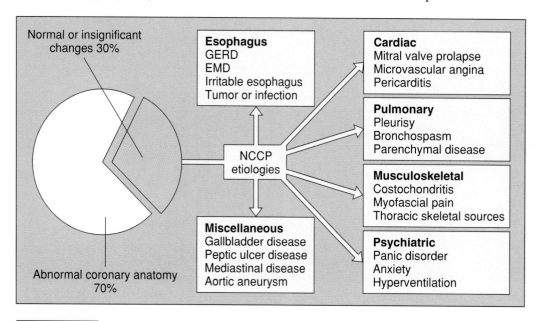

FIGURE 9-2.

Coronary versus noncoronary chest pain. Coronary arteriography demonstrates abnormal anatomy in about 70% of patients with chest pain. The remaining patients have their symptoms arising from diverse origins, including esophageal, cardiac, pulmonary, psychiatric, musculoskeletal, and other causes. In patients with noncardiac chest pain (NCCP) referred for esophageal testing, about 50% are found to have an associated esophageal cause [7,26,53,54]. EMD—esophageal motor disorder; GERD—gastroesophageal reflux disease.

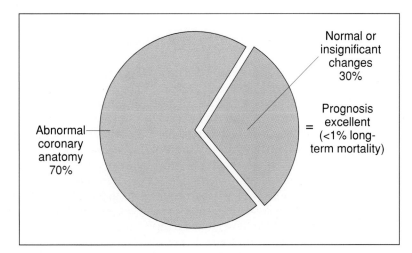

FIGURE 9-3.

Prognosis in patients with angina-like symptoms and normal coronary anatomy at cardiac catheterization is excellent. In a 10-year follow-up study, the incidence of cardiac death was 0.6% [1]. This was confirmed in a study of over 4000 patients with noncardiac chest pain (NCCP) observed for 7 years with a mortality rate less than 1% from cardiac causes [3]. The importance of searching for a cardiac cause before reassuring the patient of the benign nature of esophageal NCCP was emphasized in a small study in which 8 of 8 patients (100%) with "definite" esophageal pain were alive at a 4-year follow-up whereas 2 of 8 patients (25%) with "probable" esophageal pain had died [55].

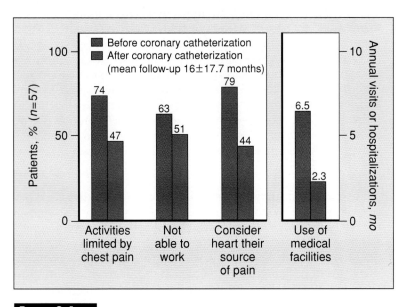

FIGURE 9-4.

Follow-up of functional status of patients with unexplained chest pain and normal coronary arteriograms in 57 patients who had

been told that their hearts were normal, the source of their chest pain was noncardiac, and that no limitation was needed on physical activity. They were evaluated at a follow-up interval of 16 to 7.7 months [4]. Large numbers of these patients still described their activities to be limited by chest pain, were unable to work, and continued to believe the heart was the source of their chest discomfort. There was a significant reduction in patient use of medical facilities compared with rates of use before the cardiac catheterizations. A similar decrease in chest pain hospitalizations was found in another group of patients with noncardiac chest pain (NCCP), the majority of whom demonstrated persistence of symptoms. An improved functional status was found in those patients with a defined or presumed esophageal cause of symptoms [56]. The overall decline in hospitalizations suggests an ability for esophageal testing to reduce overall health care costs for patients with NCCP who are reassured about the noncardiac etiology of their symptoms, although a significant number of the tested patients did not remember or understand the explained results of their esophageal investigations and continued to believe themselves to be disabled by cardiac disease. (*Adapted from* Ockene *et al.* [4].)

CHARACTERISTICS OF ESOPHAGEAL CHEST PAIN

TABLE 9-1. CLASSIC SYMPTOMS OF ANGINA PECTORIS MAY BE INDISTINGUISHABLE FROM THOSE ARISING FROM ESOPHAGEAL CAUSES

Esophageal Chest Pain Usually:

Produces pressure-like squeezing or burning

Can radiate to neck, jaw, back, or arms

May persist minutes to hours

May be sharp and severe

Resolves or abates often spontaneously when treated with antacids or nitrates

Features in the History That Help to Distinguish Esophageal Pain from Cardiac Pain:

Atypical response to exercise

Pain that continued as a background ache

Retrosternal pain without lateral radiation

Pain that disturbed sleep

Presence of certain esophageal symptoms (*eg.*, heartburn, regurgitation, dysphagia)

TABLE 9-1.

Characteristics of esophageal chest pain. Consecutive patients presenting with chest pain on an emergency basis were interviewed before they were fully investigated; features tending to favor a cardiac or esophageal source were identified [16,57]. Although 83% of the esophageal group described having associated symptoms of heartburn, regurgitation, dysphagia, and vomiting, a finding confirmed by Hewson and coworkers [15], these symptoms were also experienced by 46% of patients with chest pain ultimately ascribed to a cardiac source. Although the chest pain of esophageal origin is often described as nonexertional, exercise-induced gastroesophageal reflux does occur with reproduction of angina-like chest pain in patients with normal coronary anatomy [27].

MECHANISMS OF ESOPHAGEAL CHEST PAIN

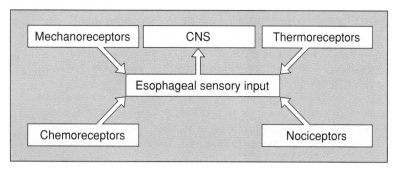

FIGURE 9-5.

Mechanisms of esophageal chest pain. Sensation from the esophagus travels to the central nervous system (CNS) by pathways of the sympathetic and parasympathetic systems, and involves stimulation of esophageal chemoreceptors, mechanoreceptors, thermoreceptors, and nociceptors [58]. The specific mechanisms producing esophageal chest pain are not well understood. Investigation has centered on the evaluation of esophageal sensitivity to chemical and mechanical stimuli; the finding that multiple stimuli may produce identical symptoms in some individuals with chest pain has led to the acceptance of the concept of an *irritable esophagus* [59,60]. Although acid sensitivity from gastroesophageal reflux is believed to be a source of noncardiac chest pain (NCCP), the

relationship between acid reflux events and symptoms is poor, with the majority of reflux events not found to cause symptoms during prolonged pH monitoring [17]. A potential role of more proximal esophageal acid exposure in causing chest pain is suggested by a recent study [61], which also suggested that patients with chest pain without heartburn symptoms differ from those who have these symptoms by having lower overall acid-reflux parameters. Although the temperature of an ingested bolus may alter esophageal motility, warmth increases speed and frequency of peristaltic contractions [62], whereas cold results in a relative paralysis and distention of the distal esophagus [63], it has not been clearly shown that patients with NCCP have altered temperature-induced sensitivity when compared with asymptomatic controls. It had been proposed that hyperosmolarity of ingested substances could be a mechanism for production of chest symptoms, but infusion of a hypertonic liquid failed to produce chest pain in at least one study of patients with NCCP [64]. Sensitivity to mechanical stimuli has been demonstrated with intraesophageal balloon distention studies in patients with NCCP, a positive test result providing reproduction of usual pain symptoms with inflation of the balloon. Acute distention as a mechanism for pain has been suggested from a study of dysfunction of the belch reflex in some individuals [20]. Esophageal myoischemia has been proposed as a possible mechanism for pain when intense esophageal contactile activity might interrupt the usual intramural blood flow [18].

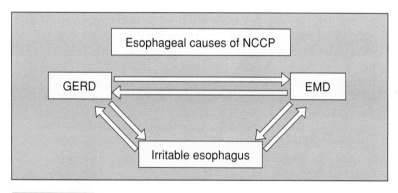

FIGURE 9-6.

Mechanisms of esophageal chest pain: issues. Acid reflux may induce esophageal motility changes with possible chest symptoms, but it also may provoke bronchial or cardiac reflexes involved in

pain sensation from the chest. Patients with noncardiac chest pain (NCCP) often have documented esophageal motility disorders, but the relationship between abnormal contraction patterns and pain symptoms is not well understood. Motility disturbances found at the time of stationary esophageal testing are most often asymptomatic; motility changes documented at prolonged monitoring are also often not symptomatic. Some have suggested that these changes in motility should be viewed as an epiphenomenon of chronic chest pain [34], rather than causative of symptoms. In patients with NCCP simultaneously monitored for acid reflux and dysmotility, many patients are discovered to have multiple causes to explain their symptoms [36,65], suggesting esophageal sensitivity to various stimuli is capable of producing identical chest pain symptoms (the *irritable esophagus*, previously mentioned) [60,66]. EMD—esophageal motility disorders; GERD—gastroesophageal reflux disease.

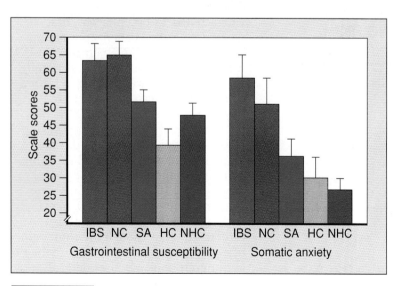

FIGURE 9-7.

Psychologic factors in noncardiac chest pain (NCCP). This figure shows the results of the average score for values (plus or minus the

standard error of the mean) on the Millon Behavioral Health Inventory scales of gastrointestinal susceptibility and somatic anxiety for five study groups: irritable bowel syndrome (IBS); nutcracker esophagus (NC); structural esophageal abnormalities—rings or esophagitis (SA); hospital healthy controls (HC); and nonhospital healthy controls (NHC). Subjects in the NC and IBS groups scored significantly higher ($P < 0.05$) on both scales than did all other subject groups. This pattern suggests that these patients react to psychologic stress with frequent and severe gastrointestinal symptoms and display hypochondriacal tendencies and unusual amounts of fear about bodily dysfunction.

Patients with gastroesophageal reflux disease whose symptoms correlate poorly with acid-reflux events differ significantly in their psychosocial profiles from those with good symptom–reflux association, showing more trait anxiety and hysteria, and having less adequate social support structures; these factors may be important in the etiology of their symptoms and in their management [67].

Unlike patients with IBS, patients with NCCP are less likely to have been sexually or physically abused; however, those who had been abused had significantly altered pain perception, higher levels of functional disability, and greater number of psychiatric disorders [68]. (*Adapted from* Richter [24].)

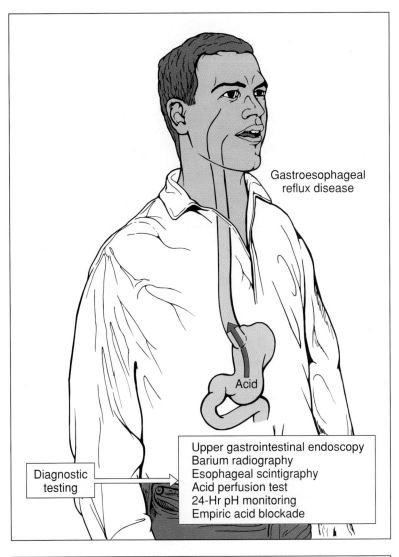

FIGURE 9-8.

Diagnostic testing to determine the relationship of gastroesophageal reflux disease (GERD) to noncardiac chest pain (NCCP). GERD is the most commonly identified esophageal cause of NCCP and data from 24-hour ambulatory pH monitoring show abnormal acid reflux in about half of patients [7,15,26,27]. Barium radiographic studies and upper gastrointestinal endoscopy may identify structural lesions from GERD that may be associated with chest pain symptoms; upper endoscopy has been shown to be a useful tool in identifying patients with acid-related upper gastrointestinal disease in whom acid-perfusion studies were negative [69]. Although esophageal scintiscanning can detect gastroesophageal reflux noninvasively with excellent sensitivity and can quantify amounts of reflux [70], it has not gained wide usage clinically for the detection of GERD in NCCP evaluations and remains mostly a research tool. For most patients, investigation for GERD will involve upper esophageal endoscopy, with mucosal biopsy to check for histologic reflux changes if endoscopically normal, followed by acid-perfusion testing with or without prolonged ambulatory esophageal pH monitoring.

Gastroesophageal reflux disease

Acid

Diagnostic testing

Upper gastrointestinal endoscopy
Barium radiography
Esophageal scintigraphy
Acid perfusion test
24-Hr pH monitoring
Empiric acid blockade

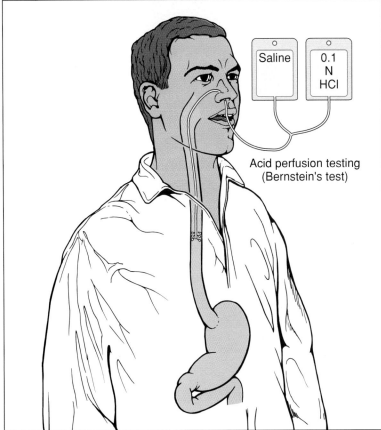

FIGURE 9-9.

Acid-perfusion (Bernstein) test. As originally described by Bernstein and Baker [71], a patient is seated upright with a nasogastric tube placed into the midesophagus and, with the patient blinded to the administration, normal saline solution and dilute hydrochloric acid (0.1 N HCl) are alternatively infused into the esophageal lumen. A positive test result is one in which acid infusion produces the patient's usual chest pain, whereas infusion of saline does not and in fact, may relieve the symptoms provoked by the acid. The cause of pain from acid perfusion of the esophagus has been attributed to triggered chemoreceptors, induction of dysmotility, or acid sensitivity of normal and inflamed mucosa.

Saline

0.1
N
HCl

Acid perfusion testing
(Bernstein's test)

TABLE 9-2. SUMMARY OF PUBLISHED EXPERIENCES WITH ACID-PERFUSION TEST (GER)

FIRST AUTHOR, YR	GER PATIENTS	CONTROLS	SENSITIVITY	SPECIFICITY
Bernstein, 1958	19/22 (86%)	1/21 (5%)	86%	95%
Siegel, 1963	25/25 (100%)	0/25 (0%)	100%	100%
Bennett, 1966	28/29 (97%)	6/15 (40%)	97%	60%
Benz, 1972	29/29 (100%)	3/21 (14%)	100%	86%
Battle, 1973	37/89 (42%)	0/24 (0%)	42%	100%
Behar, 1976	68/77 (88%)	3/20 (15%)	88%	85%
Breen, 1978	23/27 (85%)	7/14 (50%)	85%	50%
Total	229/298 (77%)	20/140 (14%)	77%	86%

Only results of studies with control subjects and heartburn as clinical endpoint are shown here.

TABLE 9-2.

Sensitivity and specificity measurements for the acid-perfusion test in patients with gastroesophageal reflux. GER—gastroesophageal reflux. (*Adapted from* Richter [72].)

TABLE 9-3. SUMMARY OF PUBLISHED EXPERIENCES WITH ACID-PERFUSION TEST (NCCP)

FIRST AUTHOR, YR	NCCP PATIENTS	AP+	SENSITIVITY	SPECIFICITY
Nasrallah, 1987	51	12%	—	—
Ghillebert, 1990	50	36%	—	—
Janssens, 1984	60	27%	15%	70%
De Caestecker, 1988	60	35%	59%	74%
Humeau, 1990	38	26%	30%	75%
Hewson, 1989	71	49%	59%	59%
Richter, 1991	75	20%	26%	85%

TABLE 9-3.

Sensitivity and specificity of the acid perfusion test in patients with noncardiac chest pain (NCCP). Experience with acid-perfusion testing in patients with NCCP has revealed good specificity but poor sensitivity, especially when compared with prolonged ambulatory monitoring [73]. AP+—positive result from acid-perfusion test. (*Adapted from* Bruley des Varannes [59].)

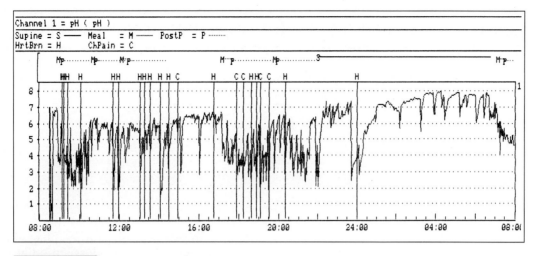

FIGURE 9-10.

Ambulatory esophageal pH monitoring can reveal correlation of symptoms and acid-reflux events. Small, compact devices are in use for continuous intraesophageal recording from 2-mm flexible pH probes placed transnasally with the distal recording tip at 5 cm above the lower esophageal sphincter. Downloading of the stored recorded data permits a correlation of symptoms and reflux events (pH dropping to 4 or less). Parameters of total esophageal acid exposure time, total number of reflux events, duration of reflux episodes, upright versus supine acid reflux, and relationship to meal intake are determined. A symptom index can be calculated by dividing the total number of chest pain episodes into the number of them associated with acid reflux. A positive symptom score may be found in some patients in whom the other reflux parameters were normal; this helps to direct therapy.

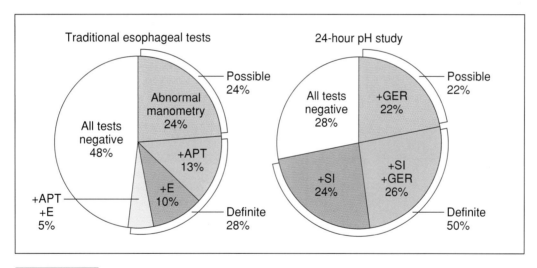

FIGURE 9-11.

Comparison between the diagnostic yield of traditional esophageal tests and 24-hour esophageal monitoring in 100 consecutive patients with noncardiac chest pain (NCCP). An esophageal test was defined as *definitely* identifying the esophagus as a cause of chest pain if provocative testing replicated the patient's usual chest pain or the patient's sponta-neous chest pain correlated with episodes of acid reflux (positive symptom index) during 24-hour pH monitoring. Abnormal stationary manometry or acid-reflux parameters without associated chest pain only suggested the esophagus as a *possible* cause of the symp-toms. Esophageal pH monitoring with symptom index was significantly superior ($P <$ 0.001) to traditional esophageal tests in definitively identifying the esophagus as a cause of chest pain symptoms. +APT—positive acid perfusion test; +E—positive edrophonium test; +GER—abnormal acid-reflux parameters; +SI—positive symptom index. (*Adapted from* Richter [74].)

TABLE 9-4. COMPARISON OF TEST RESULTS IN PATIENTS WITH NONCARDIAC CHEST PAIN (*N*=17)

	OMEPRAZOLE, 80MG	24-HR pH SYMPTOM INDEX	BERNSTEIN TEST	PLACEBO
Sensitivity (13)	69%	92%	46%	7.7%
Specificity (4)	75%	100%	50%	25%
Predictive value (+)	75%	100%	75%	25%
Predictive value (–)	43%	80%	78%	7.7%

TABLE 9-4.

Single-dose omeprazole as a test for noncardiac chest pain (NCCP). In patients with either biopsy-proven esophagitis or positive symptom index to indicate an esophageal acid–related NCCP, the single-dose omeprazole test had similar efficacy to identify an acid sensitive esophagus as 24-hour pH monitoring with symptom index; it was superior to the Bernstein test [30]. A single 80-mg dose of omeprazole relieved chest pain symptoms in 10 of 17 patients with NCCP compared with 1 of 17 treated with placebo (*P* < 0.015) in this pilot study. Similar results for improvement of symptoms in patients with gastroesophageal reflux disease (GERD) and NCCP treated with high-dose ranitidine have been reported [31]. In a study of patients with nutcracker esophagus found at time of manometry, 35% had evidence of abnormal reflux and 83% of these patients obtained significant improvement of symptoms following 8 weeks of medical antireflux therapy, with less frequent pain episodes, fewer number of days with pain, and diminished pain severity [75]. (*Adapted from* Squillace [30].)

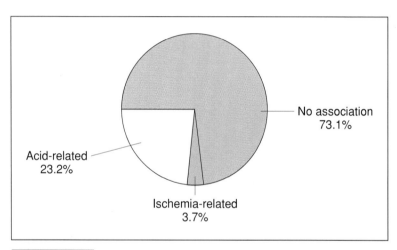

FIGURE 9-12.

Reflux-associated chest pain is also common in patients with demonstrated obstructive coronary artery disease. As demonstrated in this figure, prolonged esophageal pH monitoring combined with simultaneous (Holter) cardiac monitoring defined the percentage of pain episodes attributed to acid reflux or myocardial ischemia in 30 patients with 164 episodes of chest pain [32]. Of these patients, 20 (67%) had at least one episode of chest pain related to an acid-reflux event, and nearly 75% of patients had improvement in chest pain with the use of acid-supressive therapy. (*Adapted from* Singh *et al* [32].)

TABLE 9-5. ESOPHAGEAL MOTILITY DISORDERS IN NONCARDIAC CHEST PAIN

Achalasia
    Absent peristalsis in esophageal body*
    Incomplete LES relaxation*
    Hypertensive LES[†]
    Elevated intraesophageal pressures relative to gastric pressure[†]
Diffuse esophageal spasm
    Simultaneous contractions (>10% of wet swallows)*
    Intermittent normal peristalsis*
    Repetitive or prolonged contractions[†]
    High-amplitude and spontaneous contractions[†]
    LES hypertensive with or without incomplete relaxation[†]
Nutcracker esophagus
    Normal peristalsis*
    High-amplitude contractions*
    Long-duration contractions[†]
Hypertensive LES
    Elevated resting LES pressure*
    Normal LES relaxation*
    Normal peristalsis*
Nonspecific esophageal motility disorder (NEMD)
    Abnormal motility other than already noted*
    Nontransmitted contractions[†]
    Multiple-peaked contractions[†]
    Incomplete LES relaxation[†]
    Prolonged contractions[†]

*Required for diagnosis. [†]Associated findings.

TABLE 9-5.

Esophageal motility disorders in noncardiac chest pain. LES—lower esophageal sphincter.

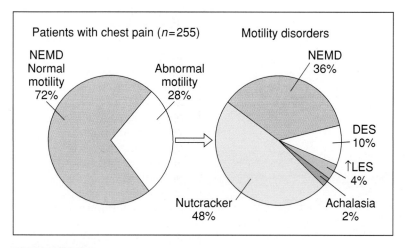

FIGURE 9-13.

Abnormal esophageal motility was present in 255 (28%) of 910 patients in whom noncardiac chest pain (NCCP) was evaluated [9]. Most of these patients had nutcracker esophagus or nonspecific motility disorders; the other primary motor disorders of achalasia, hypertensive lower esophageal sphincter, and diffuse eophageal

spasm were found less commonly. These findings have been confirmed by others [26,53,76].

Although some of the motor disorders may directly relate to causation of pain through mechanisms of spasm and distention, most investigators now consider the esophageal motility disorders to be an epiphenomenon found in patients with chronic chest pain or as a response to stress [34,35]. Contributing to this changing view are data that demonstrate that pain is most often *not present* during stationary manometry when abnormal motor events are recorded; it is the minority of patients undergoing ambulatory motor studies who have a motility disorder during an episode of pain [11]. The findings that successful resolution of chest pain symptoms may occur in the absence of any significant change in the underlying esophageal motor abnormalities [78], and that esophageal motility disorders may be treated with little effect on chest pain symptoms [79] have encouraged questions about the etiologic role of motor disorders in NCCP. Of further interest is the finding that 35% of patients with nutcracker esophagus were shown to have evidence of gastroesophageal reflux disease and that acid-suppressive therapy improved symptoms in 83% [75]. DES—diffuse esophageal spasm; LES—hypertensive lower esophageal sphincter; NEMD—nonspecific esophageal motility disorders. (*Adapted from* Richter [77].)

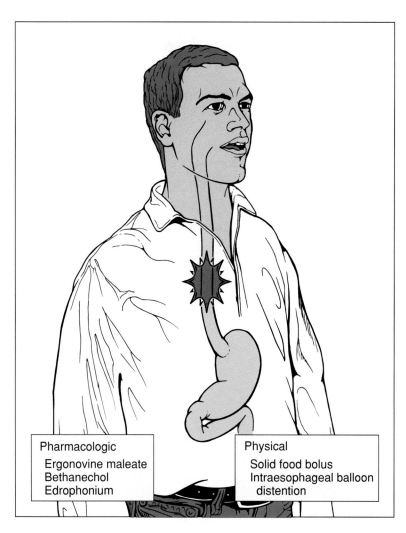

FIGURE 9-14.

Provocative testing attempts to reproduce esophageal chest pain while patients are undergoing stationary evaluations. Provocative testing can increase the yield of esophageal causes over baseline testing, as seen in Figure 9-15. Issues in the interpretation of provocative testing include that the provoked chest pain may not be the same as spontaneous chest pain and a baseline dysmotility does not predict positive provocative tests. Historically, ergonovine maleate and bethanecol were used as esophageal provocative agents; however, they are limited in their usefulness by causing significant side effects (*eg*, coronary spasm, headache, nausea, pain at the injection site, sweating) [37,38]. The most frequently used esophageal provocative test is parenteral administration of edrophonium, a cholinesterase inhibitor, which produces increased esophageal contraction amplitude and duration in normals and patients with noncardiac chest pain (NCCP). A positive test result is one in which reproduction of the patient's usual chest discomfort occurs while the patient swallows water, within minutes of the edrophonium intravenous injection, but not following injection of a saline placebo. The edrophonium challenge test is believed to be specific for the esophagus, produces few side effects, and provokes chest pain in 20% to 30% of patients with NCCP [39,40]. The interaction between patient and test administrator may influence the results of edrophonium provocative testing in patients with NCCP, demonstrating the powerful influence of coaching on the outcome of the study [80].

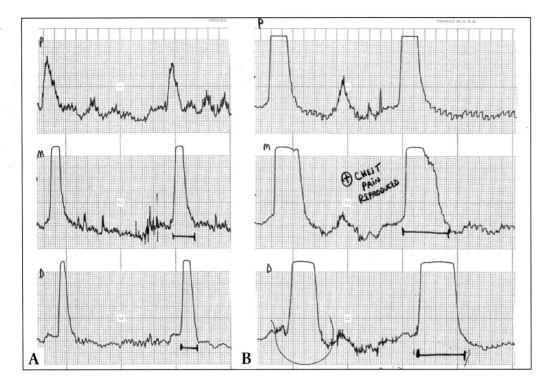

FIGURE 9-15.

Result of edrophonium testing in a patient with noncardiac chest pain. Edrophonium given as 80 mcg/kg body weight intravenously. Although an increase in amplitude and duration of esophageal contractions may be seen in anyone following administration of edrophonium, the reproduction of the patients' usual chest pain makes this a positive test. **Panel A** equals baseline; **panel B** equals edrophonium. P—proximal; M—middle; D—distal.

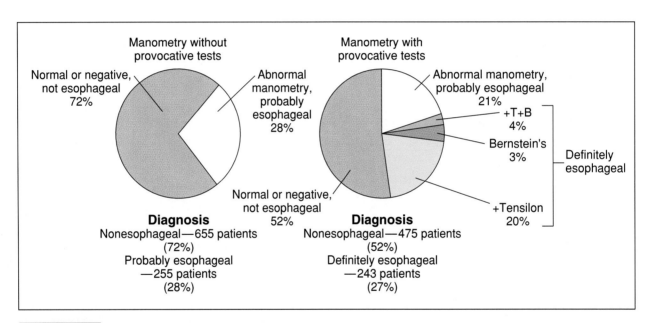

FIGURE 9-16.

Diagnostic yield of esophageal testing in 910 consecutive patients with noncardiac chest pain [9]. Manometry alone identified the esophagus as a "probable" cause of chest pain, based on abnormal stationary motility patterns, in 28% of patients. Acid-perfusion and edrophonium (Tensilon [T]) provocative testing definitely reproduced esophageal chest pain in 27%, and thus increased the overall yield of esophageal causes to 48%. B—Bernstein's test. (*Adapted from* Richter [72].)

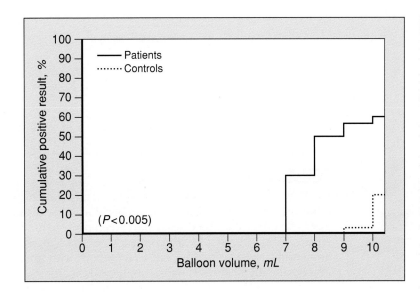

FIGURE 9-17.

Response to intraesophageal balloon distention in 30 noncardiac chest pain (NCCP) patients and 30 controls. In all, 60% of patients with NCCP experienced pain with balloon distention compared with only 20% of controls developing chest pain with this provocative test [21]. The patients with NCCP developed pain at smaller distention volumes than controls, suggesting a lower pain threshold to esophageal distention, or altered nociception. This heightened visceral awareness is similar to that seen in patients with irritable bowel syndrome in whom distention of the rectosigmoid colon by balloon inflation provoked abdominal pain at smaller balloon volumes than those volumes that produced pain in healthy controls [81]. (*Adapted from* Richter [72].)

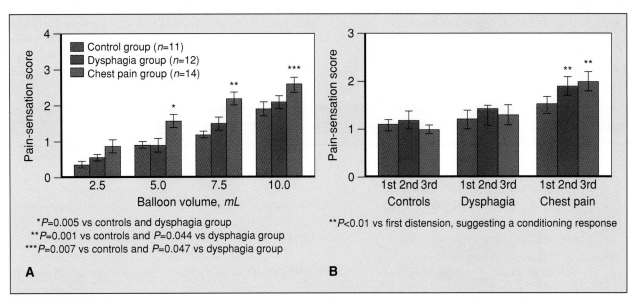

FIGURE 9-18.

A–B, Repeated esophageal balloon distension: effect on esophageal sensitivity. Pain-sensation scores varied directly with balloon volume, and mean pain scores were significantly higher for the chest pain group. In the controls and dysphagia group, pain-sensation scores were not significantly different between the first, second, or third distension at a given volume. In the chest pain group, however, pain-sensation scores increased significantly following repeated balloon distension using the same volume, suggesting a conditioning phenomenon associated with a visceral sensory abnormality. (*Adapted from* Paterson [22].)

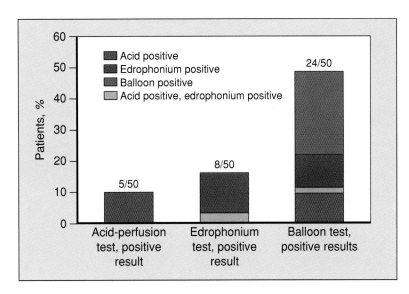

FIGURE 9-19.

Chest pain response to provocative testing [41]. Intraesophageal acid perfusion produced chest pain in 5 of 50 patients (10%) whereas intravenous edrophonium produced pain in 8 of 50 patients (16%). Overall, with one patient positively responding to both acid perfusion and edrophonium, these two tests identified an esophageal cause in 12 of 50 patients (24%). A positive result of a balloon distention test ocurred in 11 of these patients as well as identifying an additional 13 patients, increasing the diagnostic yield of esophageal causes to 48% (24 of 50 patients). (*Adapted from* Barrish [41].)

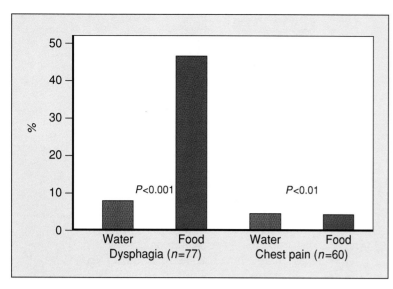

FIGURE 9-20.

Percentage of patients with a motility abnormality in the esophageal body during water swallows or food ingestion. Solid bolus ingestion significantly increased the percentage of symptomatic motor abnormalities in patients with dysphagia, but for patients with noncardiac chest pain the solid food challenge did not increase the rare reporting of symptoms that followed water ingestion [82]. (*Adapted from* Allen [82].)

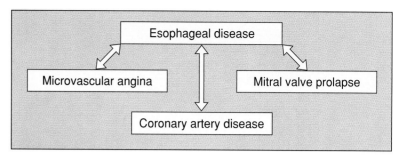

FIGURE 9-21.

Esophageal causes of chest pain may coexist in patients with demonstrated cardiac disease. Esophageal motility disorders and gastroesophageal reflux disease have been documented in from 10% to 67% of patients with abnormal coronary arteriograms and angina-like chest pain [32,83,84]. In patients with microvascular angina and atypical chest pain, esophageal disorders can be documented in 23% to 75% [43,85,86]. From 52% to 86% of patients with chest pain and documented mitral valve prolapse are shown to have esophageal disorders as evidenced by routine and provocative testing [87–89]. Interestingly, gastroesophageal reflux may lower the anginal threshold in some patients [90]; some investigators have shown esophageal acid perfusion to induce electrocardiographic changes of myocardial ischemia [91], although two recent reports do not support this finding [32,92].

TABLE 9-6A. EVALUATION OF 281 PATIENTS WITH NONCARDIAC CHEST PAIN

FIRST AUTHOR, YR	NO. OF PATIENTS TESTED	24-HOUR pH/PRESSURE RECORDING SHOWED ≥1 PAIN EPISODE IN RELATION TO, %			PROVOCATION TEST, %			OVERALL ASSESSMENT, %		
		ACID	ABNORMAL MOTILITY	BOTH	ACID	EDROPHONIUM	BALLOON	ACID SENSITIVITY	MECHANO SENSITIVITY	IRRITABLE ESOPHAGUS
Janssens, 1986	60	7	13	15	27	ND	ND	20	8	20
Peters, 1988	24	21	17	17	35	50	ND	25	29	29
Soffer, 1989	20	30	5	15	10	0	ND	30	5	15
Hewson, 1990	45	24	11	11	33	53	ND	13	22	44
Ghillebert, 1990	50	26	8	4	36	32	5	26	8	26
Humeau, 1990	45	20	ND	ND	10	15	38	16	21	12
Nevens, 1991	37	11	3	3	38	19	8	19	8	22
Total	281	18%	10%	10%	28%	30%	19%	20%	14%	24%

TABLE 9-6.

A–B, Identical esophageal noncardiac chest pain (NCCP) may be induced by a variety of stimuli: the irritable esophagus concept. Some patients experience their usual chest pain when (1) induced by acid reflux; (2) at a time of abnormal motor activity with no accompanying reflux; (3) following edrophonium challenge; or (4) during intraesophageal balloon distention. This sensitivity to a variety of stimuli producing identical chest symptoms has been termed *irritable esophagus* [60,66], a concept also applied to hypersensitivity of the esophagus to stimuli not producing symptoms in healthy controls. Details from long-term monitoring studies of 281

(*continued on next page*)

TABLE 9-6B. CRITERIA FOR PATIENTS WITH CHEST PAIN OF ESOPHAGEAL ORIGIN

PATIENT GROUP	CHARACTERISTIC
Acid-sensitive esophagus	Spontaneous pain episodes related to acid reflux (with or without accompanying motor disorders)
Mechano-sensitive esophagus	With or without positive result of acid perfusion test
	Spontaneous pain episodes related to motility disturbances without reflux
	With or without positive result of edrophonium test
Irritable esophagus	With or without positive result of balloon distention test
	Some spontaneous pain episodes related to reflux, others related to abnormal motility without reflux
	Spontaneous pain episodes related to acid reflux, and positive edrophonium test with or without balloon distention test
	Spontaneous pain episodes related to abnormal motility without reflux, and positive acid perfusion test
	Both acid perfusion test and edrophonium with or without balloon distention test positive

TABLE 9-6. (*CONTINUED*)

patients with NCCP show an acid-sensitive esophagus in 20%, a mechanosensitive esophagus in 14%, and an irritable esophagus in 24% [23]. This heightened sensitivity to various stimuli is also noted in patients with irritable bowel syndrome [93] and suggests that an altered nociception contributes to increased symptom-reporting. (*Adapted from* Janssens [23].)

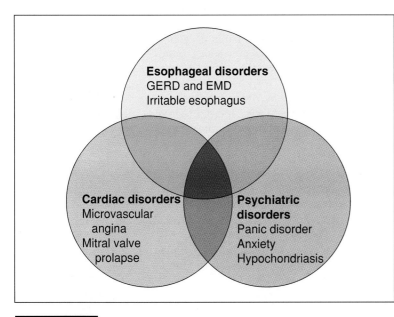

FIGURE 9-22.

Emerging overlap concept of altered pain sensitivity. Patients with panic disorders score high in measures of anxiety and hypochondriasis, and panic attack symptoms overlap with those of chest pain of esophageal origin and microvascular angina having fear of dying, shortness of breath, choking or smothering sensation, palpitations, chest pain or discomfort, sweating, faintness, dizziness, and nausea, among others. Patients with microvascular angina have been shown to frequently have demonstrable esophageal motility disorders and heightened visceral awareness of acid exposure and esophageal distension. Abnormal nociception may link esophageal with coronary smooth muscle sensitivity; patients with microvascular angina frequently have their pain provoked during injection of intracoronary contrast media and, as has been pointed out, patients with chest pain of esophageal origin may have heightened sensitivity to esophageal distension with balloon provocation. Investigators have shown a co-occurrence that is common between panic disorder symptoms and mitral valve prolapse. This is not likely cause and effect, but rather a heightened sensitivity in the susceptible patient. A generalized disorder of smooth muscle sensitivity gives rise to the "irritable person," manifesting itself with symptoms referable to the esophagus, the bowel, the heart, or other organ systems. These various symptoms arise as physiologic responses to stress. A comprehensive approach to diagnosis and treatment in the patient with atypical chest pain is mandatory. GERD—gastroesophageal reflux disease; EMD—esophageal motility disorders.

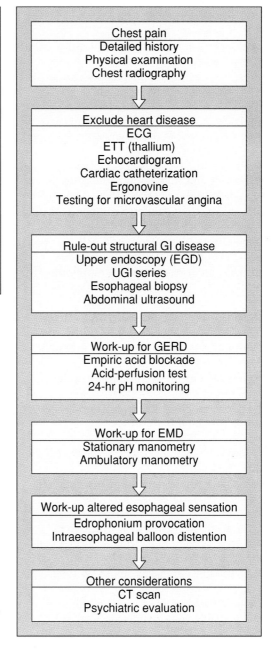

FIGURE 9-23.

Diagnostic approach to patients presenting with chest pain. CT—computed tomography; CXR—chest x-ray (radiography); EGD—esophagogastroduodenoscopy; ETT—exercise tolerance test; GERD–gastroesophageal reflux disease; GI—gastrointestinal.

REFERENCES

1. Chambers J, Bass C: Chest pain with normal coronary anatomy: A review of natural history and possible etiologic factors. *Prog Cardiovasc Dis* 1990, 33:161–184.

2. Wielgosz AI, *et al.*: Unimproved chest pain in patients with minimal or no coronary disease: A behavioral phenomenon. *Am Heart J* 1984, 108:67–72.

3. Kemp HG, *et al.*: The anginal syndrome associated with normal coronary arteriogram: Report of a six-year experience. *Am J Med* 1973, 54:735–742.

4. Ockene IS, *et al.*: Unexplained chest pain in patients with normal coronary arteriograms: A follow-up study of functional status. *N Engl J Med* 1980, 30:1249–1252.

5. Ward BW, *et al.*: Long-term follow-up of symptomatic status of patients with non-cardiac chest pain: Is diagnosis of esophageal etiology helpful? *Am J Gastroenterol* 1987, 82:215–218.

6. Swift GL, *et al.*: A long-term clinical review of patients with oesophageal pain. *Q J Med* 1991, 295:937–944.

7. DeMeester TR, *et al.*: Esophageal function in patients with angina-like chest pain and normal coronary angiogram. *Ann Surg* 1982, 196:488–498.

8. Kline M, *et al.*: Esophageal disease in patients with angina-like chest pain. *Am J Gastroenterol* 1982, 75:116–123.

9. Katz PO, *et al.*: Esophageal testing in patients with non-cardiac chest pain and/or dysphagia. *Ann Intern Med* 1987, 106:593–597.

10. Breumelhof R, *et al.*: Analysis of 24-hour esophageal pressure and pH data in unselected patients with noncardiac chest pain. *Gastroenterology* 1990, 99:1257–1264.

11. Ghillebert G, *et al.*: Ambulatory 24-hour intraesophageal pH and pressure recordings v provocation tests in the diagnosis of chest pain of oesophageal origin. *Gut* 1990, 31:738–744.

12. Hewson EG, Dalton CB, Richter JE: Comparison of esophageal manometry, provocative testing, and ambulatory monitoring in patients with unexplained chest pain. *Dig Dis Sci* 1990, 35:302–309.

13. Lam HG, *et al.*: Acute non-cardiac chest pain on a coronary care unit: A diagnostic challenge. *Gastroenterology* 1990, 98:74A.

14. Smout AJPM, *et al.*: Ambulatory esophageal monitoring in noncardiac chest pain. *Am J Med* 1992, 92(Suppl 5A):74s–80s.

15. Hewson EG, *et al.*: Twenty-four-hour esophageal pH monitoring: The most useful test for evaluating noncardaice chest pain. *Am J Med* 1991, 90:576–583.

16. Alban-Davies H, *et al.*: Angina-like chest pain: Differentiation for cardiac pain by history. *J Clin Gastroenterol* 1985, 7:477–481.

17. DeMeester TR, *et al.*: Patterns of gastroesophageal reflux in health and disease. *Ann Surg* 1976, 184:459–470.

18. MacKenzie J, *et al.*: Oesophageal ischemia in motility disorders associated with chest pain. *Lancet* 1988, 2:592–595.

19. Meyer GW, Castell DO: Human esophageal response during chest pain induced by swallowing cold liquids. *JAMA* 1981, 246:2057–2059.

20. Kahrilas PJ, Dodds WJ, Hogan WJ: Dysfunction of the belch reflex. *Gastroenterology* 1987, 93:818–822.

21. Richter JE, Barish CF, Castell DO: Abnormal sensory perception in patients with esophageal chest pain. *Gastroenterology* 1986, 91:845–852.

22. Paterson WG, Wang H, Vanner SJ: Increasing pain sensation to repeated esophageal balloon distension in patients with chest pain of undetermined etiology. *Dig Dis Sci* 1995, 40:1325–1331.

23. Janssens JP, Vantrappen G: Irritable esophagus. *Am J Med* 1992, 92(5A):27s–32s.

24. Richter JE, *et al.*: Psychological comparison of patients with nutcracker esophagus and irrritable bowel syndrome. *Dig Dis Sci* 1986, 31:131–138.

25. Beitman BD: Panic disorder in patients with angiographically normal coronary arteries. *Am J Med* 1992, 92(5A):33s–40s.

26. De Caestecker JS, *et al.*: The oesophagus as a cause of recurrent chest pain: Which patients should be investigated and which tests should be used? *Lancet* 1985, 2:1143–1146.

27. Schofield PM, *et al.*: Exertional gastroesophageal reflux: A mechanism for symptoms in patients with angina pectoris and normal coronary angiograms. *Br Med J* 1987, 294:1459–1461.

28. Hewson EG, *et al.*: The prevalence of abnormal esophageal test results in patients with cardiovascular disease and unexplained chest pain. *Arch Intern Med* 1990, 150:965–969.

29. Wiener GJ, *et al.*: The symptom index: A clinically important parameter of ambulatory 24-hour esophageal pH monitoring. *Am J Gastroenterol* 1988, 83:358–361.

30. Squillace SJ, Young MF, Sanowski RA: Single dose omeprazole as a test for noncardiac chest pain [Abstract]. *Gastroenterology* 1993, 104:A197.

31. Stahl WG, *et al.*: Diagnosis and treatment of patients with gastroesophageal reflux and noncardiac chest pain. *South Med J* 1994, 87:739–742.

32. Singh S, *et al.*: The contribution of gastroesophageal reflux to chest pain in patients with coronary artery disease. *Ann Intern Med* 1992, 117:824–830.

33. Herrington JP, Burns TW, Balart LA: Chest pain and dysphagia in patients with prolonged peristaltic contractile duration of the esophagus. *Dig Dis Sci* 1984, 29:134–140.

34. Dalton CB, Castell DO, Richter JE: The changing faces of the nutcracker esophagus. *Am J Gastroenterol* 1988, 83:623–628.

35. Anderson KO, *et al.*: Stress: A modulator of esophageal pressures in healthy volunteers and non-cardiac chest pain patients. *Dig Dis Sci* 1989, 34:83–91.

36. Janssens J, Vantrappen G: Ambulatory intraesophageal pH and pressure measurements. *Front Gastrointest Res* 1994, 22:176–187.

37. Eastwood GL, *et al.*: Use of ergonovine to identify esophageal spasm in patients with chest pain. *Ann Intern Med* 1981, 94:768–771.

38. Nostrant TT: Provocation testing in noncardiac chest pain. *Am J Med* 1992, 92:56s–64s.

39. Dalton CB, *et al.*: The edrophonium provocative test in non-cardiac chest pain: Evaluation of testing techniques. *Dig Dis Sci* 1990, 35:1445–1451.

40. Richter JE, *et al.*: Edrophonium: A useful provocative test for esophageal chest pain. *Ann Intern Med* 1985, 103:14–21.

41. Barish CF, Castell DO, Richter JE: Graded esophageal balloon distension: A new provocative test for non-cardiac chest pain. *Dig Dis Sci* 1986, 31:1292–1298.

42. Deschner WK, *et al.*: Intraesophageal balloon distention versus drug provocation in the evaluation of noncardiac chest pain. *Am J Gastroenterol* 1990, 85:938–943.

43. Cannon RO, *et al.*: Coronary flow reserve, esophageal motility, and chest pain in patients with angiographically normal coronary arteries. *Am J Med* 1990, 88:217–220.

44. Cannon RO, *et al.*: Abnormal cardiac sensitivity in patients with chest pain and normal coronary arteries. *J Am Coll Cardiol* 1990, 16:1359–1366.

45. Cannon RO, *et al.*: Imipramine in patients with chest pain despite normal coronary angiograms. *N Engl J Med* 1994, 330:1411–1417.

46. Wooley CF: From irritable heart to mitral valve prolapse: British army medical reports, 1860 to 1870. *Am J Cardiol* 1985, 55:1107–1109.

47. Jarcho S: Functional heart disease in the Civil War (DaCosta, 1871). *Am J Cardiol* 1959, 29:809–817.

48. Osler W: Principles and Practice of Medicine. New York: D. Appleton and Company; 1982.

49. Hertz AF: The Sensitivity of the Alimentary Canal. London: Oxford University Press; 1911.

50. Plummer HS, Vinson PP: Cardiospasm: A report of 301 cases. *Med Clin North Am* 1921, 5:335–369.

51. Schmidt CD, *et al.*: The value of the esophageal motility test in evaluation of thoracic pain problems. *Dis Chest* 1962, 41:303–314.

52. Benjamin SB, Gerhardt DC, Castell DO: High amplitude peristaltic contractions associated with chest pain and/or dysphagia. *Gastroenterology* 1979, 77:478–483.

53. Brand DL, Martin D, Pope CE: Esophageal manometrics in patients with angina-like chest pain. *Am J Dig Dis* 1977, 22:300–304.

54. Chobanian SJ, *et al.*: Systematic evaluation of patients with noncardiac chest pain. *Arch Intern Med* 1986, 146:1505–1508.

55. Alban-Davies H, Rhodes J: Follow-up of patients with esophageal angina. *JAMA* 1986, 255:2021.

56. Rose S, Achkar E, Easley KA: Follow-up of patients with noncardiac chest pain: Value of esophageal testing. *Dig Dis Sci* 1994, 39:2063–2068.

57. Alban-Davies H: Anginal pain of esophageal origin: Clinical presentation, prevalence and prognosis. *Am J Med* 1992, 92:5s–10s.

58. Lynn RB: Mechanisms of esophageal pain. *Am J Med* 1992, 92:11s–19s.

59. Bruley des Varannes S, Galmiche JP: Evaluation of esophageal sensitivity. *Front Gastrointest Res* 1994, 22:344–365.

60. Vantrappen G, Janssens J: What is irritable esophagus: Another point of view. *Gastroenterology* 1988, 94:1092–1093.

61. Waring JP, *et al.*: Unexplained chest pain: Is proximal reflux playing a role [Abstract]? *Gastroenterology* 1995, 108:A253.

62. Winship DH, Viegas de Andrade SR, Zboralske FF: Influence of bolus temperature on human esophageal motor function. *J Clin Invest* 1970, 49:243–250.

63. Kaye MD, Kilby AE, Harper PC: Changes in distal esophageal function in response to cooling. *Dig Dis Sci* 1987, 32:22–27.

64. Nasrallah SM, Hendrix EA: Comparison of hypertonic glucose to other provocative tests in patients with noncardiac chest pain. *Am J Gastroenterology* 1987, 82:406–409.

65. Peters LJ, *et al.*: Spontaneous non-cardiac chest pain: Evaluation by 24-hour ambulatory motility/pH monitoring. *Gastroenterology* 1988, 94:878–886.

66. Vantrappen G, Janssens J, Ghillebert G: The irritable esophagus: A frequent cause of angina-like chest pain. *Lancet* 1987, 1:1232–1234.

67. Johnston BT, *et al.*: Acid perception in gastro-oesophageal reflux disease in dependent on psychosocial factors. *Scand J Gastroenterol* 1995, 30:1–5.

68. Scarinci IC, *et al.*: Altered pain perception and psychosocial features among women with gastrointestinal disorders and history of abuse: A preliminary model. *Am J Med* 1994, 97:108–118.

69. Hsia PC, *et al.*: Utility of upper endoscopy in the evaluation of noncardiac chest pain. *Gastrointest Endosc* 1991, 37:22–26.

70. Fisher RS, *et al.*: Gastroesophageal (GE) scintiscanning to detect and quantitate GE reflux. *Gastroenterology* 1976, 70:301–308.

71. Bernstein LM, Baker LA: A clinical test for esophagitis. *Gastroenterology* 1958, 34:760–781.

72. Richter JE: Provocative tests in esophageal diseases. *Front Gastrointest Res* 1994, 22:188–208.

73. Richter JE, *et al.*: Acid perfusion test and 24-hour esophageal pH monitoring with symptom index: Comparison of tests for esophageal acid sensitivity. *Dig Dis Sci* 1991, 36:565–571.

74. Richter JE: Chest Pain and Gastroesophageal Reflux Disease. In *Ambulatory Esophageal pH Monitoring: Practical Approach and Clinical Applications.* Edited by Richter JE. New York: Igaku-Shoin; 1991:115–128.

75. Achem SR, *et al.*: Chest pain associated with nutcracker esophagus: A preliminary study of the role of gastroesophageal reflux. *Am J Gastroenterology* 1993, 88:187–192.

76. Janssens J, Vantrappen G, Ghillebert G: 24-hour recording of esophageal pressure and pH in patients with noncardiac chest pain. *Gastroenterology* 1986, 90:1978–1984.

77. Richter JE, Bradley LA, Castell DO: Esophageal chest pain: Current controversies in pathogenesis, diagnosis, and therapy. *Ann Intern Med* 1989, 110:66–78.

78. Clouse RE, *et al.*: Low dose trazodone for symptomatic patients with esophageal contraction abnormalities: A double-blind, placebo-controlled trial. *Gastroenterology* 1986, 92:1027–1036.

79. Richter JE, *et al.*: Oral nifedipine in the treatment of non-cardiac chest pain patients with the nutcracker esophagus. *Gastroenterology* 1987, 93:21–28.

80. Rose S, *et al.*: Interaction between patient and test administrator may influence the results of edrophonium provocative testing in patients with noncardiac chest pain. *Am J Gastroenterol* 1993, 88:20–24.

81. Whitehead WE, *et al.*: Irritable bowel syndrome: Physiologic and psychological differences between diarrhea-predominant and constipation-predominant patients. *Dig Dis Sci* 1980, 25:404–413.

82. Allen ML, *et al.*: Water swallows versus food ingestion as manometric tests for esophageal dysfunction. *Gastroenterology* 1988, 95:831–833.

83. Svensson O, *et al.*: Oesophageal function and coronary angiogram in patients with disabling chest pain. *Acta Med Scand* 1978, 204:173–178.

84. Gacia-Pulido J, *et al.*: Esophageal contribution to chest pain in patients with coronary artery disease. *Chest* 1990, 98:806–810.

85. Ducrotte PH, *et al.*: Coronary sinus lactate estimation and esophageal abnormalities in angina with normal coronary angiograms. *Dig Dis Sci* 1985, 29:305–310.

86. Cattau EL, *et al.*: Esophageal motility disorders in patients with abnormalities of coronary flow reserve and atypical chest pain [Abstract]. *Gastroenterology* 1987, 92:A1339.

87. Spears PF, Kock KL: Esophageal disorders in patients with chest pain and mitral valve prolapse. *Am J Gastroenterol* 1986, 951–954.

88. Kock KL, *et al.*: Esophageal dysfunction and chest pain in patients with MVP: A prospective study utilizing provocative testing during esophageal manometry. *Am J Med* 1989, 86:32–38.

89. Hewson EG, *et al.*: The prevalence of abnormal esophageal test results in patients with cardiovascular disease and unexplained chest pain. *Arch Intern Med* 1990, 150:965–969.

90. Alban-Davies H, *et al.*: Oesophageal stimulation lowers exertional angina threshold. *Lancet* 1985, 1:1011–1014.

91. Mellow MH, *et al.*: Esophageal acid perfusion in coronary artery disease: Induction of myocardial ischemia. *Gastroenterology* 1983, 83:306–312.

92. Wani M, Hishon S: ECG recording during changes in oesophageal pH. *Gut* 1990, 31:127–128.

93. Tack J, *et al.*: Is the irritable colon really irritable [Abstract]? *Gastroenterology* 1989, 96:A499.

Chapter 10

Therapeutic Esophageal Endoscopy

R. LEE MEYERS

EUGENE M. BOZYMSKI

The advances in therapeutic endoscopy over the last two decades have been impressive and rapid. One can expect that progress in endoscopic therapy will continue and that esophageal disease will be the target of much of that therapy. The esophagus being a long, relatively narrow, tubular structure that transports food from the oropharynx to the stomach is subject to numerous pathologic processes which tend to provoke symptoms that lead the patient to a physician and often then to a gastroenterologist. For example, the proximity of the squamous mucosa of the distal esophagus to the stomach render it susceptible and vulnerable to acid-peptic injury, which may result in a symptomatic peptic stricture. Also, the collateral circulation that develops in the setting of portal hypertension may result in esophageal varices which frequently can present with life threatening hemorrhage. Malignant disease of the esophagus, unfortunately, usually presents late, and the gastroenterologist is often involved in the palliation of patients with these tumors.

The first therapeutic procedures involving the esophagus were dilations of esophageal strictures with various forms of "bougies" (eg, wax candles, whalebones, etc.) and have been performed for centuries. In this century, surgery had been the standard approach to the majority of esophageal disorders (with the notable exception of strictures). Although the first flexible fiberoptic endoscopy was done in 1957, only in the last three decades has therapeutic endoscopy directed toward the esophagus become more widely practiced. This of course was due in large part to advances in the endoscope itself and also the technology one was able to bring to the esophagus with accessories through the biopsy channel. Endoscopic techniques and accessories for dealing with esophageal disease have continued to develop and evolve so that many disorders involving the esophagus can be primarily treated most effectively and safely by the physician through the endoscope.

Through-the-scope balloon dilators and endoscopically placed wires for the guided dilator technique are relatively new and have just flourished since the mid-1980's. Likewise, sclerotherapy, which is now being challenged and replaced in large part by rubber band ligation of varices, has only been generally practiced since the early 1980's. Current new techniques that are exciting include expandable metal stents for the palliation of esophageal malignancy, local injection of botulinum toxin for achalasia, and possibly alcohol injection and photodynamic laser therapy for cancer. We are hoping that advances will be forthcoming to help us manage patients with Barrett's esophagus more easily.

Undoubtedly, new methods will continue to develop as expertise with current techniques accumulates and technology evolves. This chapter provides an overview of currently applied techniques of therapeutic endoscopy involving the esophagus and its diseases. Emphasis is placed on practical considerations as well as on newer techniques that appear to represent significant advances in the treatment of esophageal disorders.

■ TYPICAL ESOPHAGEAL DISORDERS

TABLE 10-1. SYMPTOMS ASSOCIATED WITH ESOPHAGEAL DISORDERS

Acid-peptic strictures
Heartburn—long standing
Dysphagia—solids > liquids

Other benign strictures
Stable symptoms
Absence of reflux symptoms
Solids > liquids
History of radiation treatment
History of esophageal surgery
Corrosive substance ingestion

Malignant strictures
Progressively worsening dysphagia
Tobacco-alcohol history
Older age
Weight loss
Dysphagia—solids > liquids
Odynophagia
Remote history of corrosive ingestion

Achalasia or other motility disorder
Solid and liquid dysphagia at the onset and intermittent
    weight loss
Regurgitation
Aspiration and pulmonary symptoms
Chest pain
Widened mediastinum on chest radiography
Air-fluid level on chest radiography; absent gastric
    air bubble

TABLE 10-1.

The patient's history in esophageal disorders. In general, the history is most important in the evaluation of patients with esophageal disease. Dysphagia is the symptom which most often prompts the patient with a stricture to seek treatment from a physician. The history provides more significant information than the physical examination regarding the type of stricture present. For example, long-standing reflux symptoms with dysphagia for solid foods suggests a benign, peptic stricture. Progressive dysphagia with weight loss with a history of tobacco and alcohol use is more suggestive of an esophageal malignancy. Interestingly, patients with esophageal cancer often only recall a relatively short (2 months or shorter) duration of dysphagia. Odynophagia may be an earlier symptom in some patients. Schatzki's ring is the most common cause of dysphagia with the severity of symptoms based on both the diameter of the ring and on the size of the ingested bolus. Initially dysphagia is intermittent in these patients and is marked by increasingly frequent episodes of solid food (usually meat and/or bread) impaction that either eventually passes or is intentionally regurgitated by the patient. Food impactions that require endoscopic removal may occur.

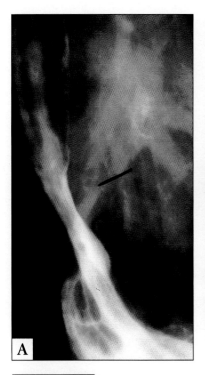
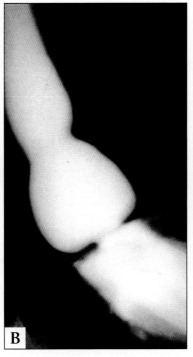
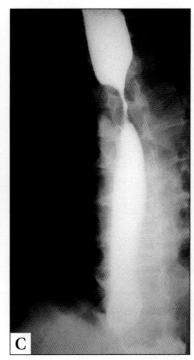
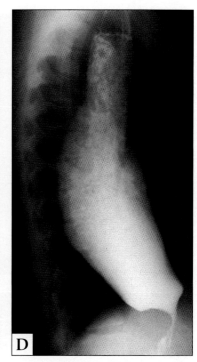

FIGURE 10-1.

Use of contrast radiography in preparation for therapeutic esophageal endoscopy. Contrast radiography is an important part of the work-up of a patient with dysphagia and provides the best measure of lumen caliber. In addition to defining the location of the lesion and probable cause, it also helps clarify the best therapeutic approach, including the method of dilation, the need for fluoroscopic guidance, the need for biopsies or brushings, and aids in follow-up examinations. Barium esophagram may also identify a motility disorder as the cause of the dysphagia. Esophagrams demonstrating peptic stricture (**A**), Schatzki's ring (**B**), malignant stricture (**C**), and achalasia (**D**).

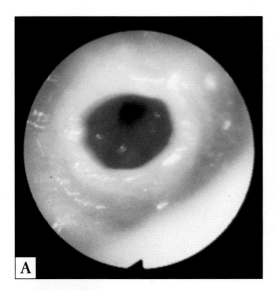
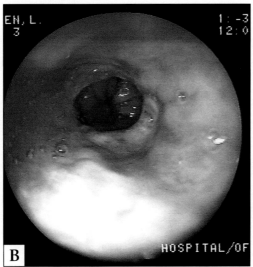
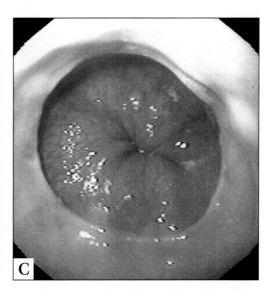

FIGURE 10-2.

Endoscopic appearance of benign strictures. Acid-septic strictures and Schatzki's rings are the most common strictures requiring dilation. Although in most instances endoscopic examination allows obvious distinction between the two, variation in air insufflation and the differences in magnification over short distances between the lower esophageal sphincter and the endoscope can make the assessment of the lower esophagus difficult in some patients. A subtle peptic stricture may be missed endoscopically, or, alternately, may be confused with a Schatzki's ring. Contrast radiology can be a more sensitive technique for demonstrating subtle rings and strictures and for calibrating the lumen more precisely. **A–C,** Endoscopic photographs of several Schatzki's rings; **D–G,** peptic strictures. Note the esophageal pseudodiverticula proximal to the peptic stricture in Figures 10-2f and 10-2g. Their presence

(continued on next page)

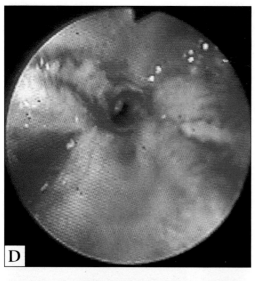

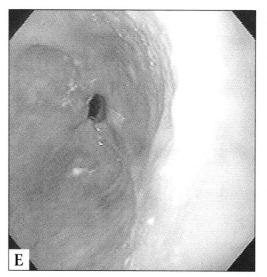

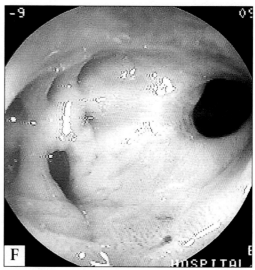

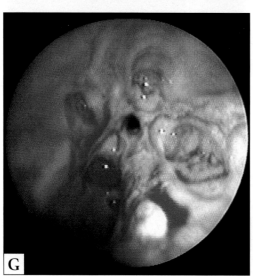

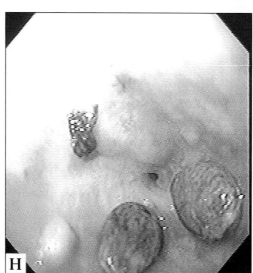

FIGURE 10-2. (CONTINUED)

increases the risk of unguided dilatation of the esophagus and mandates the use of a guidewire technique. **H**, Tight anastomotic stricture (suture at 10 o'clock) and "watermelon esophagus" viewed endoscopically. The watermelon seeds and kernel of corn provide a reference for the pinhole quality of this stricture.

DILATORS

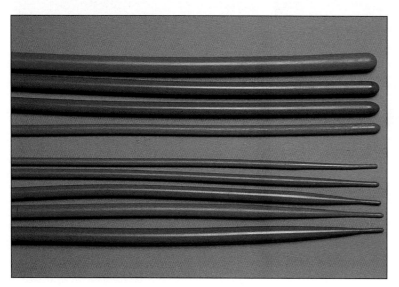

FIGURE 10-3.

Types of dilators: Hurst/Maloney. Mercury-filled rubber bougies, first used by Hurst in 1915, have a blunt tip. Mercury is used for the inner core because it provides an optimal balance between rigidity and flexibility, although its weight is helpful as well. Tungsten is being used to replace the mercury in some dilators. Maloney was the first to describe the tapered tip version of this type of bougie, which has become popular. No studies compare the safety and efficacy of the two. Some clinicians, however, believe that the Maloney version is easier for patients to swallow and is better suited for introducing the dilator into smaller strictures. On the other hand, because of its smaller tip, the Maloney model has a greater chance of becoming misdirected (*eg*, into a small esophageal diverticulum or becoming coiled in a large hiatal hernia sac). Some believe that the Hurst dilator is the dilator of choice for therapy of a Schatzki ring because it provides more of a "bursting" effect rather than a stretching of the ring. Both types of dilators are shown in the figure.

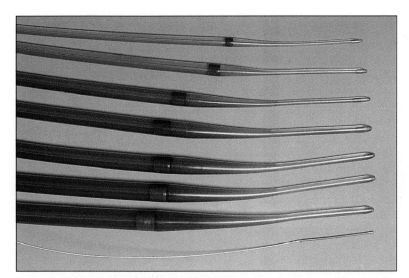

FIGURE 10-4.

Types of dilators (wire-guided): Savary/Eder-Puestow. Management of esophageal strictures improved in 1955 when Puestow developed a guide-wire technique involving the passage of a steel wire beyond the stenosis with subsequent passage of successively larger metal olives over the wire with the assistance of a carrier device. In 1980, Savary and Coll developed a flexible, tapered polyvinyl dilator with a hollow central core that permitted direct passage of the dilator over a guidewire. By the middle and latter 1980s, Savary dilators had largely replaced Eder-Puestow dilators as the instrument of choice when dilation over a guidewire is required because of their ease of passage and the fact that by necessity they must follow the guidewire. A range of Savary dilators is shown.

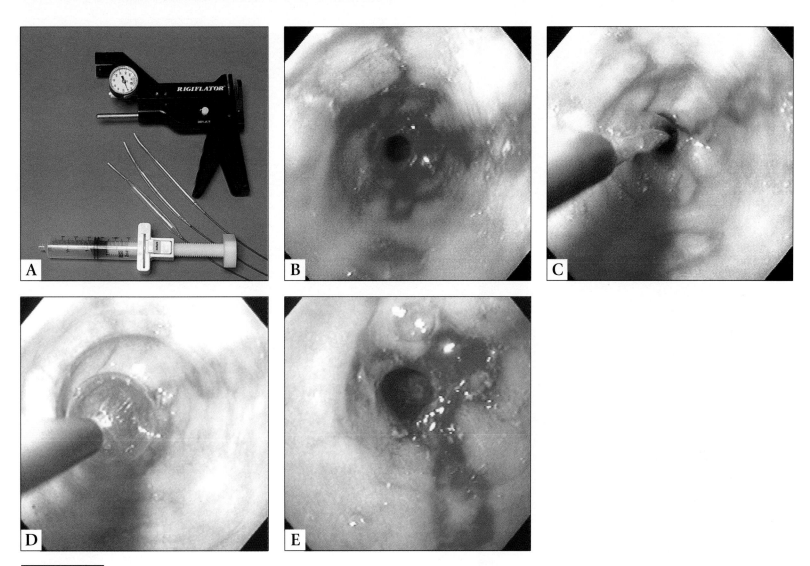

FIGURE 10-5.

Types of dilators: balloons. Balloon dilators are an additional option for the endoscopist approaching an esophageal stricture. They may be placed over a guidewire or through the scope (TTS). Theoretically, balloons have the advantage of being safer because of the radial application of force and elimination of the shearing effect of rigid dilators. Moreover, dilation can be performed under direct visualization using the TTS balloon. Recent balloon innovations facilitating their use include longer balloons that avoid the tendency for slippage with inflation, and new, high-pressure balloons that should provide a truer diameter for the dilation of more resistant strictures. In the limited number of randomized studies comparing Savary-type dilators with balloon dilators, they appeared equally safe. Efficacy, as assessed by symptom improvement and luminal patency, has been variably reported in the literature favoring either technique [1–3]. A, range of available balloons and an inflation gun. B–E, a peptic stricture before and after balloon dilation, thus demonstrating the direct visualization that is possible with the TTS technique.

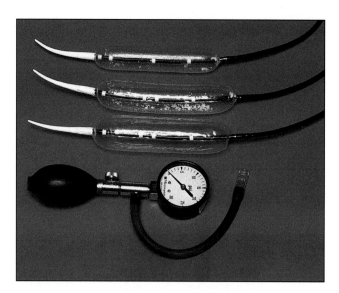

FIGURE 10-6.

Pneumatic balloon dilators for achalasia. Dilation of the lower esophageal sphincter with a pneumatic balloon is generally the therapy chosen for achalasia. Successful dilation entails rupturing of some of the circular muscular layer of the esophagus [4]. The newer polyethylene balloons are currently the most readily available, and range in size from 30 to 40 mm; they are passed over a guidewire. There are different recommendations regarding the technique of pneumatic dilatation for achalasia. There does not appear to be an increased risk associated with longer periods of inflation (up to 1 to 2 minutes), although we prefer a shorter duration (5 to 10 seconds). Risk of perforation increases with performing the initial dilation with larger balloons, and a 30-mm balloon should always be used as the first dilator [5]. Pictured are the range of pneumatic dilator balloons and a manometer for insufflation.

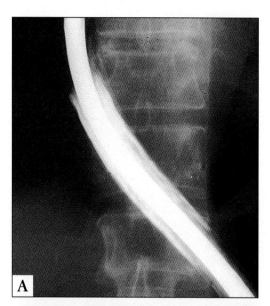

A

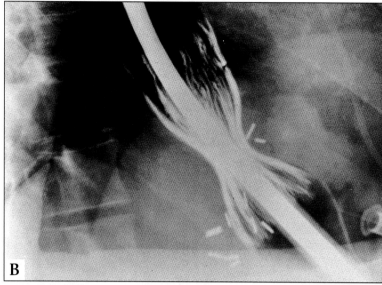

B

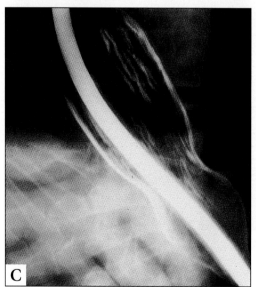

C

FIGURE 10-7.

A–C, Pneumatic balloon dilators for achalasia. To perform a pneumatic dilation the balloon is positioned fluoroscopically so that it straddles the lower esophageal sphincter near the level of the diaphragm. The balloon is then inflated creating an hourglass appearance under fluroscopic visualization until either one or both sides of the waist of the hour-glass are obliterated. Typically, this requires 9 to 15 psi. We also prefer to obtain a contrast study as soon as the patient is alert enough to swallow to rule out a perforation (risk = 0.6%–11%). This can usually be done within minutes of completing the dilation. If a noncontained perforation occurs, early detection with prompt surgical repair is required. Many perforations after pneumatic dilation are contained and can be managed conservatively with intravenous antibiotics, nasogastric decompression, and thoracic surgery consultation [6].

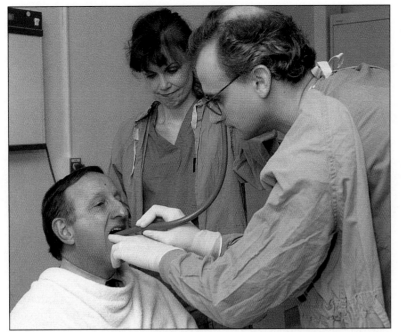

FIGURE 10-8.

Dilation techniques: Hurst/Maloney type. If the stricture is well-defined radiographically, or, if it has been recently dilated, then a nonendoscopically guided dilation can be performed, and, in most cases, no sedation is required. The patient sits upright, the posterior pharynx is anesthetized, and the neck is flexed forward. The patient is asked to swallow and the bougie is advanced with the strong hand. With the index and middle finger of the guide hand placed on the hard palate, the dilator is passed between the two fingers through the stricture. The tactile feel of the dilation is important and the amount of resistance should be noted. A "pop" or "give" is often felt. The "rule of threes" remains a useful guideline. This states that the clinician should not attempt to pass more than three successively larger dilators than the first size that met resistance. If, however, there is a considerable amount of blood on any dilator, the procedure should generally be immediately terminated. Even if the patient has been sedated for endoscopy, it is preferable to have the patient sitting upright because this position appears to facilitate correct passage of the dilator (compared with a higher rate of misdirected passage demonstrated by fluoroscopy when the patient remains in the left lateral decubitus position [10]).

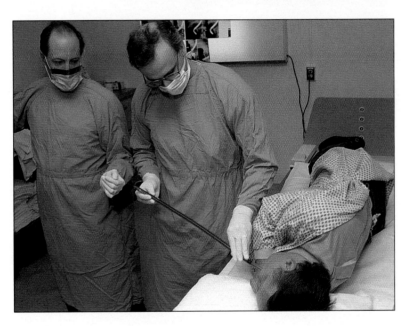

FIGURE 10-9.

Dilation techniques: guidewire technique. In a Savary dilation, the first step is placement of the guidewire beyond the stricture. This may be done endoscopically or with fluoroscopy. In either case, the patient is usually in the left lateral decubitus position. With endoscopic placement, if the stenosis is traversible with the endoscope, the wire is passed under direct visualization into the antrum and the endoscope is withdrawn while the assistant advances, or exchanges, the wire in corresponding increments. If the endoscope cannot be advanced beyond the stricture, then wire placement should be guided by fluroscopy. Impregnated markings on the guidewire aid in maintaining a stationary wire position, which is essential throughout the procedure. The rule of threes is applied, as successively larger dilators are passed. The dilator should be passed gently, holding it much like a pencil and advancing with movement of the wrist. After passage of the final dilator, the wire and dilator are removed together as a single unit.

RISK OF BACTEREMIA

TABLE 10-2. RISK OF BACTEREMIA

	NO. OF PATIENTS	MEAN INCIDENCE, %	RANGE, %
EGD	785	4	0–11
EGD/dil	95	45	0–54
Sclerotherapy	129	18	5–52
Laser therapy	35	29	0–40

TABLE 10-2.

Risk of bacteremia in therapeutic esophageal endoscopy. Incidence of bacteremia associated with therapeutic gastrointestinal procedures involving the esophagus is relatively high compared with simple diagnostic upper endoscopy. Thus, it is rational to use antibiotic prophylaxis in higher risk procedures in susceptible individuals, even though only a handful of endoscopically related cases of endocarditis have been reported. The table demonstrates the range of bacteremia measured by surveillance blood cultures obtained after a surgical procedure in several pooled studies [8]. Current recommendations by the American Heart Association and the American Society for Gastrointestinal Endoscopy identify a prosthetic heart valve, previous endocarditis, and surgically created systemic-pulmonic shunts as high-risk lesions that require prophylaxis [9]. Lower risk lesions for which prophylaxis may be given include hypertrophic cardiomyopathy, most congenital lesions, acquired valvular dysfunction, and mitral valve prolapse with a murmur. Prophylaxis is not generally warranted in other settings unless accompanied by a significant immune deficiency. The recommended regimen for intravenous prophylaxis is ampicillin (2 g) and gentamycin (1.5 mg/kg up to 80 mg maximum dose) with vancomycin substituted for penicillin allergic patients or oral amoxicillin as an alternative for low-risk patients.

BOTULINUM TOXIN FOR ACHALASIA

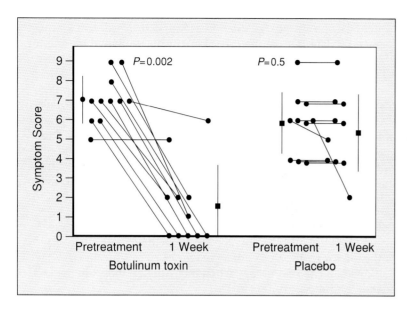

FIGURE 10-10.

Intrasphincteric injection of botulinum toxin for the treatment of achalasia. An innovation in the treatment of achalasia is the endoscopic injection of botulinum toxin in the region of the lower esophageal sphincter (LES). The toxin binds presynaptically and prevents release of acetylcholine, thus causing local paresis and hypotonia of the LES. The complications appear to be minimal; however, the effects tend to be less lasting compared with pneumatic dilation. In the only placebo-controlled trial, the treatment group had improved symptom scores at 1 week (shown in figure), lower LES pressures, and improved esophageal emptying (measured by scintigraphy) compared with the placebo group. Ultimately, all patients were treated and the response rate after the initial injection was 90% with 66% still in remission at 6 months [7]. The tendency for botulinum toxin's effects to wane with time requiring repeated injections makes it a less than ideal treatment for the younger patient. Its primary use will probably be in the elderly patient who is at high surgical risk if perforation occurs following pneumatic dilation. Laparoscopic myotomy is a good alternative in many patients with achalasia. (*Adapted from* Paricha *et al.* [7].)

ESOPHAGEAL FOREIGN BODIES

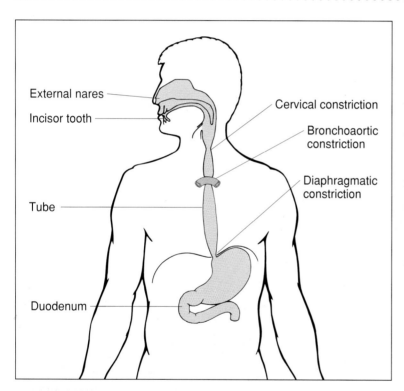

FIGURE 10-11.

Esophageal foreign bodies. In the last two decades endoscopy has become the method of choice in the management of esophageal foreign bodies, although a trial of sublingual nitroglycerin and intravenous glucagon is warranted. At times this will allow the offending bolus to pass. The most common location of the impaction is the distal esophagus at the level of the diaphragm; however, compressions at the level of the cricopharyngeus, aortic arch, and left main-stem bronchus may also be the site of impaction. It is also helpful to identify foreign bodies as sharp or dull, pointed or blunt, and toxic or nontoxic (*eg*, batteries). Also, food-related impactions should be distinguished. If the foreign body is known, in vitro simulation may be helpful in choosing the right accessory for use during the procedure.

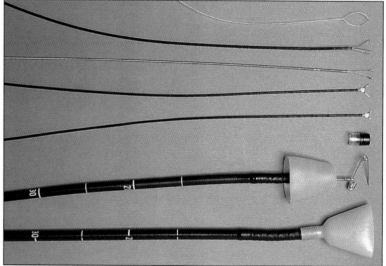

FIGURE 10-12.

Esophageal foreign bodies. A variety of devices that may assist the endoscopist in the retrieval of esophageal foreign bodies exist. For sharp and pointed objects, attention must be given to protection of the mucosa on withdrawal. Occasionally, the object must be pushed into the stomach and reoriented before removal. The hood adapter or the overtube can provide protection for sharp tipped objects. Coins cannot be adequately grasped with the routine forceps and require alligator forceps or coin retrieval forceps. An awareness of the resistance of the upper esophageal sphincter and a firm grasp on the object are required because aspiration of a partially removed foreign body can occur. Pictured are a snare, tripod, several forceps, banding adaptor, and the hood adaptor (the hood covers the sharp object as the hood is drawn through the lower esophageal sphincter).

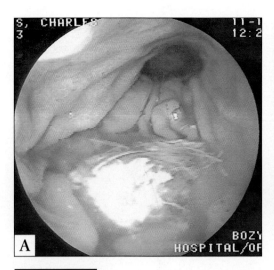
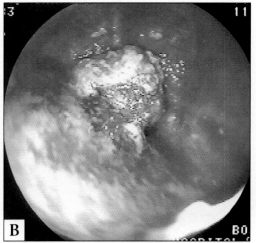

FIGURE 10-13.

Esophageal foreign bodies: food impactions. In the adult population, the most commonly encountered esophageal "foreign body" is impacted food. Techniques for removal include: gentle forward pressure with the scope only if there is lumen visualized; forceful targeted flushing of the bolus with water; piecemeal removal with the forceps using the overtube (if retrieval is attempted early on, the bolus tends to be easier to remove in a single or larger clumps); suction using a simultaneously passed nasogastric (NG) tube with endoscopically directed placement of the NG tube over the bolus before applying suction; and use of the endoscopic variceal band ligator adaptor to generate a larger suction force than possible with the scope alone (also used with the overtube). If one can ascertain the direction of the lumen and advance the scope under direct vision (much like advancing a sigmoidoscope over stool in the colon) into the stomach, the food sometimes follows. Definitive dilation should generally not be carried out in this acute setting, but, rather, the patient should be reexamined at a later date and appropriate therapy undertaken at that time. **A,** a meat bolus lodged in the esophagus; **B,** it is gently pushed into the stomach with the tip of the endoscope.

PALLIATION OF ESOPHAGEAL CANCER

TABLE 10-3. PALLIATIVE OPTIONS IN THE TREATMENT OF ESOPHAGEAL CANCER

ENDOSCOPIC OPTIONS	NONENDOSCOPIC OPTIONS
Dilation	Surgery
Placement of a prosthesis	Radiation
Laser ablation	Chemotherapy
Photodynamic therapy	Nutritional
Alcohol injection	
Placement of a feeding tube	

TABLE 10-3.

Palliative options in the treatment of esophageal cancer.

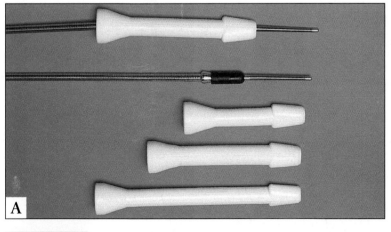
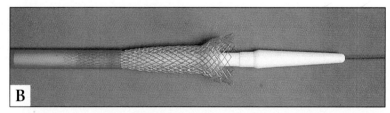
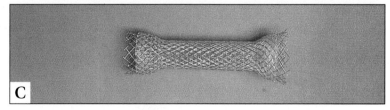

FIGURE 10-14.

Prosthetic devices and stents. Endoscopically placed stents have not emerged as a superior method of palliation; however, they appear to be as effective as other treatments. Their role in treating malignant tracheo esophageal fistulas is well established, indeed they are the treatment of choice. With the development of the newer, metallic, self-expandable stents, the use of esophageal prostheses may become more common. A variety of stents is available in different lengths and diameters. **A,** Atkinson stents and insertion rod. **B–C,** Expandable metal stent with a silicon-coated membrane is depicted, partially deployed and still contained within the sheath (**panel B**) and fully expanded (**panel C**). The membrane helps to prevent tumor ingrowth and allows adequate treatment of a fistula.

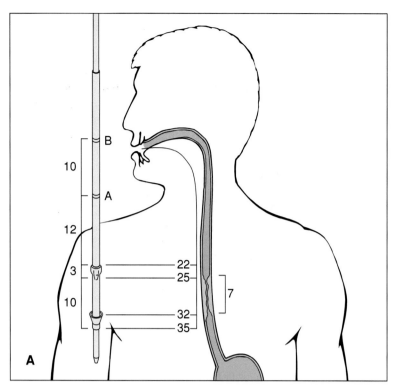

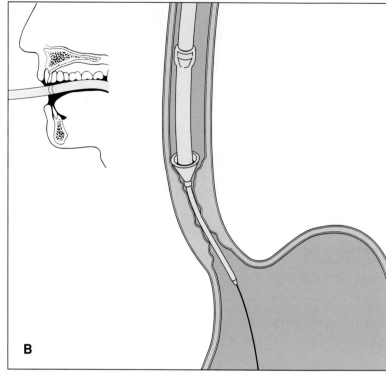

FIGURE 10-15.

Technique: Placement of a rigid prosthetic stent. Before stent placement, the tumor margins should be precisely measured during endoscopy and the lumen should be dilated up to 15 to 17 mm (several sessions are generally required). **A,** Measuring the tumor and correctly marking the pusher tube. **B–C,** Placement of the prosthesis. A smaller Savary dilator passed over a guidewire is advanced beyond the stricture and acts as a guide for the prosthesis that is advanced with a pusher tube. With the use of fluroscopic guidance and the pre-marked pusher tube, the stent is positioned with the proximal and distal flange approximately three cm beyond the tumor margins. Before insertion of the prosthesis, a thin string is tied through a small hole to the end of the proximal flange to allow for withdrawal if necessary during the insertion. After successful placement, the string is removed [13]. (*Adapted from* Fleischer *et al.* [13].)

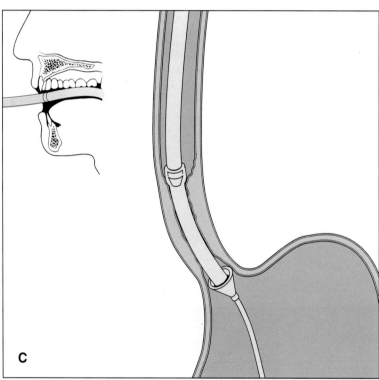

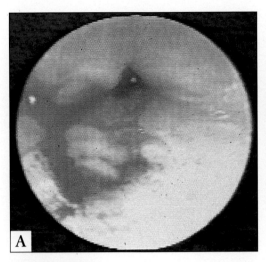 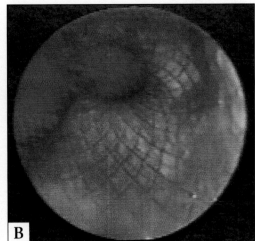 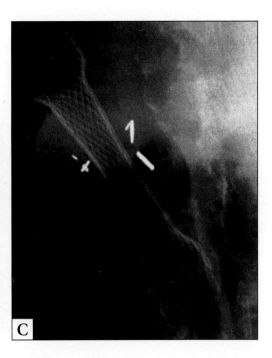

FIGURE 10-16.

FIGURE 10-16.

Techniques: Expandable metallic stents. Self-expanding metallic stents are relatively new and may increase the use of stenting to palliate patients with esophageal cancer. They have several advantages over traditional stents. Their small pre-expansion diameter requires less dilation before stent placement and permits easier placement. Their post-expansion diameter is generally larger than rigid stents and, therefore, should provide more effective relief of dysphagia and longer stent patency. In the only prospective, randomized trial to date comparing expandable stents with rigid stents, the expandable metal stents were more cost-effective and had fewer complications [14]. In these models, tumor ingrowth through the mesh was a problem, although some more recent models are coated with synthetic membranes designed to prevent this. If tumor ingrowth or overgrowth at the margins occurs, then it is often treatable with laser or additional stent placement. Although metal stents are easier to place than traditional stents, initially after expansion, they are difficult to reposition, and, therefore, should only be placed by experienced physicians. **A–B,** Endoscopic views of an esophageal tumor before and after stent placement. **C,** Radiograph demonstrating the expanded stent in the esophagus.

TABLE 10-4. ENDOSCOPIC PALLIATION OF MALIGNANT DISEASE

FAVORABLE FOR LASER TX	UNFAVORABLE FOR LASER TX
Length shorter than 6 cm	Length greater than 10 cm
Straight segment of esophagus	High cervical esophagus
Mucosal, exophytic, polypoid	Submucosal
Recurrent tumor after esophagogastrectomy near the anastomosis	

TABLE 10-4.

Endoscopic palliation of malignant disease: laser therapy. Endoscopically delivered laser therapy can be used in the palliation of esophageal cancer. With experienced operators, luminal patency is generally achieved in 90% of appropriately selected patients in two to three sessions. Functional improvement, however, is less, typically ranging from 70% to 80%. Selection of suitable lesions to treat with laser is determined by the exophytic appearance on endoscopy, distal location, and a straight segment of the esophagus; the total length of the lesion should be less than 6 cm.

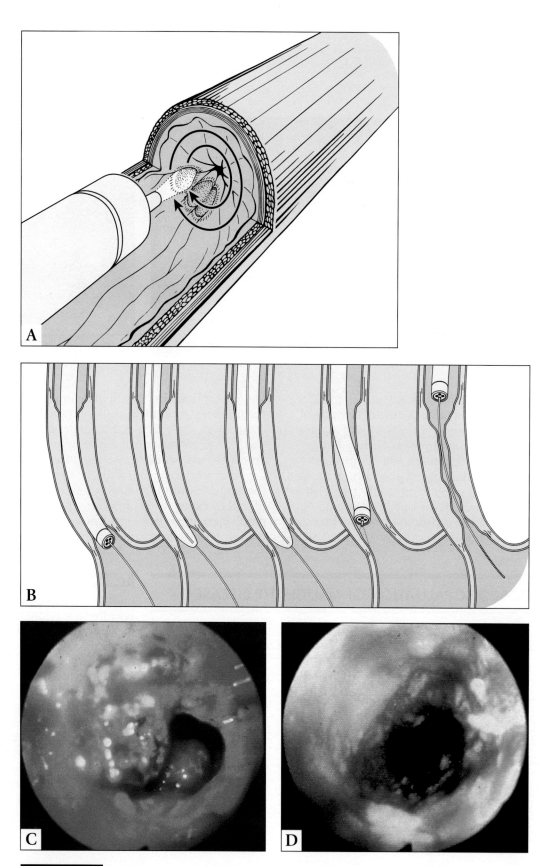

FIGURE 10-17.

Endoscopic laser treatment of esophageal cancer: Technique. This procedure can generally be done with intravenous conscious sedation rather than general anesthesia. Two strategies for laser application exist. The initially developed method involves application of the laser beam with concentric destruction of tumor proceeding from the lumen to the wall, proximally to distally as much as possible during a single session (**A**). Progression to the distal portion of the tumor may be limited by the formation of edema with this method. The second, and more preferred, technique involves application of laser distal to proximal (**B**). If feasible, a guidewire is first placed distal to the lesion into the stomach; several Savary dilators are passed to facilitate maneuverability of the scope during the treatment. This latter method generally requires fewer treatment sessions. **Panel C** and **panel D** demonstrate an exophytic tumor obstructing the esophagus and a patent lumen established after laser treatment.

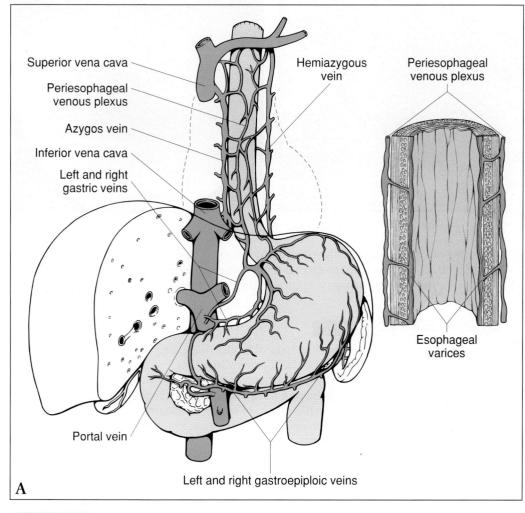

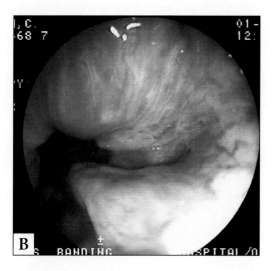

FIGURE 10-18.

Pathogenesis of esophageal varices. Esophageal (and gastric) varices are enlarged veins that are part of the extensive collateral circulation that can develop in the setting of portal hypertension (A). In normal individuals, almost 100% of portal venous flow (approximately 1 L/min) is recoverable in the hepatic vein, whereas in the patient with cirrhosis up to 87% may be directed into collateral flow. Although varices can develop in many areas, they are most problematic in the esophagus (and proximal stomach), wherein life-threatening hemorrhage may occur. Increased portal venous pressure is most commonly secondary to cirrhosis from a variety of causes, but can be caused by noncirrhotic liver disease or from extrahepatic causes. Systemic vasodilation with decreased vascular resistance and the formation of a hyperdynamic circulation may also play a role in the development of portal hypertension and subsequent varices. It has been estimated that this increased flow is responsible for 40% of the increase, and that resistance to flow is responsible for 60% of the increase in portal pressure in cirrhosis. B, Active hemorrhage from a distal esophageal varix with a sclerotherapy injector at the 7-o'clock position. (A, *From* Waye [17]; with permission.)

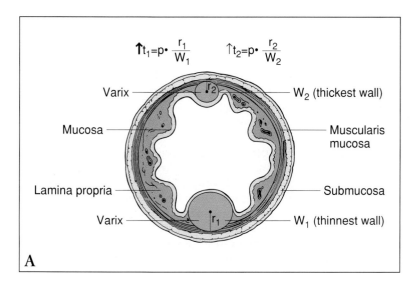

FIGURE 10-19.

Factors involved in variceal hemorrhage. The lifetime risk for bleeding from esophageal varices has been estimated at 10% to 67% with the probable risk being from 30% to 40%. Multiple factors have been proposed to identify varices at higher risk for hemorrhage. A portal pressure of at least 12 mmHg appears to be necessary for the development of varices and for significant hemorrhage. Higher pressures, however, do not correlate with greater bleeding risk. Variceal size appears to have some predictive value, and perhaps wall thickness does as well, particularly in how they contribute to wall tension (t). Wall tension in larger varices will be greater than in smaller varices with the same intravariceal pressure (p). Wall tension also varies inversely with the thickness of the variceal wall (w). These relationships are demonstrated in the modification of Laplace's law shown in **panel A** [15,16].

(*continued on next page*)

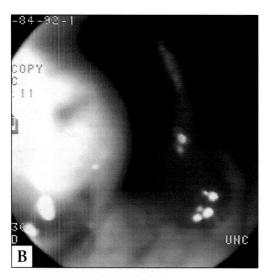

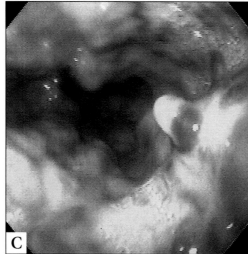

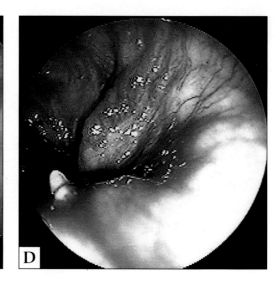

FIGURE 10-19. (*CONTINUED*)

"Red color" signs also appear to portend a greater risk of bleeding; when seen on large varices they are particularly worrisome (**panels B, C, and D**). They represent "varices on varices" and probably correspond histologically with dilated intraepithelial venules. Also note the fibrin-platelet plugs (**panel C** and **panel D**) which identify the site of recent hemorrhage and provide useful information to the endoscopist.

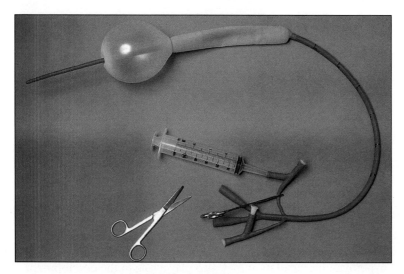

FIGURE 10-20.

Options in acute variceal hemorrhage. Endoscopic therapy is useful in the management of acute variceal hemorrhage. Other options include medical treatment, direct tamponade with a Sengstaken-Blakemore tube or a Minnesota tube (pictured above), placement of an intrahepatic shunt, or surgery. Vasoactive drugs such as vaso-pressin and nitroglycerin, octreotide, and terlipressin are effective in the acute setting in decreasing bleeding by lowering portal pressures. Some gastroenterologists feel that concurrent use of vasoactive drugs during endoscopic treatment of acute bleeding improves visualization and outcome, although this has not been proven. Despite all these options, the 1-year survival rate after initial hemorrhage has changed little over the last 40 years, and remains about 40%.

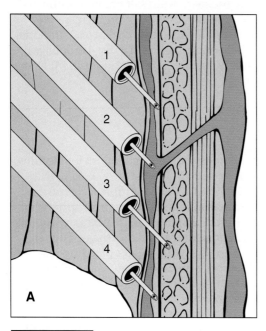

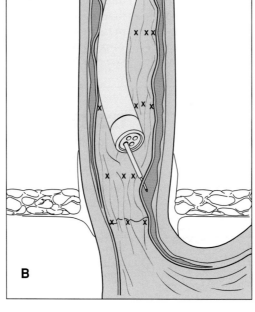

FIGURE 10-21.

Endoscopic sclerotherapy. Sclerotherapy has been widely used over the last 15 years as an effective treatment for acute variceal hemorrhage and for prophylaxis for recurrent hemor-

rhage after the initial bleeding episode has stopped. Both paravariceal and intravariceal injection techniques have been recommended. Regardless of the location of the external puncture, the depth of needle penetration may be difficult to control and may range from intravariceal to submucosal, or into the muscular layer, the latter perhaps predisposing to deeper ulceration (**panel A**). The preferred technique is for injections of 1 to 2 mL of sclerosant into the varix starting as distally in the esophagus as possible (near or just below the esophageal-gastric junction) and in a circumferential route. Injections are then repeated 2 to 5 cm more proximally (**panel B**). The total volume of scleroscent should not exceed 20 mL per session, above which rate the incidence of complications may increase. No particular sclerosant has emerged as consistently superior (sodium tetradecyl, ethanolamine oleate, absolute ethanol, and sodium morrhuate are agents available in the United States). (*Adapted from* Waye [17].)

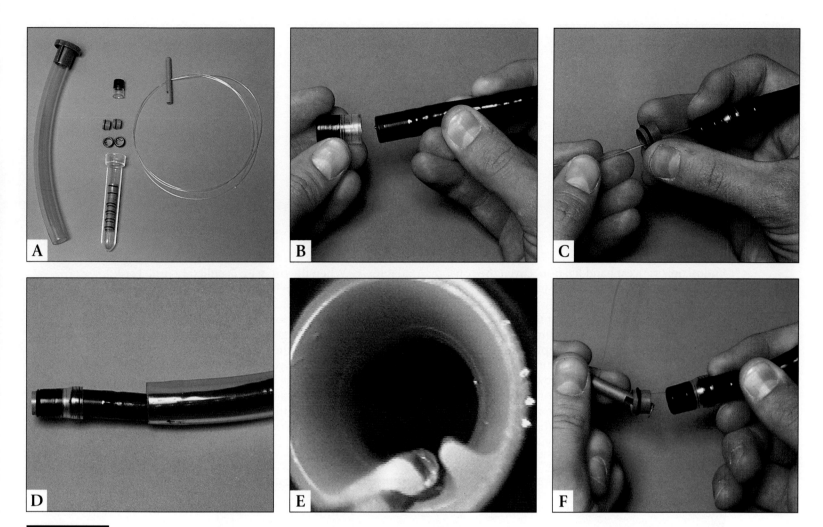

FIGURE 10-22.

Endoscopic variceal band ligation (EVL). Endoscopic variceal band ligation is an alternate method to treat varices. It is based on the technique used for elastic band ligation of internal hemorrhoids. The equipment is relatively inexpensive and easily used with most endoscopes. This figure demonstrates the technique for preparing for EVL: **A,** all the accessory equipment necessary for banding. An overtube is required for the frequent insertion of the endoscope that is required in reloading and placing successive bands. **B,** The outer cylinder adapter is placed on the tip of the endoscope. **C,** The trip wire is threaded through the biopsy port and connects to the notch on the band holder (inner cylinder). **D,** "Loaded" scope ready for banding. **E,** Endoscopic view of the loaded scope. Note that tripwire is oriented to approximately a 5-o'clock position (wire should be in line with the aspiration port). **F,** The hooker is used to facilitate removal of "fired" inner cylinder for reloading.

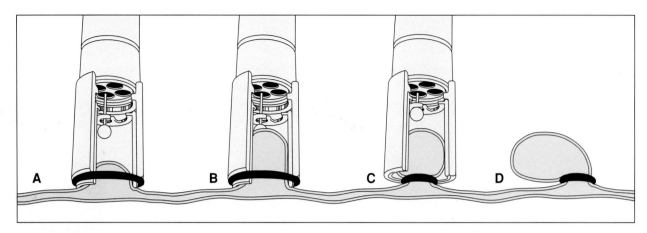

FIGURE 10-23.

Endoscopic variceal band ligation. Given the constriction of the endoscopic field with the adapter in place, the clinician should initially survey the involved region of the esophagus without the adaptor and then plan the sites and order of banding. Targeting should be similar to that for sclerotherapy, that is, initially low, near the gastroesophageal junction, and circumferential, then banding more proximally. **A,** When the target varix is identified, the tip of the adaptor should be brought into contact with the varix (filling the endoscopic field). **B,** Suction is then applied, which should draw the varix and overlying mucosa into the adaptor. **C,** When the trip wire is pulled (a firm, brisk tug works best), the preloaded inner cylinder is drawn into the adaptor (outer cylinder), thus causing the release of the band around the varix. **D,** Several small puffs of air should be given to free the mucosa from the adaptor gently as the endoscope is withdrawn. The banded varix may contain all or part of the submucosal varix. The development of a multiple band ligator device, which can be used without an overtube, should decrease the necessary manipulations and improve the procedure. (*Adapted from* Goff [18].)

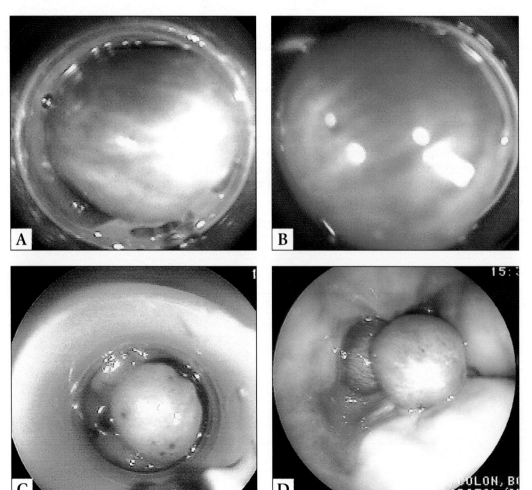

FIGURE 10-24.

Endoscopic variceal band ligation. **A–D,** Endoscopic views of variceal band ligation that correspond to the sequence of steps discussed in Figure 10-23.

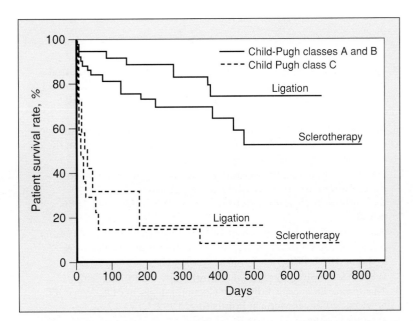

FIGURE 10-25.

Comparison of the efficacy of endoscopic variceal band ligation (EVL) and esophageal sclerotherapy (ES). EVL has been compared with ES in two randomized, controlled trials [19,20]. The survival rates compare the two treatment modalities stratified according to severity of liver disease, rated by Child-Pugh class [19]. In patients with less severe liver disease (classes A and B, upper lines in graph), treatment with banding was associated with improved survival. The efficacy in cessation of active bleeding, length of hospital stay, and transfusion requirement for the initial bleeding was comparable in both groups. The incidence of nonbleeding complications (*eg*, pneumonia, esophageal ulceration, stricture formation) was lower in the EVL group and probably contributes to the improved survival. Complete obliteration of varices occurs more quickly with EVL (average one to two fewer sessions). Some groups have advocated combination ligation and sclerotherapy at the same session, reporting even more rapid variceal eradication [21]. The recent availability of multiple-band ligators that can be used without an overtube is a distinct advantage. (*Adapted from* Stiegman *et al.* [19].)

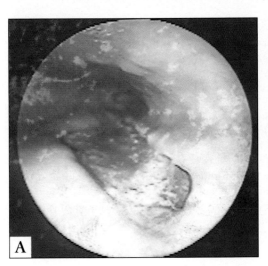

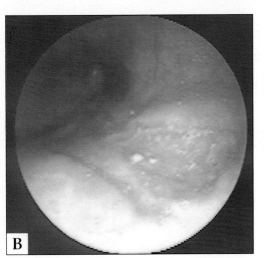

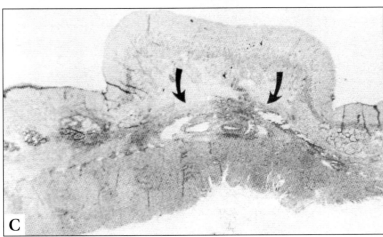

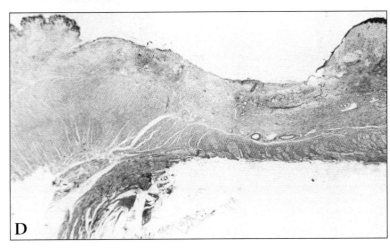

FIGURE 10-26.

Complications of endoscopic treatment of varices. The overall complication rate from sclerotherapy is from 10% to 20%. Local complications include stricture formation (3% to 5%) and perforation (rare, < 1%). The incidence of esophageal ulceration approaches 100% and should not be considered a complication unless it leads to stricture, perforation, or persistent dysphagia. **A–B,** A deep sclerotherapy-induced ulcer 1 week after injection (**panel A**) and 4 weeks after injection (**panel B**) with substantial healing (this patient developed a symptomatic stricture). Banding has been reported to cause less severe ulceration because the muscularis propria may not be injured, which may occur with deeper injections [22]. **C,** Histologic sections of the banded mucosa and submucosa. **D,** The same ulcer healing at 7 days with an intact muscularis. Nonlocal complications of sclerotherapy include pulmonary complications (*eg,* pneumonitis, pleural effusion, and aspiration), transient bacteremia (5% to 50% of cases), and bleeding from collateral vessels [21,23]. Rarer complications include infarcts of the spinal artery and distal large vessel thrombosis. A complication unique to banding is perforation from passage of the overtube. The risk of this problem is reduced by passage of the overtube with an obturator (*eg,* a Hurst dilator) that fills the lumen of the overtube to avoid pinching the esophageal wall. (**C** and **D,** *From* Stiegman *et al.* [22]; with permission.)

REFERENCES

1. Saeed ZA, Winchester CB, Ferro PA, *et al.*: Prospective randomized comparison of polyvinyl bougies and through-the-scope balloons for dilation of peptic strictures of the esophagus. *Gastrointest Endosc* 1995, 41:189–195.

2. Cox JGC, Winter RK, Maslin SC, *et al.*: Balloon or bougie for dilation of benign oesophageal stricture? An interim report of a randomized controlled trial. *Gut* 1988, 29:1741–1747.

3. Shemesh E, Czerniak A: Comparison between Savary-Gilliard and balloon dilatation of benign esophageal strictures. *World J Surg* 1990, 14:518–522.

4. Graham DY: Treatment of benign and malignant strictures of the esophagus. In *Therapeutic Gastrointestinal Endoscopy.* Edited by Silvis SE. New York: Igaku-Shoin, 1990:1–41.

5. Kadakia SC, Wong RK: Graded dilation using rigiflex achalasia dilators in patients with primary esophageal achalasia. *Am J Gastroenterol* 1993, 88:34–38.

6. Bozymski EM: Dilatation of the esophagus: pneumatic. In *Manual of Gastroenterologic Procedure.* Edited by Drossman DA. New York: Raven Press, 1993:180–184.

7. Paricha PJ, Ravich WJ, Hendrix TR, *et al.*: Intrasphincteric botulinum toxin for the treatment of achalasia. *N Engl J Med* 1995, 322:774–778.

8. Fleischer DE, Neu HC: Recommendations for antibiotic prophylaxis before endoscopy. *Am J Gastroenterol* 1989, 84:1488–1491.

9. Dajani A, Bisno A, Chung K, *et al.*: Prevention of bacterial endocarditis: Recommendations by the American Heart Association. *JAMA* 1990, 264:2919–2922.

10. Ho BH, Cass O, Katsman RJ, *et al.*: Fluoroscopy is not necessary for Maloney dilation of chronic esophageal strictures. *Gastrointest Endosc* 1995, 41:11–14.

11. Wang KK, Geller A: Photodynamic therapy for early esophageal cancers: Light versus surgical might. *Gastroenterology* 1995, 108:593–596.

12. Chung SC, Leong HT, Choi CY, *et al.*: Palliation of malignant esophageal obstruction by endoscopic alcohol injection (Abstract). *Gastrointest Endosc* 1992, 38:231.

13. Fleischer DE: Treatment of esophageal and other gastrointestinal cancers. In *Techniques in Therapeutic Endoscopy.* Edited by Geenen J, Fleischer DE, Waye JD. New York: Gower Medical Publishing, 1992:4.1–4.34.

14. Knyrim K, Wagner HJ, Bethge N, *et al.*: A controlled trial of an expansile metal stent for palliation of esophageal obstruction die to inoperable cancer. *N Engl J Med* 1993, 329:1302–1307.

15. Polio J, Groszmann RJ: Hemodynamic factors involved in the development and rupture of oesophageal varices: A pathophysiologic approach to treatment. *Semin Liver Dis* 1986, 6:318.

16. Kaplowitz N: Pathophysiology of portal hypertension. In *Liver and Biliary Diseases.* Edited by Kaplowitz N. Baltimore: Williams & Wilkins, 1992:499–503.

17. Waye JD: Esophageal variceal sclerotherapy. In *Techniques in Therapeutic Endoscopy.* Edited by Geenen J, Fleischer DE, Waye JD. New York: Gower Medical Publishing, 1992:3.1–3.12.

18. Goff JS: Esophageal varices. *Gastroenterol Endosc Clin North Am* 1994;4:747–771.

19. Stiegman GV, Goff J, Michaletz-Onody P, *et al.*: Endoscopic sclerotherapy as compared with endoscopic ligation for bleeding esophageal varices. *N Engl J Med* 1992, 326:1527–1532.

20. Lane L, El-Newihi HM, Migkovsky B, *et al.*: Ligation compared with sclerotherapy for the treatment of bleeding esophageal varices. *Ann Intern Med* 1993, 119:1.

21. Reville RM, Goff JS, Stiegmann GV, *et al.*: Combination endoscopic variceal ligation and low volume sclerotherapy for bleeding esophageal varices: A faster route to variceal eradication? (Abstract). *Gastrointest Endosc* 1991, 37:243.

22. Stiegman GV, Sun JH, Hammond WS: Results of experimental endoscopic esophageal varix ligation. *Am Surg* 1988, 54:105–108.

23. Sivak MV, Blue MG: Endoscopic sclerotherapy of esophageal varices. In *Therapeutic Gastrointestinal Endoscopy.* Edited by Silvis SE. New York: Igaku-Shoin, 1990:42–97.

Chapter 11

Surgery of the Esophagus

■ SURGICAL ANATOMY OF THE ESOPHAGUS

BERNARD M. JAFFE

The esophagus courses from the pharynx to the stomach and is divided arbitrarily into four segments. The pharyngoesophagus is that segment which intervenes between the laryngopharynx and the upper border of the cricopharyngeus muscle. This latter structure represents the esophageal introitus. The cervical esophagus begins at the inferior border of the first thoracic vertebral body and extends caudally for 5 to 6 cm. The thoracic esophagus spans the posterior mediastinum. It includes the bronchoaortic constriction and the superior and inferior dilations above and below. A second constriction is present at the diaphragm. The abdominal esophagus extends for 1 to 6 cm below the diaphragm and ends at the esophagogastric junction. This segment of the esophagus includes the lower esophageal sphincter. The arterial supply and venous and lymphatic drainage (*see* Figs. 11-1 and 11-2) are critical to successful surgery of the esophagus.

■ ESOPHAGEAL PERFORATION AND HIATAL HERNIAS

Two major types of esophageal defects are perforation (*see* Figs. 11-3 to 11-5) and hernias (*see* Figs. 11-6 to 11-13). Of the four major etiologies of esophageal perforation (*see* Fig. 11-3), the most common are spontaneous and iatrogenic causes. Esophageal perforation continues to carry significant rates of morbidity and mortality.

Esophageal, or hiatal, hernias occur as sliding or paraesophageal hernias. Sliding hiatal, or type I, hernias do not create symptoms and do not warrant therapy. On the other hand, gastroesophageal reflux occurs primarily in patients with hiatal hernias. Operative therapy for gastroesophageal reflux is indicated for reflux esophagitis (*ie*, not merely reflux) when medical treatment has failed or when the patient is noncompliant.

Paraesophageal, or type II, hiatal hernias differ significantly from the sliding variety. As displayed in Figure 11-7, the following occurs in paraesophageal hernias: the esophagogastric junction remains in the normal location; a true peritoneal hernial sac is present; structures other than the stomach (eg, spleen, splenic flexure, omentum, etc.) can herniate above the diaphragm; there is an associated incidence of gastric volvulus; compression at the hiatus can cause ischemic necrosis of the herniated viscera. In further contrast with sliding hernias, all paraesophageal hernias require repair whether they are symptomatic or not.

Paraesophageal hernia repairs require anatomic correction of the specific abnormalities involved. This mandates reduction of the stomach and all herniated viscera, excision of the hernial sac in its entirety, and anatomic closure of the defect in the hiatus, both anterior and posterior to the esophagus. This final component is the most difficult because the muscular crura are severely attenuated. By anchoring the posterior position of the crural closure to the arcuate ligament, however, successful repair can consistently be accomplished. Rates of recurrence average 10% to 15%, significantly higher than those for repairs of sliding hiatal hernias.

Some controversy exists about the need for simultaneous Nissen fundoplication during paraesophageal hernia repair. One argument offered by proponents is that some patients have gastroesophageal reflux preoperatively, which warrants operative correction. The absence or presence of reflux should be assessed before repair is undertaken and fundoplication should be performed only in patients with complications such as esophagitis. Some surgeons further argue that the Nissen procedures are protective if the repair fails and the patient develops a sliding hiatal hernia [1]. Fundoplication should not be performed prophylactically, however; rather, the focus should be on meticulous care to prevent recurrent herniation.

■ ESOPHAGEAL OBSTRUCTION

Dysphagia is the characteristic symptom of esophageal obstruction. The obstruction can be functional in origin, as in achalasia and esophageal diverticular diseases, or mechanical, as a result of fibrous stricture or malignant luminal occlusion. Aggressive therapy is indicated under both circumstances, because unless the obstruction is relieved, the patient cannot eat nor clear salivary secretions.

Achalasia

Techniques for diagnosing achalasia are described elsewhere in this volume. For most patients, hydrostatic balloon dilation is appropriate initial therapy. Surgery (Heller myotomy) is reserved for those patients in whom dysphagia recurs after two dilations, those who wish immediate definitive therapy, and those who have a hiatal hernia with or without a history of reflux esophagitis. Myotomy provides excellent results in curing achalasia (see Figs. 11-14 and 11-15). In the series of 468 patients reported by Okike and colleagues [2], the opera-

tive mortality rate was 0.2%; only 1% of patients had mucosal perforation.

Esophageal diverticula

Esophageal diverticula (see Figs. 11-16 and 11-17) occur as Zenker's diverticula, traction diverticula, or epiphrenic diverticula. Pharyngoesophageal, or Zenker's, diverticula are the most common types. Because they are caused by a muscular abnormality, myotomy plays a major role in their treatment.

Traction diverticula occur in the middle third of the esophagus and result from adhesion to inflammatory lymph nodes at the carina. These lesions usually do not cause dysphagia, but when they do, they are best treated by excision with staple closure of the defect with or without sutures. Myotomy is not necessary.

Like Zenker's diverticula, epiphrenic diverticula are caused by muscular hyperplasia, and treatment requires myotomy.

Benign esophageal strictures

Reflux esophagitis is the most common cause of esophageal strictures (see Fig. 11-18). Fibrosis following caustic ingestion is another cause. Alkaline material, such as lye, causes esophageal mucosal necrosis and induces a severe inflammatory response. The end results of this process may be fibrosis and luminal obliteration. Ingested acid generally affects the stomach far more than it does the esophagus. Consequently, gastric, rather than esophageal, obstruction generally occurs.

Both these lesions, reflux–induced and caustic ingestion-induced strictures, are associated with an increased incidence of carcinoma. In reflux disease, malignancy may occur in areas of Barrett's esophagus or in gastric mucosal esophageal metaplasia. In patients with Barrett's esophagus, endoscopic surveillance with mucosal biopsy is indicated to identify the premalignant state, or high-grade dysplasia, in areas of the intestinal type of adenomatous metaplasia.

The goal of treatment for benign esophageal strictures is to provide an adequate lumen through which food and salivary secretions readily pass. This may be accomplished by stricturoplasty (see Fig. 11-19) or by resection and reanastomosis.

Esophageal carcinoma

The incidence of esophageal carcinoma is increased in patients with a history of caustic ingestion, Barrett's esophagus, achalasia, and combined heavy smoking and drinking. Ingested nitrosamines have also been incriminated in the pathogenesis of esophageal malignancy.

The predominant symptoms of esophageal carcinoma relate to luminal obstruction. Virtually all patients describe dysphagia, but weight loss, regurgitation, cough, and chest pain are also common manifestations. The only successful treatment of esophageal carcinoma is surgical excision.

Physical examination of affected patients is generally normal, and any findings (cervical lymphadenopathy, Horner's syndrome, vocal cord paralysis, or hepatomegaly) attest to the presence of extensive disease.

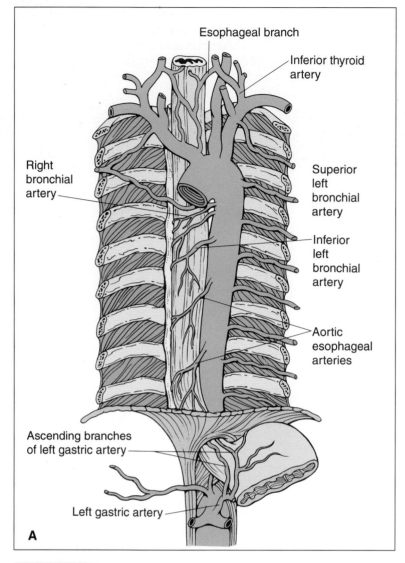

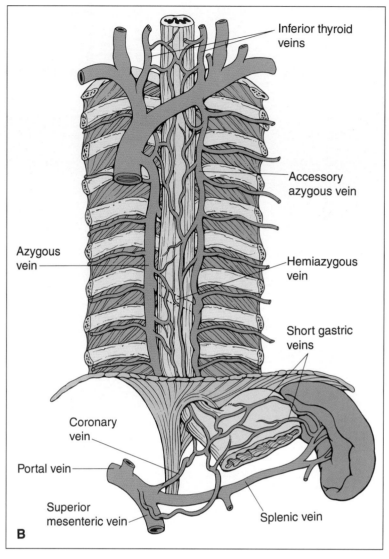

FIGURE 11-1.

A, Arterial supply of the esophagus. The tenuous nature of the arterial supply accounts for some of the technical problems with esophageal surgery. As shown, the arteries are derived from multiple sources. The major vascular supply, however, comes directly from the aorta. **B**, Venous drainage of the esophagus. Venous drainage parallels the arterial supply. Major vessels include the inferior thyroid and azygous, hemiazygous, and coronary veins. The proximal esophagus drains into the systemic circulation whereas the distal esophagus drains through the portal system. (*Adapted from* Rothberg *et al.* [6].)

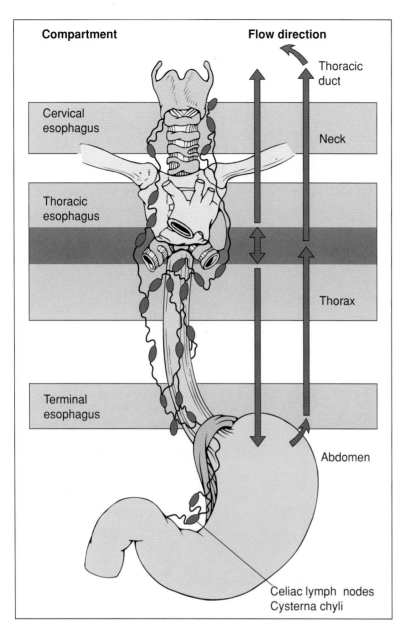

Compartment   **Flow direction**

Cervical
esophagus

Thoracic
esophagus

Terminal
esophagus

Thoracic
duct

Neck

Thorax

Abdomen

Celiac lymph nodes
Cysterna chyli

FIGURE 11-2.

Lymphatic drainage of the esophagus is pertinent to the treatment of esophageal carcinoma. Lymph flow is bi-directional at the level of the bifurcation of the trachea. In addition to the paraesophageal nodes, lesions distal to that anatomic juncture drain distally, including into the celiac nodes, whereas proximal lesions drain cephalad to the cervical nodes. (*Adapted from* Liebermann-Meffert [7].)

ESOPHAGEAL PERFORATION

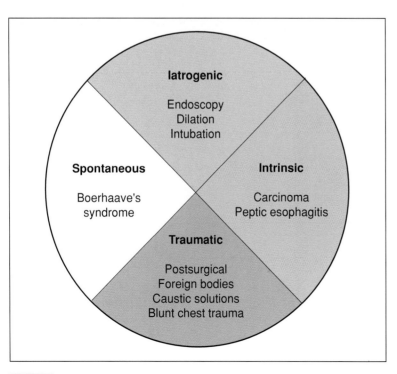

Iatrogenic

Endoscopy
Dilation
Intubation

Spontaneous

Boerhaave's
syndrome

Intrinsic

Carcinoma
Peptic esophagitis

Traumatic

Postsurgical
Foreign bodies
Caustic solutions
Blunt chest trauma

FIGURE 11-3.

Causes of esophageal perforation. Spontaneous perforation of the distal esophagus, or Boerhaave's syndrome, is the most common cause. The frequency of iatrogenic perforation, however, is increasing as exploration of the esophagus with instruments becomes more common. Postsurgical perforation, or leakage following esophageal resection, occurs with an incidence of approximately 5%. Perforation in areas of malignancy and peptic esophagitis is rare, even in the presence of ulceration.

Early recognition of perforation is critical to successful therapy. The predominant symptoms include chest pain, nausea, vomiting (occasionally with hematemesis), and shortness of breath. Physical findings include fever, tachycardia, cervical crepitus, mediastinal crunch, decreased breath sounds over the left chest, and abdominal tenderness and guarding.

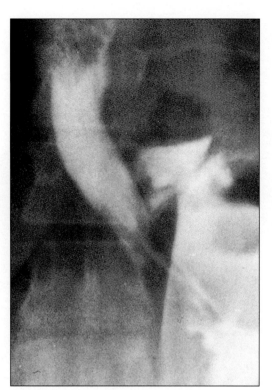

FIGURE 11-4.

Radiographic diagnosis of esophageal
perforation. Chest radiography may reveal
air with or without fluid in the left pleural
space. There may also be free air under the
diaphragm if the perforation is low. The
diagnosis is confirmed by Gastrografin
(Squibb, Princeton, NJ) swallow, which
demonstrates extravasation from the
esophageal lumen. (*From* Skinner [8];
with permission.)

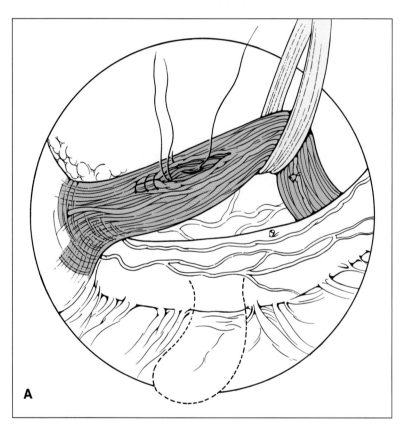

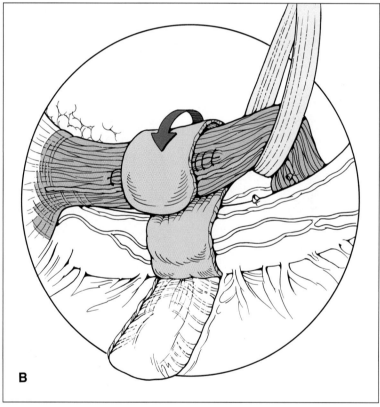

FIGURE 11-5.

This figure demonstrates repair of esophageal perforation. The
principles of therapy include operative closure of the perforation
buttressing with a patch of pleura and/or intercostal muscle. **A,**
Esophageal closure and selection of the buttressing flap; **B,** wrap-
ping the closure. Pleural drainage with two large-bore chest tubes
and gastrostomy are also performed.

Perforation of the esophagus mandates surgical correction to
prevent or minimize the severity of mediastinitis. For example, if
the esophagus cannot be closed because of a tumor or if the
diagnosis of perforation is made after 24 hours or more, cervical
esophagostomy should be performed to divert the saliva from
the perforation. Despite advances in operative management and
antibiotic therapy, esophageal perforation carries a significant
mortality rate (10% to 15% with prompt management; 50%
if treatment is delayed longer than 24 hours). (*Adapted from*
Skinner [9].)

Sliding hiatal hernias

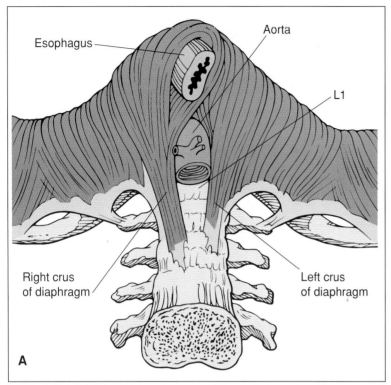
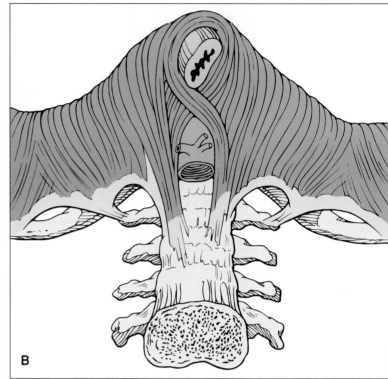
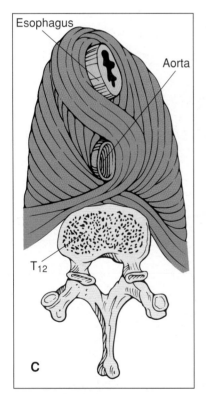
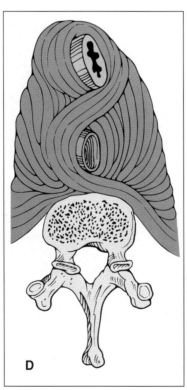
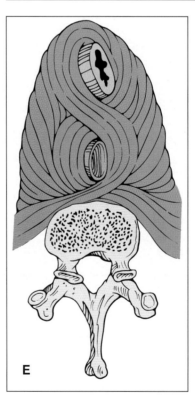
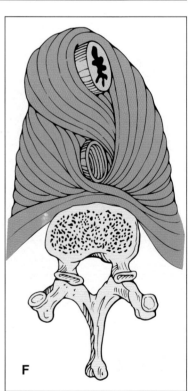

FIGURE 11-6.

The anatomy of the esophageal hiatus. The esophageal hiatus is a complex and highly variable structure; this accounts for some of the developmental problems resulting in hiatal hernias. Most commonly, the right crus of the diaphragm constitutes both limbs of the hiatal ring. Almost 40% of the time, however, the ring includes components from both right and left crura (**A**). Finally, a variety of patterns and configurations exist in the remaining patients (**B–F**). No relationship exists between the crural pattern of derivation of the hiatus and the development of hiatal hernias. On the other hand, this variability adds to the complexity of repair of the hiatus, when indicated. (*Adapted from* Gray *et al.* [10].)

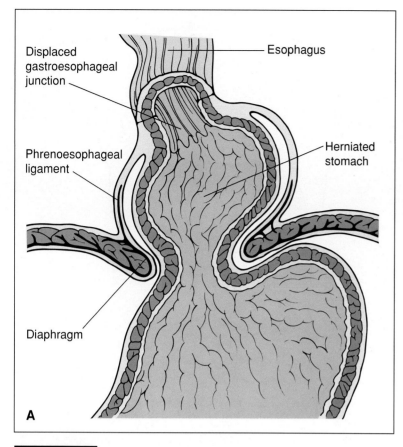

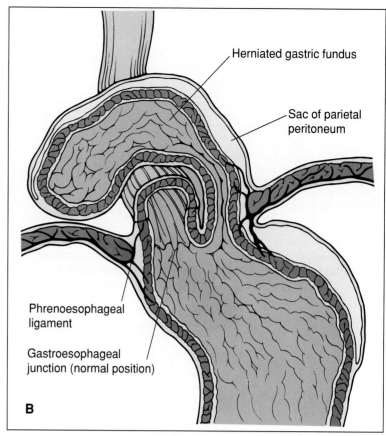

FIGURE 11-7.

Types of hiatal hernia. In a type I, or axial or sliding hiatal hernia, the endoabdominal fascia relaxes, allowing a portion of the gastric fundus to slide through the hiatus into the mediastinum (A). The phrenoesophageal membrane remains intact and there is no hernial sac. In a type II, or paraesophageal hernia, the esophagogastric junction is at the normal site and there is a true hernial sac (B). (*Adapted from* Gray *et al.* [11].)

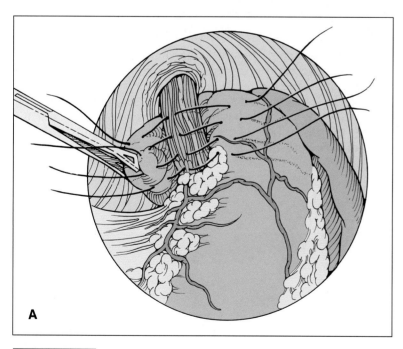

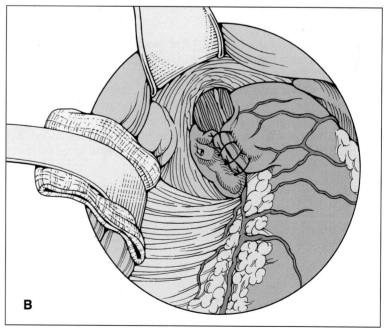

FIGURE 11-8.

Various operative procedures have been derived to treat gastro-esophageal reflux and to relieve reflux esophagitis. Each attempts to recreate the esophagogastric angle of His, but varies in technical details. The most commonly used procedure is the transabdominal Nissen fundoplication. The Nissen procedure creates a 360-degree wrap of gastric fundus around the esophagus. This is facilitated by division of the short gastric vessels. Gastric wall is passed behind the esophagus to permit the wrap. To prevent "slipping" of the wrap, the esophageal wall is incorporated in the repair (A). Once completed (B), the procedure recreates the angle of His and works equally well if the esophagogastric junction is above or below the diaphragm. (*Adapted from* Skinner [12].)

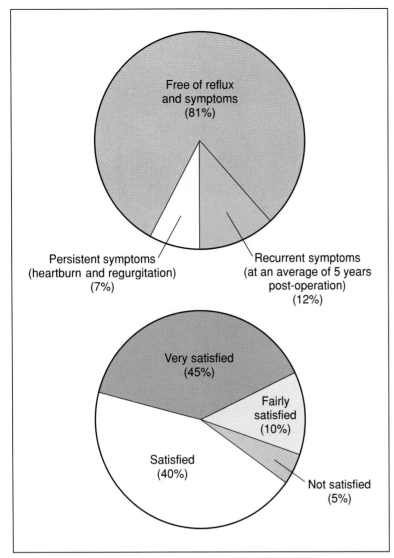

FIGURE 11-9.

Results of Nissen fundoplication 10 years after surgery. The results of transabdominal fundoplication for gastroesophageal reflux are excellent [1]. The most frequent postoperative side effects are change in mastication (food is chewed more completely), excessive flatus, and difficulty in belching. When the operation is performed using a 40-Fr bougie, dysphagia is a rare complication. For patients with simultaneous duodenal ulcer disease, a parietal cell vagotomy can readily be added without any increase in morbidity.

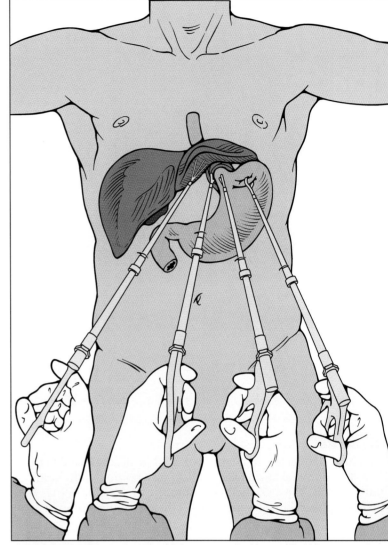

FIGURE 11-10.

Laparoscopic Nissen procedure. Rather than a single incision, the laparoscopic procedure is carried out through four 1-cm ports. Hospitalization and recuperation times are considerably shorter than after the open procedure. Although the early results seem encouraging, the follow-up has not been long enough to document whether the success rates of the two procedures are comparable. (*Adapted from* Hinder [13].)

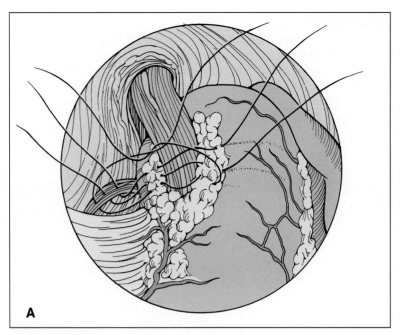

A

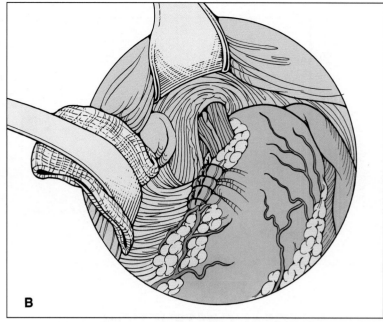

B

FIGURE 11-11.

Technique of the Hill repair of reflux esophagitis. This procedure has two major goals: (1) maintaining the gastroesophageal junction below the diaphragm by anchoring the superior margin of the gastrohepatic ligament to the arcuate ligament, the strong band of fascia which crosses in front of the aorta; and (2) "calibrating" the cardia by narrowing it at the base of the esophagus to increase the lower esophageal sphincter pressure by 40 to 50 mm Hg. **A**, Suture placement in the stomach and crus; **B**, completed procedure. Although this procedure is effective, it is technically demanding and suitable only for surgeons with considerable experience in its use. (*Adapted from* Skinner [14].)

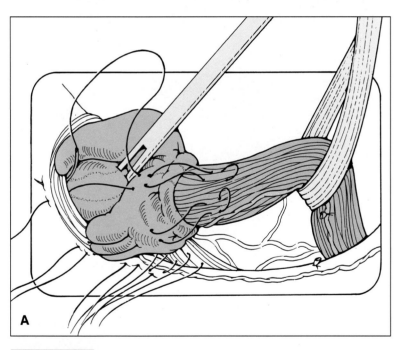

A

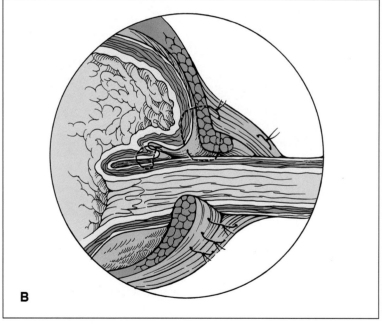

B

FIGURE 11-12.

Technique of the Belsey Mark IV repair of reflux esophagitis. This transthoracic procedure creates the equivalent of a 270-degree gastroesophageal wrap. This is accomplished using two rows of sutures. The initial layer sutures the upper cardia to the lower esophagus for three quarters of their combined circumference (**A**); this recreates the equivalent of the angle of His. The second row passes through the more distal gastric cardia and the under-surface of the diaphragm to ensure that the newly created valve is maintained within the abdomen (**B**). The hiatus is also narrowed to its normal size using posterior crural sutures. By careful placement of sutures the vagi can readily be spared, avoiding the need for pyloroplasty or pyloromyotomy. (*Adapted from* Skinner [15].)

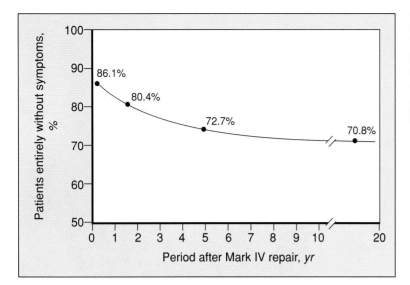

FIGURE 11-13.

Results of the Belsey Mark IV repair. The Belsey Mark IV repair is acknowledged to be the most successful transthoracic antireflux operation. In a study of 209 patients, 86% were cured within the first 3 months and 70% remained free of symptoms 10 or more years postoperatively. The longevity of this procedure is one of its major advantages. (*Adapted from* Hiebert and O'Mara [16].)

ESOPHAGEAL OBSTRUCTION

Achalasia

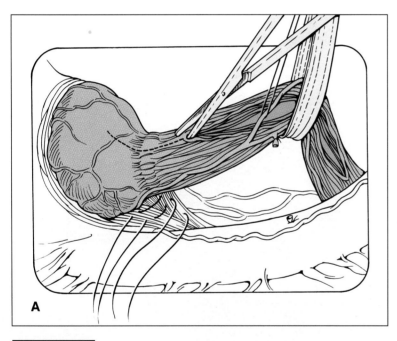

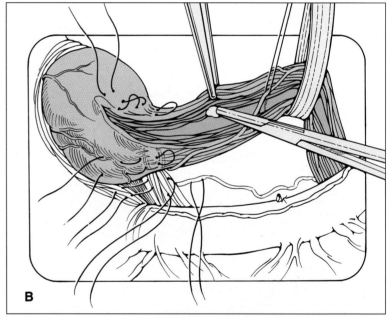

FIGURE 11-14.

Heller myotomy as therapy for achalasia. **A,** It is vital that both circular and longitudinal muscles are completely divided and that the mucosa bulges freely. The myotomy must be carried either to the aortic arch or high enough on the esophagus to include all thickened smooth muscle. The distal extent of the gastric component is controversial. There is no question that extending the myotomy for 1 to 2 cm into the stomach lowers the rate of recurrent achalasia. This incision also greatly increases the risk of reflux, however. **B,** Some surgeons advocate long myotomy and the routine addition of the Belsey Mark IV antireflux operation. I am not a proponent of this combined procedure. If properly performed, a myotomy carried just onto the gastric side of the gastroesophageal junction relieves the characteristic obstructive symptoms without rendering the lower esophageal sphincter incompetent and inducing reflux as a new problem. In performing the Heller myotomy the surgeon must avoid two pitfalls: injury to the vagus nerves and incision through the mucosa into the esophageal lumen. (*Adapted from* Skinner [17].)

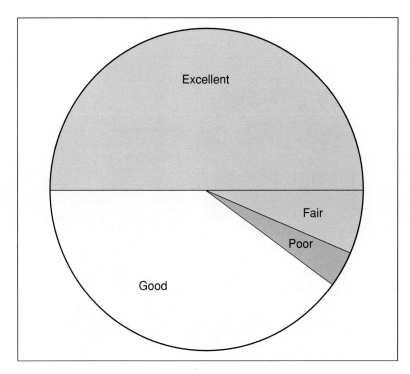

FIGURE 11-15.

Results of myotomy as therapy for achalasia. Overall, 85% of patients have consistently good to excellent outcomes [2], significantly higher than the results achieved with balloon dilation. More importantly, less than 2% of patients have poor postoperative results [2].

Diverticula

Zenker's diverticula

TABLE 11-1. SYMPTOMS OF ZENKER'S DIVERTICULA, %

Oropharyngeal dysphagia	98
Regurgitation of undigested food	85
Episodes of aspiration	61
Weight loss	36
Noisy deglutition	20
Halitosis	25
Hoarseness	13

TABLE 11-1.

Symptoms of Zenker's diverticula. The constellation of Zenker's diverticula is so characteristic that the diagnosis can generally be made on clinical grounds alone. Virtually all patients have dysphagia, more from the hypertrophic muscle than the pouch itself. Regurgitation and aspiration are secondary to esophageal obstruction. Although only one fourth of patients have halitosis, it is quite characteristic. This manifestation is due to stasis of food within the diverticula. (*Adapted from* Duranceau [3].)

FIGURE 11-16.

Pharyngoesophageal or Zenker's diverticula are caused by inflammation and fibrosis of the cricopharyngeus muscle, resulting in increased upper esophageal sphincter and intrapharyngeal pressures. Attempts by the hypopharynx to overcome resistance at the esophageal introitus causes extrusion of esophageal mucosa posteriorly just above the cricopharyngeus muscle. Diverticula tend to protrude to the left side of the neck twice as frequently as to the right. Regardless of their size, these diverticula are rarely palpable on physical examination. Endoscopy is contraindicated because of the risk of perforation. After the diagnosis has been confirmed by barium swallow, surgery is indicated. Zenker's diverticula are best approached by a left cervical incision along the anterior border of the sternocleidomastoid muscle. The sac should be isolated and dissected back to its origin. Myotomy of the cricopharyngeus muscle should be performed for 2 to 3 cm up onto the hypopharynx and caudally to the level of the thoracic inlet. After the myotomy has been completed, diverticula of 2 cm or less in diameter disappear spontaneously with no further therapy. Larger sacs should be suspended vertically by suturing the dome of the sac to the pharyngeal wall. The alternative approach, suturing the diverticulum to the prevertebral fascia, is associated with a significantly higher rate of infection. Only rarely is the sac so large that resection (rather than suspension) is indicated. This can safely be accomplished using either a staple or suture closure of the mucosal defect. (*Adapted from* Duranceau [18].)

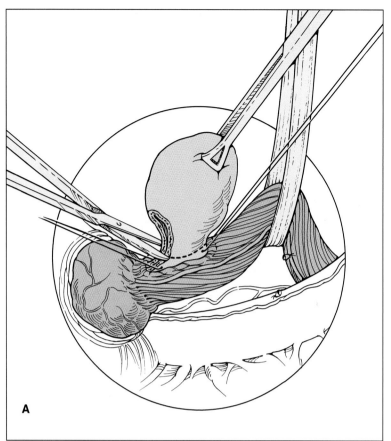
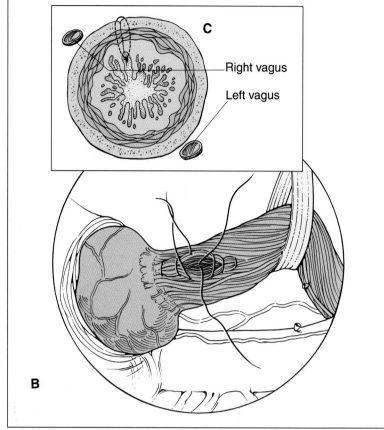

FIGURE 11-17.

Surgical treatment of epiphrenic diverticula. Epiphrenic diverticula result from motor disorders at the lower esophageal sphincter. Elevated intraluminal pressure caused by muscular hyperplasia and contraction extrudes the mucosa between longitudinal muscle fibers. The most common location is on the right side of the supradiaphragmatic esophagus, just posterior to the vagus nerve. Because of the associated motor disorder, the predominant symptom is dysphagia. Repair requires myotomy as a vital component of the procedure.

The approach is through a left thoracotomy. After the esophagus is detached by dissection from the mediastinal tissues it is rotated 90 degrees to provide access to the right side of the organ. The sac is isolated and cleared of attenuated muscle fibers. The sac should be excised back to normal tissue (**A**) and the esophagus closed in two layers (**B**), taking care to protect the adjacent vagus nerves (**C**). After the diverticulectomy has been completed, the esophagus is allowed to return to its normal position and a myotomy is performed, as it is for achalasia. The results of diverticulectomy plus myotomy for epiphrenic diverticulum are quite good. Dysphagia is cured in 75% to 80% of patients whereas symptoms improve in the remainder. The complication rate is low, and less than 5% of candidates develop reflux or perforation following operation. (*Adapted from* Skinner [19].)

Benign strictures

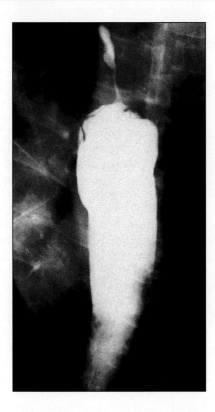

Figure 11-18.

Benign esophageal stricture. Benign strictures most commonly result from long-standing reflux esophagitis. Most younger patients have a long history of symptomatic reflux; the stricture, therefore, represents a failure of pharmacologic management. In contrast, strictures may be the first manifestation of reflux esophagitis in the elderly. Prevention is the key to the management of esophageal strictures. When strictures develop despite appropriate conservative therapy, attempts should be made to dilate them, accepting some risk of perforation. Operative repair is indicated only for patients with nondilatable fibrous strictures.

Although strictures are easy to identify on barium swallow, the distinction between benign and malignant may be quite subtle. Shouldering and irregularity of adjacent mucosa, which are characteristic of cancer, also commonly occur with benign strictures. Computed tomographic scanning often provides important diagnostic information, as does endoscopic ultrasonography. Because the treatment of malignant strictures is so different from that of the benign variety, every attempt must be made (by endoscopy and multiple biopsies) to identify cancer preoperatively. If a malignancy is initially identified during operative stricture repair, any chance of curing the patient is lost.

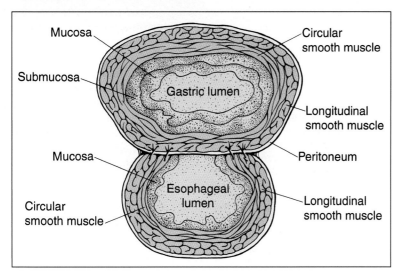

Figure 11-19.

Stricturoplasty. Distal strictures can readily be treated by making a full-thickness longitudinal incision through the strictured esophagus onto the very proximal stomach. This assures adequate luminal volume. The defect is closed by suturing the serosal surface of the stomach over the defect as a patch. The use of the gastric wall accomplishes two objectives: it bridges the defect without compromising the luminal diameter and recreates the angle of His, thus preventing gastroesophageal reflux.

Organ	Technique	Anastomoses, no	Inherent possible morbidity	Upper limit of usefulness	Disadvantages
Stomach	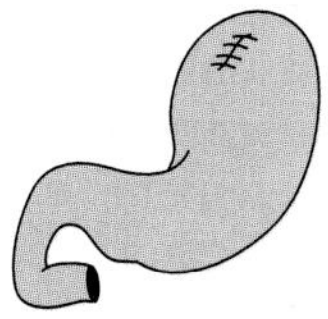	1	+	Cervical esophagus and pharynx	Bulky Reflux risk
Greater curvature tube	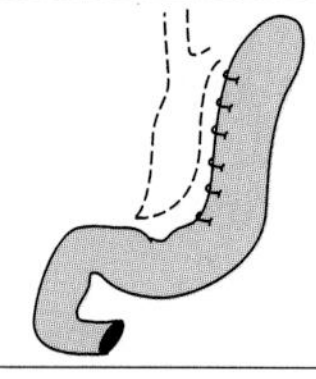	1	+	Cervical esophagus and pharynx	Reflux risk
Reversed gastric tube	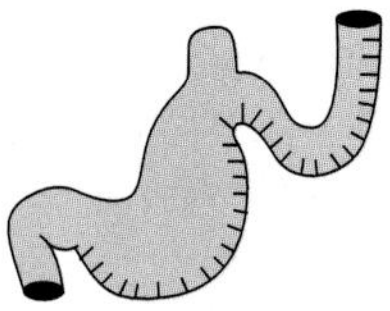	1	+++	Cervical esophagus and pharynx	Long suture line; limited blood supply
Nonreversed gastric tube	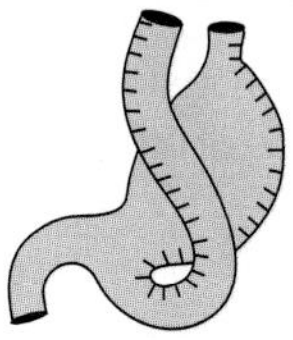	1	++	Lower cervical esophagus	Long suture line
Right colon	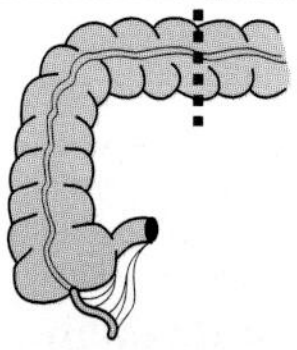	3	+++	Lower cervical esophagus	Thin-walled; bulky; short pedicle
Left colon	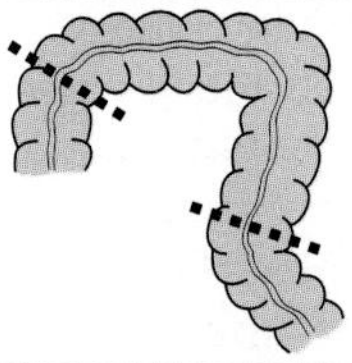	3	++++	Most versatile organ or use at any level; lower third to Pharynx	Extensive operation; redundancy over time
Jejunum	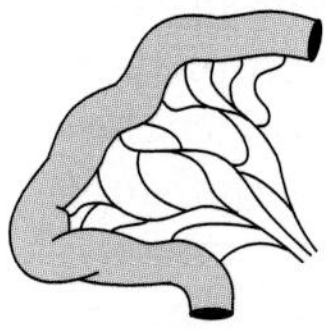	2 (Roux-en-y loop) 3 (Interposition)	++	Lower third	Limited graft length without revision of pedicle or bowel
Free graft	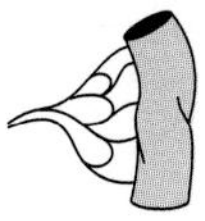	5 (2 microvascular)	+++++	Pharynx and cervical esophagus	Microvascular anastomoses required

FIGURE 11-20.

Types of esophageal replacement. Resection of the strictured area leaves a gap, usually of at least several centimeters, between the cut ends of the stomach and esophagus. The various techniques developed to bridge this deficit can be divided into two broad approaches: partial bypass of the esophagus using a thoracic upper anastomosis and total esophageal bypass with a cervical anastomosis. Thoracic bypasses are significantly simpler to perform but they subject the patient to the considerable risks of an intrapleural esophageal anastomosis. Cervical conduits are more complex to create and run a higher risk of ischemia. Leakage from the cervical esophagus, however, is far less mortal and significantly easier to control than an intrathoracic leak.

A number of organs have been used. The stomach can be mobilized directly and sutured to the cervical esophagus or constructed as a tube. Both right and left colon can be used, as can the jejunum. Free flaps of jejunum sutured using microsurgical techniques are effective and can be used to bridge gaps within the chest.

Although all these techniques are useful in specific circumstances, I prefer to use the stomach for intrathoracic anastomoses. The gastric blood supply is so extensive that ischemia is extremely rare, even when the left gastric and gastroepiploic arteries are divided. Anastomoses between the cut end of the thoracic esophagus and a newly created orifice in the anterior gastric wall (the proximal gastric suture line is closed) are relatively easy to perform. They also permit simultaneous creation of a Nissen wrap using the remaining gastric cardia; this procedure requires two separate incisions. The abdominal component permits mobilization of the stomach and performance of either pyloroplasty or pyloromyotomy, necessary because the vagi are invariably divided during esophagectomy. The resection, reanastomosis, and antireflux procedure are accomplished via thoracotomy. When total esophageal bypass is required, I prefer to use right colon passed through a substernal tunnel (See Figs. 11-21 and 11-22). (Adapted from Hiebert and Bredenberg [20].)

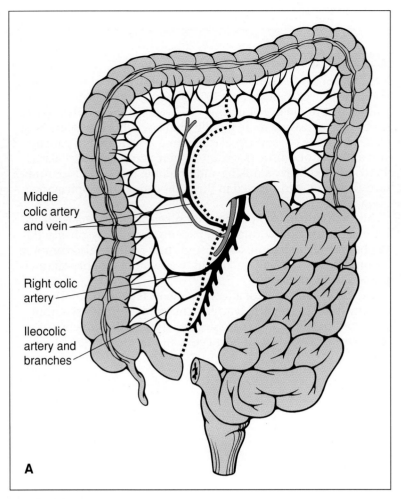

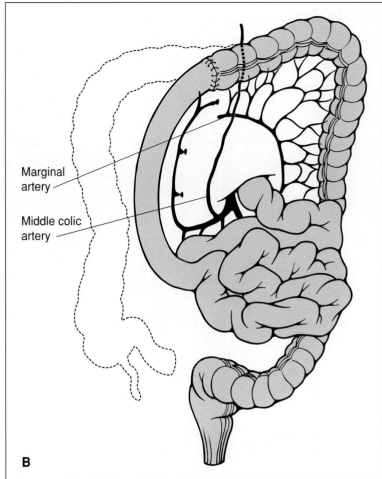

FIGURE 11-21.

Technique of right colon bypass. **A,** By carefully preserving the marginal artery of Drummond a viable bypass can be constructed based on the middle colic artery and vein. **B,** The colon is divided and passed behind the stomach through the lesser sac into the anterior or posterior mediastinum. Intestinal continuity is restored by ileo-transverse colostomy. (*Adapted from* Clowes *et al.* [21].)

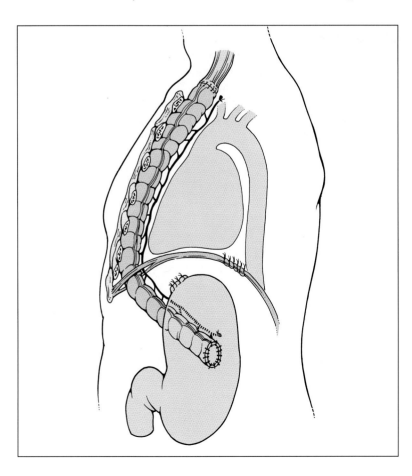

FIGURE 11-22.

Position of the substernal colon bypass. The right colon usually provides adequate length to reach the distal cervical esophagus. Whenever possible, I prefer to anastomose the cervical esophagus to the very distal ileum because it ensures a better size match. Although this bypass uses isoperistaltic colon, emptying the segment is accomplished predominantly by gravity. Colon bypasses are durable procedures that are associated with low anastomotic stricture rates and surprisingly few symptoms. (*Adapted from* Skinner [22].)

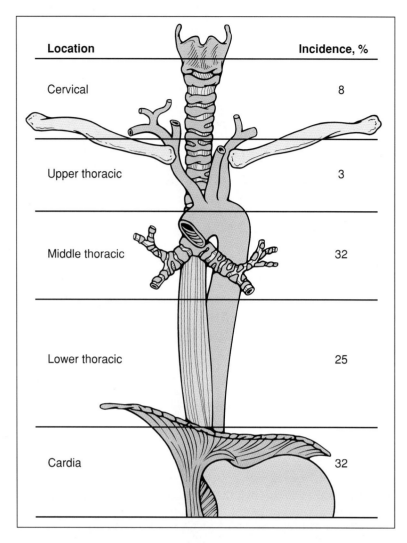

Location	Incidence, %
Cervical	8
Upper thoracic	3
Middle thoracic	32
Lower thoracic	25
Cardia	32

FIGURE 11-23.

Sites of esophageal carcinoma. Note the relative rarity of very proximal lesions, which account for only 10% of esophageal malignancies. In contrast, the frequency of finding carcinoma at the esophagogastric junction is increasing more rapidly than any other site in the body.

The incidence of esophageal carcinoma is increased in patients with a history of caustic ingestion, Barrett's esophagus, achalasia, and combined heavy smoking and drinking. Ingested nitrosamines have also been incriminated in the pathogenesis of esophageal malignancy.

The predominant symptoms of esophageal carcinoma relate to luminal obstruction. Virtually all patients describe dysphagia, but weight loss, regurgitation, cough, and chest pain are also common manifestations. The only successful treatment of esophageal carcinoma is surgical excision.

Physical examination of affected patients is generally normal, and any findings (cervical lymphadenopathy, Horner's syndrome, vocal cord paralysis, or hepatomegaly) attest to the presence of extensive disease. (*Adapted from* Peters and DeMeester [23].)

TABLE 11-2. HISTOPATHOLOGY OF TUMORS IN 1048 PATIENTS PRESENTING WITH CANCER OF THE ESOPHAGUS AND CARDIA, WHO WERE SEEN BETWEEN JULY 1982 AND JANUARY 1992

Squamous cell carcinoma	820
Adenocarcinoma	177
Mucoepidermoid carcinoma	19
Anaplastic (small-cell) carcinoma	16
Leiomyosarcoma	4
Lymphoma	2
Melanoma	2
Carcinosarcoma	1
Unclassified	7

TABLE 11-2.

Histopathology. The histopathology of esophageal malignancies confirms the predominance of squamous cell carcinoma. Adenocarcinoma accounts for almost 20% of tumors and arises either from the esophagogastric junction or in areas of Barrett's adenomatous metaplasia. (*Adapted from* Fok *et al.* [24].)

TABLE 11-3. FUNCTIONAL GRADES OF DYSPHAGIA

Grade	Definition	Incidence at diagnosis, %
I	Eats normally	11
II	Requires liquids with meals	
III	Able to take semisolids but unable to take any solid food	30
IV	Able to take liquids only	40
V	Unable to take liquids, but able to swallow saliva	7
VI	Unable to swallow saliva	12

TABLE 11-3.

Classification of dysphagia. Takita and colleagues [4] have characterized the grades of dysphagia. Symptoms range from normal ability to eat (grade I) to unable to swallow saliva (VI). Seventy percent of patients fall into grades III and IV and are unable to tolerate solid foods. (*Adapted from* Peters and DeMeester [25].)

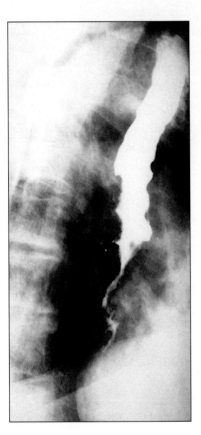

FIGURE 11-24.

Barium study in esophageal carcinoma. The diagnosis of esophageal carcinoma can usually be made by barium swallow. The characteristic abnormalities include shouldering and irregularity of esophageal involvement because of submucosal invasion in both directions from the intraluminal mass. Endoscopy, biopsy, and computed tomographic scanning of the chest and upper abdomen are other essential components of the work-up. If the lesion is at the level of the carina or higher, bronchoscopy should also be performed to rule out invasion of the respiratory tree. Staging of esophageal malignancy is performed at the time of operation (*see* Figs. 11-25 and 11-26). (*From* Casson [26]; with permission.)

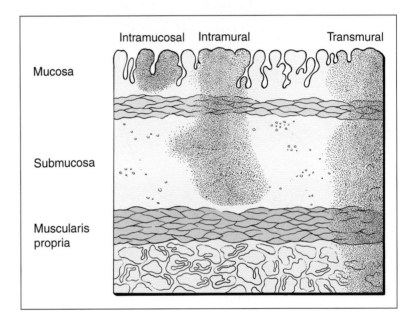

FIGURE 11-25.

Invasion of esophageal carcinoma. In staging of esophageal malignancies the T descriptor is based on the depth to which the invasion of T1 lesions is confined to the mucosa or submucosa, T2 to the muscularis, T3 to the adventitia, and T4 to invasion into surrounding structures. (*Adapted from* DeMeester *et al.* [27].)

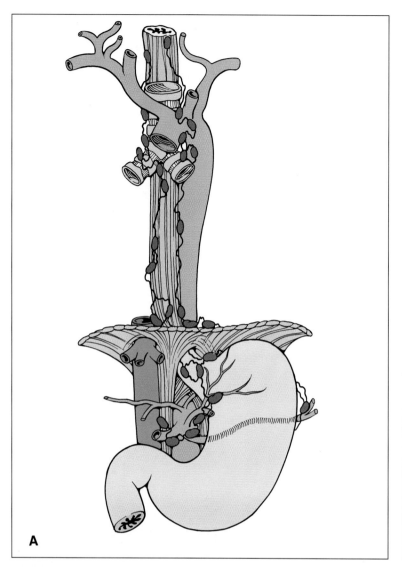

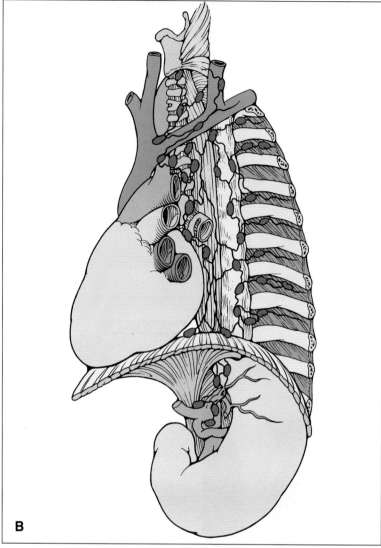

FIGURE 11-26.

A–B, Lymph node involvement. Identification of lymph node involvement is best characterized by mapping of the cervical, mediastinal, and subdiaphragmatic areas. This information is useful in predicting survival rates as well as in directing radiation therapy. (*Adapted from* Casson [28].)

TABLE 11-4. TNM STAGING SYSTEM FOR ESOPHAGEAL CARCINOMA

DEFINITION OF TNM

Primary tumor (T)

TX	Primary tumor cannot be assessed
T0	No evidence of primary tumor
Tis	Carcinoma in situ
T1	Tumor invades lamina propria or submucosa
T2	Tumor invades adventitia
T4	Tumor invades adjacent structures

Regional lymph nodes (N)

NX	Regional nodes cannot be assessed
N0	No regional node metastasis
N1	Regional node metastasis

Distant Metastasis (M)

MX	Presence of distant metastasis cannot be assessed
M0	No distant metastasis
M1	Distant metastasis

STAGE GROUPING

Stage 0	Tis	N0	M0
Stage I	T1	N0	M0
Stage IIA	T2	N0	M0
	T3	N0	M0
Stage IIB	T1	N1	M0
	T2	N1	M0
Stage III	T3	N1	M0
	T4	Any N	M0
Stage IV	Any T	Any N	M1

TABLE 11-4.

Staging of esophageal carcinoma. The final staging is based on the T and N descriptors plus information as to the presence or absence of distant metastases. (*Adapted from* Orringer [29].)

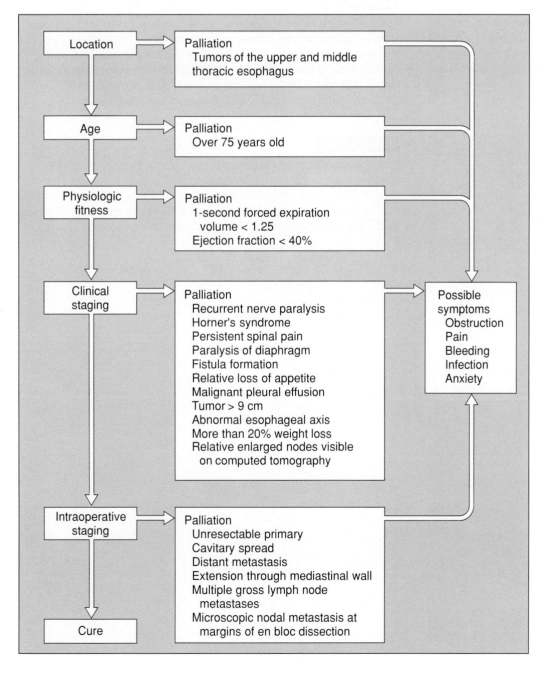

FIGURE 11-27.

Algorithm for therapeutic decisions in esophageal carcinoma. This algorithm is quite pessimistic because of the aggressiveness of esophageal carcinoma. Overall, rates of survival are poor, even with surgical resection. Palliation and a good quality of life plays a vital role in the treatment of this disease. (*Adapted from* Peters and DeMeester [30].)

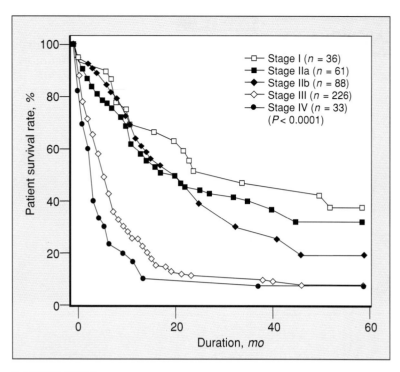

FIGURE 11-28.

Survival by stage of carcinoma. As expected, survival rates can be predicted based on the stage of malignancy. Following resection in 444 patients, median survival times were 27 months for stage 1, 19 months for stage 2, 7 months for stage 3, and 4 months for stage 4. (*Adapted from* Fok and Wong [31].)

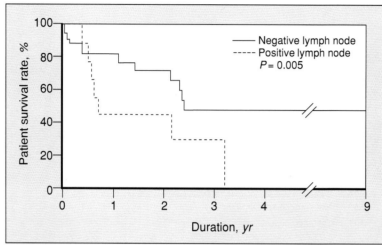

FIGURE 11-29.

Role of lymph node status in survival from esophageal carcinoma. Positive lymph nodes have enormous negative implications for survival. In 44 patients treated with preoperative radiation and chemotherapy positive lymph nodes were associated with a highly significant (*P* < 0.005) decrease in survival as compared with cohorts with no positive nodes. (*Adapted from* Vogel *et al.* [5].)

FIGURE 11-30.

Curative resection for esophageal carcinoma. In a series of 507 patients, curative resection was associated with a 5-year survival rate of 33% and a median survival time of 23 months. In contrast, the results for patients who underwent palliative resection were 6% and 7 months, respectively. (*Adapted from* Fok and Wong [31].)

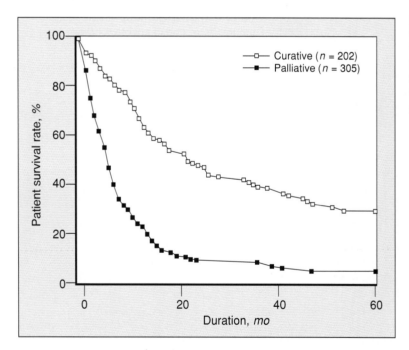

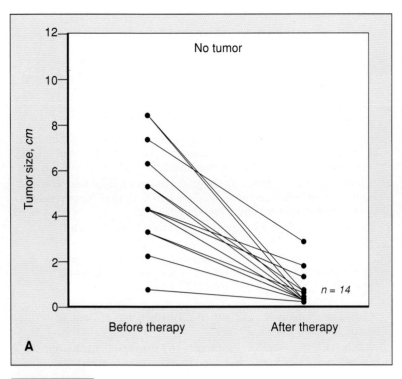

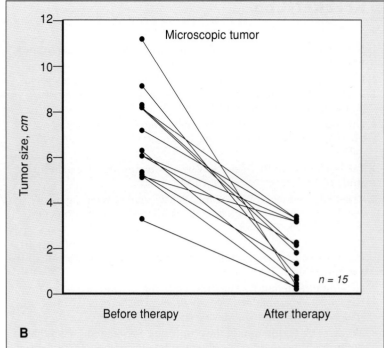

FIGURE 11-31.

Downstaging of tumor size. Because patients resected for cure fare significantly better than those operated on for palliation, preoperative radiation plus chemotherapy has been used to downstage patients by shrinking primary lesions and by sterilizing the node-bearing areas. Preoperative radiation and chemotherapy administered to 44 patients resulted in disappearance of tumor in 14 patients (**A**) and only residual microscopic tumor in 15 others (**B**). In contrast, gross carcinoma remained following therapy in 15 patients. (*Adapted from* Vogel *et al.* [5].)

TABLE 11-5. LYMPH NODE STATUS

GROUP	NO. OF PATIENTS	POSITIVE NODES	%
Adjuvant pharmacotherapy and surgery	44	10	23*
Surgery only	54	26	48
Downstage			
No tumor	14	0	0
Microscopic tumor	15	1	6.6
Gross tumor	15	9	60

*$P=0.02$.

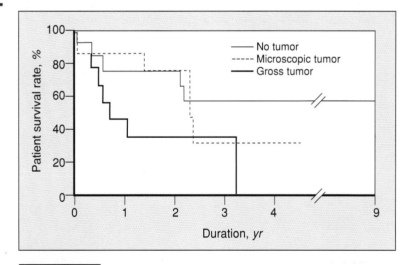

TABLE 11-5.

Lymph node status. Preoperative radiation and chemotherapy reduced the incidence of positive lymph nodes from 48% (26/54 patients) to 23% (10/44 patients). Only 1 of 29 patients (3%) with no or only a microscopic tumor had metastases to lymph nodes whereas 60% of patients in whom gross carcinoma persisted after therapy had positive lymph node involvement. (*Adapted from* Vogel *et al.* [5].)

FIGURE 11-32.

Survival rates following preoperative radiation and chemotherapy. Preoperative adjuvant therapy improved 5-year survival rates from 11% (operation alone) to 36% (operation plus preoperative radiation and chemotherapy). Among the latter group of patients there was a good correlation between tumor regression and survival. Overall, 18 of 29 patients (62%) whose specimens contained either no tumors or only microscopic tumors were still alive at last reporting. (*Adapted from* Vogel *et al.* [5].)

REFERENCES

1. Negre JB, Markkula HT, Keyrilainen O, *et al.*: Nissen fundoplication: Results at 10-year follow-up. *Am J Surg* 1983, 146:635.

2. Okike N, Payne WS, Neufeld DM, *et al.*: Esophagomyotomy versus forceful dilation for achalasia of the esophagus: Results in 899 patients. *Ann Thorac Surg* 1979, 28:119.

3. Duranceau A, Jamieson GG: Cricopharyngeal myotomy for pharyngoesophageal diverticula. *Int Trends Gen Thorac Surg* 1987, 3:358.

4. Takita H, Vincent RG, Caicedo V, *et al.*: Squamous cell carcinoma: A study of 153 cases. *J Surg Oncol* 1977, 9:547.

5. Vogel SB, Mendehall WM, Sombeck MD, *et al.*: Downstaging of esophageal cancer after preoperative radiation and chemotherapy. *Ann Surg* 1995, 221:685

6. Rothberg M, DeMeester TR: Surgical anatomy of the esophagus. In *General Thoracic Surgery*, edn. 3. Edited by Shields TW. Philadelphia: Lea and Febiger; 1989:84–85.

7. Liebermann-Meffert D: Anatomy, embryology, and histology. In *Esophageal Surgery*. Edited by Pearson FG, DeSlauriers J, Ginsberg RJ, *et al.* New York: Churchill Livingstone; 1995:10.

8. Skinner DB: Perforation of the esophagus: Spontaneous (Boerhaave's syndrome), traumatic, and following esophagoscopy. In *Textbook of Surgery*, edn. 13. Edited by Sabiston DC Jr. Philadelphia: WB Saunders; 1986:752.

9. Skinner DB: *Atlas of Esophageal Surgery*. New York: Churchill-Livingstone; 1991:179.

10. Gray SW, Skandalakis JE, McClusky DA: *Atlas of Surgical Anatomy for General Surgeons*. Baltimore: Williams and Wilkins; 1985:83.

11. Gray SW, Skandalakis JE, McClusky DA: *Atlas of Surgical Anatomy for General Surgeons*. Baltimore: Williams and Wilkins; 1985:81.

12. Skinner DB: *Atlas of Esophageal Surgery*. New York: Churchill Livingstone; 1991:131.

13. Hinder RA: Laparoscopic Nissen procedure. *Curr Tech Gen Surg* 1993, 2:1–7.

14. Skinner DB: *Atlas of Esophageal Surgery*. New York: Churchill Livingstone; 1991:137.

15. Skinner DB: *Atlas of Esophageal Surgery*. New York: Churchill Livingstone; 1991:123.

16. Hiebert CA, O'Mara OB: The Belsey operation for hiatal hernia: A twenty-year experience. *Am J Surg* 1979, 137:532.

17. Skinner DB: *Atlas of Esophageal Surgery*. New York: Churchill Livingstone; 1991:157–159.

18. Duranceau A: Pharyngeal and cricopharyngeal disorders. In *Esophageal Surgery*. Edited by Pearson FG, Deslauriers J, Ginsberg RJ, *et al.* New York: Churchill Livingstone; 1995:411.

19. Skinner DB: *Atlas of Esophageal Surgery*. New York: Churchill Livingstone; 1991:169.

20. Hiebert CA, Bredenberg CE: Selection and placement of conduits. In *Esophageal Surgery*. Edited by Pearson FG, Deslauriers J, Ginsberg RJ, *et al.* New York: Churchill Livingstone, 1995:652.

21. Clowes GHA Jr, Neville WE, Gregoire HB: Esophageal resection and replacement with a segment of colon. In *The Craft of Surgery*. Edited by Cooper P. Boston: Little, Brown; 1971:440.

22. Skinner DB: *Atlas of Esophageal Surgery*. New York: Churchill Livingstone; 1991:107.

23. Peters JH, DeMeester TR: Esophagus and diaphragmatic hernia. In *Principles of Surgery*, edn. 6. Edited by Schwartz SL, Shires GT, Spencer FC. New York: McGraw-Hill; 1994:1092.

24. Fok M, Wong J: Squamous cell carcinoma. In *Esophageal Surgery*. Edited by Pearson FG, Deslauriers J, Ginsberg J, *et al.* New York: Churchill Livingstone; 1995:572.

25. Peters JH, DeMeester TR: Esophagus and diaphragmatic hernia. In *Principles of Surgery*, edn. 6. Edited by Schwartz SL, Shires GT, Spencer FC. New York: McGraw-Hill; 1994:1094.

26. Casson AG: Staging. In *Esophageal Surgery*. Edited by Pearson FG, Deslauriers J, Ginsberg RJ, *et al.* New York: Churchill Livingstone; 1995:562.

27. DeMeester TR, Attwood SEA, Smyrk TC, *et al.*: Surgical therapy in Barrett's esophagus. *Ann Surg* 1990, 212:530.

28. Casson AG: Staging. In *Esophageal Surgery*. Edited by Pearson FG, Deslauriers J, Ginsberg RJ, *et al.* New York: Churchill Livingstone; 1995:567.

29. Orringer MB: Turns, injuries, and miscellaneous conditions of the esophagus. In *Surgery: Scientific Principles and Practice*. Edited by Greenfield LJ, Mulholland MW, Ordham KT, *et al.* Philadelphia: JB Lippincott; 1993:637.

30. Peters JH, DeMeester TR: Esophagus and diaphragmatic hernia. In *Principles of Surgery*, edn. 6. Edited by Schwartz SL, Shires GT, Spencer FC. New York: McGraw-Hill; 1994:1092.

31. Fok M, Wong J: Squamous cell carcinoma. In *Esophageal Surgery*. Edited by Pearson FG, Deslauriers J, Ginsberg J, *et al.* New York: Churchill Livingstone; 1995:576.

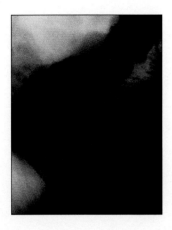

Index

Page numbers followed by *t* or *f* indicate tables or figures, respectively.

B

Bacteremia, with therapeutic endoscopy, risk of, 10.7*t*
Balloon dilators, 10.5*f*
    pneumatic, 10.6*f*
        for achalasia, 10.6*f*
    through the scope (TTS) technique for, 10.5*f*
Balloon distention, intraesophageal, as provocative test for chest
        pain, 9.3, 9.13*f*
Barium esophagram
    of achalasia, 2.3*f*, 10.3*f*
    with diffuse esophageal spasm, 2.3*f*
    and endoscopy, comparison of, 2.2*t*, 2.3*f*
    of esophageal carcinoma, 2.6*f*
    indications for, 2.2*t*
    of malignant stricture, 10.3*f*
    of peptic stricture, 10.3*f*
    of Schatzki's ring, 1.15*f*, 10.3*f*
Barium swallow
    with achalasia, 6.3*f*–6.4*f*
    in carcinoma, 11.17*f*
    with diffuse esophageal spasm, 6.7*f*
    epiphrenic diverticulum seen on, 1.20*f*
    with esophageal varices, 1.12*f*
    manometry during, 1.14*f*
    pharyngeal anatomy on, 7.4*f*
    in scleroderma, 6.10*f*
    video recording of, 1.14*f*
Barrett's epithelium, diagnosis of, endoscopy versus radiology
        for, 2.5*t*
Barrett's esophagus, 4.8*t*, 4.10–4.18
    adenocarcinoma arising in, 8.9*f*–8.10*f*
    antireflux surgery and, 4.18*f*
    dysplasia in
        histologic appearance of, 8.9*f*–8.10*f*
        histologic criteria for, 8.11*t*
    endoscopic pathology of, 4.10*f*
    histopathology of, 4.10*f*
    length of, 4.17*t*, 4.18*f*
    malignant potential of, 4.10*f*–4.11*f*
        alcohol and, 4.18*t*
        smoking and, 4.18*t*
    pathogenesis of, 4.2
    prevalence of, and patient age, 4.18*f*
    with reflux esophagitis, prevalence of, 4.9*t*
Belsey Mark IV repair
    results of, 11.10*f*
    technique of, 11.9*f*
Belsey's fundoplication, 4.15*f*
Bernstein test, 3.20, 9.2
    diagnostic yield of, with noncardiac chest pain, 9.12*f*–9.13*f*
    results with, 9.8*t*
    technique for, 9.7*f*
    as test for noncardiac chest pain, results with, 9.10*t*
Bethanechol (Urecholine)
    dosage and administration, 4.12*t*
    mechanism of action, 4.12*t*
    in provocative testing, 9.11*f*
    for reflux esophagitis, 4.12*t*
Bilirubin absorption, 3.19*f*
Bilitec probe, 3.19*f*
Bird's beak appearance, 2.3*f*, 6.3*f*

Boerhaave's syndrome, 11.4*f*
Botulinum toxin, intrasphincteric injection of, for achalasia treat-
        ment, 10.7*f*
Bougies. *See* Dilator(s)
Burn(s), corrosive, grading system for, 5.3*t*

C

Cancer. *See also* Carcinoma, esophageal
    epiglottic, 7.17*f*
    laryngeal, 7.15*f*
    pharyngeal, 7.18*f*
    of tongue base, 7.17*f*
Candida esophagitis, 5.13–5.16
    clinical features of, 5.13*f*
    diagnosis of, 5.13*f*
    endoscopic findings in, 5.15*f*–5.16*f*
    endoscopic grading of, 5.15*t*
    in HIV-infected (AIDS) patient, 5.5*f*, 5.13*f*
    pathology of, 5.14*f*
    radiologic findings in, 5.14*f*–5.15*f*
    risk factors for, 5.13*f*
    treatment of, 5.16*t*
Carafate. *See* Sucralfate
Carcinoma, esophageal, 11.2, 11.16–11.21. *See also* Adenocarcinoma;
        Squamous cell carcinoma
    alcohol and, 4.18*t*, 8.3*f*
    barium study in, 11.17*f*
    basaloid, 8.6
    clinical features of, 8.1, 11.2
    curative resection for, 11.20*f*
    diagnosis of, 2.6*f*–2.7*f*
        endoscopy versus radiology for, 2.5*t*
    esophageal narrowing caused by, 5.20*f*
    histologic types, risk factors for, 4.18*t*
    histopathology of, 11.16*t*
    incidence of, 11.2
        trends in, 4.11*f*
    invasion of, 11.17*f*
    lymph node involvement in, 11.18*f*, 11.21*f*
        diagnosis of, 2.7*f*
    midesophageal, coexisting with Zenker's diverticulum, 7.24*f*
    pathogenesis of, 11.2
    preoperative radiation plus chemotherapy for, 11.21*f*
    prognosis for, 8.1
    regression, with preoperative radiation plus chemotherapy for,
        11.21*f*
    risk factors for, 4.18*t*, 11.2, 11.16*f*
    signs and symptoms of, 11.16*f*
    sites of, 11.16*f*
    small cell, 8.8
    smoking and, 4.18*t*, 8.3*f*
    spindle cell, 8.7–8.8
    staging of, 11.17*f*–11.18*f*
    submucosal extension, 8.3*f*
    survival rates for, 11.19*f*–11.21*f*
        with preoperative radiation plus chemotherapy for, 11.21*f*
    TNM staging for, 8.4*t*, 11.17*f*–11.18*f*, 11.19*t*
    treatment of, 11.2, 11.16*f*
        algorithm for, 11.19*f*
        downstaging of tumor size in, 11.21*f*

H